Family Planning
SOURCEBOOK

Health Reference Series

First Edition

Family Planning SOURCEBOOK

Basic Consumer Health Information about Planning for Pregnancy and Contraception, Including Traditional Methods, Barrier Methods, Hormonal Methods, Permanent Methods, Future Methods, Emergency Contraception, and Birth Control Choices for Women at Each Stage of Life

Along with Statistics, a Glossary, and Sources of Additional Information

Edited by
Amy Marcaccio Keyzer

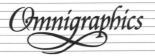

Omnigraphics

615 Griswold Street • Detroit, MI 48226

BIBLIOGRAPHIC NOTE

Edited by
Amy Marcaccio Keyzer

EdIndex, Services for Publishers, *Indexers*

Omnigraphics, Inc.

Matthew P. Barbour, *Vice President, Operations*
Laurie Lanzen Harris, *Vice President, Editorial Director*
Kevin Hayes, *Production Coordinator*
Thomas J. Murphy, *Vice President, Finance and Comptroller*
Peter E. Ruffner, *Senior Vice President*
Jane J. Steele, *Marketing Consultant*

Frederick G. Ruffner, Jr., *Publisher*
Copyright © 2001, Omnigraphics, Inc.

Library of Congress Cataloging-in-Publication Data

Family planning sourcebook: basic consumer health information about planning for pregnancy and contraception, including traditional methods, barrier methods, hormonal methods, permanent methods, future methods, emergency contraception, and birth control choices for women at each stage of life, along with statistics, glossary, and sources of additional information / edited by Amy Marcaccio Keyzer.—1st ed.
    p. cm.—(health reference series)
    ISBN 0-7808-0379-5
    1. Birth control—United States. 2. Contraception—United States. I. Keyzer, Amy Marcaccio. II. Series.

    HQ766.5.U5 F3455 2000
    363.9'6'0973—dc21

                                                                00-053029

∞

Table of Contents

Part III: An Overview of Contraception

Part IV: Traditional Methods of Contraception

Part V: Barrier Methods of Contraception

Part VI: Hormonal Methods of Contraception

Part VII: Permanent Methods of Contraception (Sterilization)

Part VIII: Emergency Contraception

Part IX: Abortion

Part X: Future Methods of Contraception

Part XI: Additional Help and Information

Preface

About This Book

According to The Alan Guttmacher Institute, almost half of the 6.3 million pregnancies in the United States each year are unintended. Yet, family planning contributes to healthy families and healthy babies. According to a report from the National Commission to Prevent Infant Mortality, infant deaths could be reduced by 10 percent, and the incidence of low birthweight babies could be reduced by 12 percent, if all pregnancies were planned. *Family Planning Sourcebook* was designed to provide women and men with objective information on family planning issues and contraceptive choices so that they can make informed decisions about the birth control that best fits into their lifestyle, value system, health situation, and stage of life.

How to Use This Book

This book is divided into parts, chapters, and sections. Parts focus on broad areas of interest, and individual chapters present topics within those areas. To help the reader locate specific information, some chapters are further subdivided into sections.

Part I: *Planning Your Family* focuses on factors to consider before starting a family, such as emotional readiness for parenthood, becoming parents later in life, pre-pregnancy health and nutrition, and the adoption option.

Part II: *Special Family Planning Issues* addresses areas of concern. It considers infertility, unintended pregnancies and attendant options available, teenage and later-age contraception and pregnancy, and health insurance coverage of contraceptives.

Part III: *An Overview of Contraception* describes and compares various methods of birth control. Comparison charts include effectiveness rates, main advantages, possible problems, how to use the method and how it actually works to prevent pregnancy, and the contraceptive's ability to reduce risk for HIV/AIDS and STIs/STDs. Statistics on contraceptive use and information about Title X, the National Family Planning Program, are also presented.

Part IV: *Traditional Methods of Contraception* focuses on family planning methods such as fertility awareness (temperature method, cervical mucus method, calendar method), abstinence, withdrawal, and breastfeeding. Chapters provide details on the effectiveness rates, benefits, disadvantages, and instructions for use for each individual method.

Part V: *Barrier Methods of Contraception* considers birth control methods such as male and female condoms, spermicides, diaphragms, and cervical caps. Effectiveness rates, advantages, disadvantages, cost, and instructions for use are detailed for each method.

Part VI: *Hormonal Methods of Contraception* describes prescription methods of birth control that use hormones to prevent pregnancy, such as the birth control pill, implants, injectables, and IUDs. Each chapter provides information on effectiveness rates, mechanism of action, benefits, risk factors, side effects, cost, and instructions for use or description of procedure provided by health care professional.

Part VII: *Permanent Methods of Contraception (Sterilization)* presents information on surgical methods of birth control, including tubal sterilization and vasectomy, as well as reversal surgery. A complete description of each medical procedure, along with the advantages and disadvantages, cost, and effectiveness rate, is included.

Part VIII: *Emergency Contraception* discusses the use of oral contraceptives or IUDs to prevent pregnancy after unprotected intercourse. This section provides background information on emergency contraception (EC), including risk factors, side effects, effectiveness rates, and instructions on how to use regular birth control pills in high dosages for EC.

Part IX: *Abortion* focuses on factors to consider before making a decision, abortion options, the long-term health risks of the procedure, and statistics on abortion.

Part X: *Future Methods of Contraception* provides information on birth control options currently under development or soon to be approved by the FDA for use in the United States.

Part XI: *Additional Help and Information* includes a glossary of family planning terms and a directory of organizations able to provide additional information.

Bibliographic Note

Family Planning Sourcebook contains documents and excerpts from publications issued by the following U.S. government agencies: Centers for Disease Control and Prevention (CDC); Department of Health and Human Services (DHHS); National Adoption Information Clearinghouse; National Center for Health Statistics; National Cancer Institute (NCI); National Institute of Child Health and Human Development (NICHD); Office of Population Affairs (OPA); and U.S. Food and Drug Administration (FDA).

In addition, this volume contains copyrighted documents from the following organizations: The Alan Guttmacher Institute; American Medical Women's Association; American Society for Reproductive Medicine; Association of Reproductive Health Professionals; AVSC International; BabyCenter, Inc.; CARAL Pro-Choice Education Fund; Family Health International; Family Planning Council; Feminist Women's Health Center; Fertilitext; Mayo Foundation for Medical Education and Research; National Abortion Federation; National Family Planning and Reproductive Health Association; Natural Family Planning Inc. New Zealand; Office of Population Research at Princeton University; Planned Parenthood® Federation of America; Population Council; Reproductive Health Outlook; and Virginia Tech University

Student Health Service Pharmacy. Materials included from the Emory University School of Medicine are not copyrighted. Copyrighted articles from the following journals are also included: *Progress in Human Reproduction* and *The Women's Quarterly*. Full citation information is provided on the first page of each chapter. Every effort has been made to secure all necessary rights to reprint the copyrighted material. If any omissions have been made, please contact Omnigraphics to make corrections for future editions.

Acknowledgements

The editor wishes to thank the many organizations listed above that provided the material presented in this volume. In addition, I would like to give special thanks to Laurie Lanzen Harris for her editorial advice; researchers Joan Margeson and Jenifer Swanson for locating those documents that were particularly elusive; Dan Harris for his technical expertise; and permissions specialist Maria Franklin.

Note from the Editor

This book is part of Omnigraphics' *Health Reference Series*. The series provides basic consumer health information about a broad range of medical concerns. It is not intended to serve as a tool for diagnosing illness, in prescribing treatments, or as a substitute for the physician/patient relationship. All persons concerned about medical symptoms or the possibility of disease are encouraged to seek professional care from an appropriate health care provider.

Our Advisory Board

The *Health Reference Series* is reviewed by an Advisory Board comprised of librarians from public, academic, and medical libraries. We would like to thank the following board members for providing guidance to the development of this series:

Dr. Lynda Baker, Associate Professor of Library and Information Science, Wayne State University, Detroit, MI

Nancy Bulgarelli, William Beaumont Hospital Library, Royal Oak, MI

Karen Imarasio, Bloomfield Township Public Library, Bloomfield Township, MI

Karen Morgan, Mardigian Library, University of Michigan-Dearborn, Dearborn, MI

Rosemary Orlando, St. Clair Shores Public Library, St. Clair Shores, MI

Health Reference Series *Update Policy*

The inaugural book in the *Health Reference Series* was the first edition of *Cancer Sourcebook* published in 1992. Since then, the Series has been enthusiastically received by librarians and in the medical community. In order to maintain the standard of providing high-quality health information for the lay person, the editorial staff at Omnigraphics felt it was necessary to implement a policy of updating volumes when warranted.

Medical researchers have been making tremendous strides, and it is the purpose of the *Health Reference Series* to stay current with the most recent advances. Each decision to update a volume will be made on an individual basis. Some of the considerations will include how much new information is available and the feedback we receive from people who use the books. If there is a topic you would like to see added to the update list, or an area of medical concern you feel has not been adequately addressed, please write to:

Editor
Health Reference Series
Omnigraphics, Inc.
615 Griswold Street
Detroit, MI 48226

The commitment to providing ongoing coverage of important medical developments has also led to some format changes in the *Health Reference Series*. Each new volume on a topic is individually titled and called a "First Edition." Subsequent updates will carry sequential edition numbers. To help avoid confusion and to provide maximum flexibility in our ability to respond to informational needs, the practice of consecutively numbering each volume has been discontinued.

Part One:

Planning Your Family

Chapter 1

Is Parenthood for You?

*—by Ann Bartz; questions developed by
BabyCenter staff with help from San Francisco
psychotherapists Ann Davidman and Denise Carlini*

For some people this is the world's easiest question—they've always been able to see themselves as parents, they have their life set up the way they want it, and they're ready to go. Others go back and forth on this one for years, or feel the need to do a little serious wobbling before taking the plunge. Some just never get the call. Wherever you are on the spectrum, even if you know you want to do it, you can make a conscious decision about whether to become a parent.

If you're having trouble deciding whether you want to have a child, or are just wondering whether you're ready to take on this lifelong project, we hope this chapter will help you get closer to a decision. One thing's for sure: No one *has* to have children. The world's not short on people to populate it, and whether to become a parent is completely up to you and whatever hopes and dreams you have for your life.

The Hardship Factor

And it's a big decision, not to be taken lightly. Being a parent is really fun, and satisfying in a way you can't fully imagine when you don't have children. *And* it's really hard work—more work than you can imagine until you've done it. It's hard because of the sheer volume of demands on your time and energy, with few breaks to refresh and recharge; it's hard because parents almost never have enough time, money, emotional support, training, or preparation to do the job they want to do; it's hard because it puts your own emotional issues squarely in your face as your children inevitably push every button you have, and it's hard because the mistakes you make—and you'll make some, for sure—affect the ones you love the most: your children.

Having a child is a major life change, and because women everywhere bear the major responsibility for raising children, it's a change that in general affects women's lives more than men's. It means adding the way society treats parents (not well) on top of the way society treats women (ditto). "Parenting—the vitally important job of raising the next generation—is treated economically almost like a hobby," says Patty Wipfler, founder of the Parents Leadership Institute in Palo Alto, California. "Women already don't get enough pay, support, or recognition for their contributions to society, and becoming a parent kind of squares that." Men as a whole are more involved as parents today than ever before, but the day-to-day housework, meal-making, emotional counseling, childcare, purchasing, and household details and logistics still tend to fall—unpaid—to the woman of the house.

That's not to say it's an easy decision for men. Both men and women face unhappy tradeoffs between work and parenthood in modern society, with women usually having to choose parenting to the detriment of work, and men usually having to choose work to the detriment of parenting. Men's patterns of workaholism, reinforced by most workplaces today, are fueled by a new sense of responsibility for the family. Long hours of work increase the sense of emotional isolation that most men deal with anyway, and many feel frustrated at not being able to be the kind of father they wish they could be.

A Reality Check

With all the romanticized images of children and parenthood floating around, hardly anyone gets a realistic idea of what it's like to be a parent before they actually become one. If you never had to carry a 5-

pound sack of flour around for a week in junior high, psychologist Harriet Lerner's *The Mother Dance: How Children Change You* can serve as an on-paper preview, or you can always get a real-life glimpse by caring for a friend's or relative's baby overnight. Or try assuming you've made the decision to have a child and then spend a week thinking about how that makes you feel and all the ways your life would change, then assume you've decided not to have one and live with that for a week.

Parenthood isn't for everyone. Maybe you've never wanted children; maybe you have other ambitions for yourself that caring for children would make impossible. "We are this wonderfully creative species," says Mindy Toomay, a fiction and cooking writer and teacher who at 47 is entirely comfortable with her decision not to have children. "But so many people never explore their creative or spiritual potential because family demands get in the way. For me it felt like it would be an impediment—it has been for a lot of people I know, particularly women." Essayist Katherine Griffin has written movingly of her choice not to have children and to pursue other dreams in *Childless by Choice*. And certainly there are instances of people becoming parents and then regretting their decision.

Then again, some people are surprised by how much they like being a parent. "I did catering during high school so I wouldn't have to babysit," says Sally Webb, now the mother of two small boys. "But I found I really love being a mom."

Most people, especially women, are brought up to expect that they'll be parents. From baby dolls to baby showers, girls and women are surrounded by images and expectations from parents, peers, religion, advertising, and the media. But the decision to be a parent is not up to your mother, your father, your friends, your church, or even any expectations you might have grown up with. It's your life, and it's up to you.

Are You Ready to Have a Baby?

The following series of questions, developed by our staff with help from San Francisco psychotherapists Ann Davidman and Denise Carlini, is designed for you to discuss with your partner or a friend, mull over on your own, write about in your journal, take to your therapist—whatever helps you take a good look at them. If you would be having a child with a partner, show these questions to your partner and see whether you would be comfortable with his or her answers. The questions are meant to be answered by both men and women.

Davidman and Carlini lead separate weekend workshops for men and women called "Motherhood: Is It for Me?" and "Fatherhood, Is It for Me?" to help people get closer to making this important decision. (You can inquire about taking their workshops by calling (415) 752-9165.) "A lot of our work is helping people to understand their ambivalence so they can move on to the next step of making a decision," says Davidman. "We've found that ambivalence can be a result of emotional issues the person isn't completely aware of, such as unresolved grief."

They suggest you start by asking **What do you want for you?** This is regardless of your current situation, regardless of what you might have to go through to get what you want, such as finding a partner if you want one. If you think you might want a child, don't even ask yourself at this point how that will come about—whether biologically, through adoption, or whatever. Just concentrate on your personal wishes and desires.

Evaluate Your Parenting Readiness

Your Expectations

- Do you currently spend time with children? Do you enjoy it? (Whether you answer yes or no doesn't predict how you'll feel about your own children, but giving some thought to the issue can highlight some of your assumptions and attitudes about life with children.)

- What ages of children are you particularly comfortable with? What age do you gravitate toward? (If you're not comfortable with a particular age group, it may hint at issues in your own childhood that need resolving. Also, addressing this question is a good reality check: Parenthood is permanent, and you can't just raise your kids during the "fun" years.)

- What are your thoughts on the responsibilities and commitment of parenthood? (This question is just a way to help you reflect on the demands of parenting and whether you're comfortable with them.)

- How do you cope with stress? Is it something you would want your child to witness? How did you learn that method of coping? (Research shows that your level of stress can affect your children and your ability to parent effectively. If you feel you don't

6

have a good handle on managing your stress, now is a great time to start learning some new coping mechanisms.)

- What are your hopes about being a parent? What if they're not met? (Parenthood isn't all shared hugs and fits of giggling; there will be tough times and disappointments, and your children may not be what you expect. This is a good reality check question.)

- What are your fears? What if they *are* met? (You can't work out your fears in advance. Aspects of parenting are frightening—it's a big responsibility. But it can help to voice your fears and examine them now.)

- How much like your own parents do you want to be? How different do you want to be? (Our own parents are the best models we have for raising children. Some of their lessons are positive and others negative. Examine your life with your parents and think about what you can learn from their triumphs and shortcomings.)

- As a child, what messages did you get about what a parent is supposed to be? (This is another question that can help you examine your expectations of parenthood and weed out underlying assumptions that may not be useful.)

Your Family History

These questions can help you access blocked feelings that may be clouding your decision-making process. Often unresolved, possibly unrecognized, grief from earlier losses stands in the way of making big decisions—such as whether to become a parent.

- What did you enjoy about being a child? What didn't you enjoy? (If you're having trouble deciding whether you want children, it may have something to do with unresolved issues from your own childhood.)

- What did you appreciate about the parenting you received? What didn't go well? (Our own parents teach us many lessons— both positive and negative. Think about what you'd like to emulate from your own childhood and what you'd like to change.)

- Was one of your parents (or other family members) gravely ill during your childhood? Did one or both die? Have you effectively grieved this loss? (Unresolved, or even unrecognized, grief from childhood can stand in the way of making big decisions, such as whether to become a parent.)

Your Values

This set of questions will help you pinpoint the personal attitudes and values you'll bring to the role of parent. It will also help identify differences that may exist between you and your partner (if you have one).

- What would you like to pass on that you got from your parents? What wouldn't you like to pass on? (This question helps you hone in on and verbalize what you think is important to bring to the role of parent.)

- What are your priorities for your children? For example, do you want them all to have a college education? What values do you want to instill in them? (We all come to parenthood with a set of expectations, often unspoken. This question helps you clarify your hopes and dreams for your children.)

- What are your thoughts about disciplining children? Check with your partner and compare. (This is an area where partners often disagree. Talking about these issues now won't prevent future problems, but it will give you a chance to talk about setting limits and how you might go about doing so.)

Your Life and How It Could Change

Answering these will give you insight into the practical realities of your situation, which you should consider before taking on parenthood.

- Talk to people who've decided not to have children; talk to people who've decided to have children. How does what they tell you make you feel? (We're not suggesting that you base your decision on what others say, but hearing friends and relatives talk about their own parenthood choices can raise new issues for you to consider.)

- What does your support system look like? (We're not saying you need a *whole* village to raise your child, but a few people to lean on can really help. Childrearing is difficult to do on your own. Do you have a partner, or family and friends nearby that you can look to for assistance? This isn't a prerequisite for parenthood, but it's a wonderful addition.)

- What do you do when you have free time? What will you do when you don't have any? (This is one of the practical realities of parenthood. You'll never again be able to do whatever you want, whenever you want, without considering the effect on your children. They will and should become your number one priority—are you ready for that?)

- How do you think your life will change? (This is a given. Your life will change irrevocably. Most parents say it's for the better, but the effect on your time, energy, wishes and desires can be enormous. Take a moment now to seriously think about the new life you are considering.)

Chapter 2

Parenting at a Later Age

Raising kids, despite its many rewards, can be an exhausting, seemingly endless job. It's enough to give anyone gray hair. But imagine starting a family at an age when you might already have gray hair, at 40, 45, or 50? Many couples today are having babies later in life and face some unique challenges.

Why Many Couples Are Waiting

The birth rate among women older than 40 has increased by nearly half in the last 20 years. Why? Many couples have chosen to establish their careers before having children or simply didn't feel ready for the responsibility. Others didn't marry until later in life or had children from an early marriage, divorced, and then started a second family with a new partner. Also, improvement in treatments for infertility and the fact that most women over 40 are in excellent health have helped make middle-age parenting a greater possibility.

Mayo Clinic Health Oasis, August 25, 1997; © 2000 Mayo Foundation for Medical Education and Research; available at http://www.mayohealth.org/mayo/9708/htm/latemom.htm; reprinted with permission.

Should You Wait?

It's likely that older parents may be wiser, more mature, and have greater patience. They may be better focused, having achieved a lot in their careers and feel ready for the "next phase." They may be more stable financially and may have more flexibility in their careers that allow being home to parent. And one could argue that just having lived longer, older parents may have a healthier perspective on life and better coping skills to aid them in their parenting.

But on the other hand, they may have less energy than their younger counterparts. And, if older couples have spent decades establishing careers and are accustomed to structure and predictability in their lives, they may have more trouble adjusting to the unpredictable nature of children. Some may consider the normal frustrations of child-rearing as reflections of their inability (in their opinion) to be "successful" parents. Then there are the obvious concerns of living to see their children reach adulthood.

Some Tips for Older Parents

It seems, then, that the advantages and disadvantages in later-age parenting aren't clear-cut and vary depending on whom you ask. "In the end, no matter what your age, your ability to parent really comes down to you as an individual—your maturity, personality, and values," emphasizes Aria J. Bernard, R.N., parent education coordinator at Mayo Clinic, Rochester, Minnesota. Bernard offers this advice for middle-age parents:

- **Ask yourself some tough questions**—Before you decide a new baby is right for you, ask yourself if you are emotionally and physically strong enough to handle raising a child?

- **Have realistic expectations**—Babies mean change. Be prepared for what may be a great adjustment in your lifestyle. Ask yourself how a baby would fit into your current lifestyle, and how flexible could you be?

Mayo pediatrician William J. Barbaresi, M.D., echoes Bernard's concern. "Be prepared that, no matter how much reading or preparing you do, you can't control or predict every aspect of your child's development."

- **Seek out a support system**—Older couples may have less support from extended family because their own parents are even older (or may no longer be living). Meanwhile, many of their friends may already have raised their children. If you have other responsibilities—older children, parents or relatives to care for, a business to run—you may have even more reason to seek support from others going through similar phases in life. Seek out people who are willing to listen as well as offer advice.

- **Exercise, eat right, and take time for yourself**—As you age, your body's ability to bounce back after being up all night with a child or working all day and then coming home to parent may change. It's important to balance good nutrition with aerobic activity to increase your energy level while maintaining good health.

"Also it's important for parents who may feel overwhelmed with their new responsibilities to set aside some time just for themselves and for their relationship," notes Laura T. Evans, co-founder of the National Parents Association in Val Paraiso, Indiana, a volunteer organization that provides support and information for parents.

- **Make long-term financial plans**—It's very possible you may be in your retirement years at the same time you have the greatest expenses of raising a child. By planning ahead, you may provide a more secure future for your family.

- **Be prepared for other people's reactions**—When a 63-year-old woman recently gave birth for the first time, it received a lot of attention. People generally have children when they are in their 20s and 30s. That's considered the "ideal." And while people may be more accepting of older men having children, they may not feel the same about older women. You may face sex and age discrimination and being prepared with a straight-forward but non-defensive response may make things easier.

Challenging Society's Notions of the Ideal Parent

Bernard points out that advice she gives to middle-and later-age parents is really no different from what she gives to younger parents, and that there is no guarantee any parent will live to see his or her child into adulthood. And she reminds parents that once the baby arrives—despite any reservations they might have once had—they probably won't be able to imagine what their life was like before their new child.

She challenges friends and families of later-age parents to be accepting, empathetic, and supportive. "As we see more and more nontraditional families, it's important that society as a whole begin to challenge the notion of the 'ideal parent'," Bernard says. She adds: "Parenting at 20, 40, or even later takes the same basic things: nurturing love—and a sense of humor."

Chapter 3

Preconception Planning

If you've decided the time is right to get pregnant, you've likely already begun the most important work: preparing emotionally to make a life-long commitment to a child. Before conceiving, take the time to ensure that your body and your environment are equally prepared.

The Preconception Visit

Begin your preparation by scheduling an appointment to see your chosen obstetrical care provider. This visit will allow your doctor to get a picture of your overall health, and to help you map out lifestyle changes that may benefit your pregnancy. It will also serve as an excellent chance for you and your partner to ask questions and discuss concerns.

Expect a complete physical examination during your preconception visit. Your doctor will determine if you're immune to certain infections, such as rubella, that could cause serious birth defects in a developing fetus. If you're not immune, your physician may recommend immunization at least 3 months before you become pregnant. For women who have an ongoing medical condition, such as diabetes, high blood pressure, asthma, or lupus, making sure the condition is controlled before

"Preconception Planning: Take a Pregnant Pause," *Mayo Clinic Health Oasis*, November 2, 1998; © 2000 Mayo Foundation for Medical Education and Research; available at http://www.mayohealth.org/mayo/9811/htm/preconception.htm; reprinted with permission.

pregnancy is an important safeguard both for the mother and the future baby.

Your doctor will also want to know what prescription and over-the-counter medications you take, and may suggest adjustments before you conceive as well as changes that may be required after conception.

Both you and your partner should be prepared to answer a number of questions about family medical history during the preconception visit. Certain medical conditions can be inherited, such as sickle cell anemia, cystic fibrosis, and muscular dystrophy. If your family history suggests a predisposition to a serious inherited disorder, your physician may refer you to a genetic counselor, who can advise you about the potential risks and options.

Tobacco and Alcohol—What Should You Do?

Preparing for pregnancy is an excellent motivation to get healthy. Take an honest look at your habits in the following areas, and make the necessary adjustments before making a baby:

- **Smoking**—There has never been a better time to stop. Women who smoke during pregnancy tend to have babies of lower birthweight than nonsmokers, and these babies may have developmental problems. In addition, smokers have a higher incidence of miscarriages and stillbirths. It's equally important that your partner give up smoking because exposure to secondhand tobacco smoke can increase the risk of spontaneous abortion, fetal death, preterm labor, low birthweight, and sudden infant death syndrome (SIDS).

- **Alcohol consumption**—Prenatal exposure to alcohol can have severe long-term consequences in children, including mental retardation, learning disabilities, and behavioral problems. If you need an additional reason to stop drinking, remember that alcohol use may decrease your ability to have children. In a recent study, women who consumed as few as one to five alcoholic drinks per week were 50 percent less likely to conceive than non-drinking women.

  It's a good idea for your partner to reduce or terminate alcohol consumption, as well; research shows that alcohol affects both the quality and quantity of sperm.

- **Stress**—A recent study at the Mind/Body Institute at Beth Israel Medical Center suggested that stress reduction techniques such as guided imagery and deep relaxation increased conception rates among women who had sought the help of fertility specialists. And don't forget the healthiest, most reliable stress buster—exercise!

- **Nutrition**—When you become pregnant, the food you eat also will nourish your growing baby. Start making healthy changes now. Reduce your intake of empty calories, artificial sweeteners, and caffeine. Increase your intake of nutritious fare, including protein-rich foods, fruits, vegetables, grains, and dairy products. If you're overweight and want to reduce, do it before you become pregnant. Pregnancy is not the time to start a weight reduction diet.

  Before conceiving, begin taking a daily supplement of folic acid. Folic acid protects your baby against neural tube birth defects such as spina bifida (incomplete closure of the spine), anencephaly (partially or completely missing brain) and encephalocele (herniation of the brain). A daily intake of at least 400 micrograms (mcg) of folic acid—up to 800 mcg if you are trying to conceive—can reduce your baby's risk of neural tube defects by 50 percent, and may reduce your chance of miscarriage. Ask your doctor to recommend a daily dosage for you.

The Fun Part

Now that you've converted your body into a baby-friendly environment, you're ready to begin the pursuit of pregnancy. The first step: Stop using birth control. If you're on the birth control pill, your doctor may recommend using a barrier method for a few months before you attempt to conceive. Occasionally, it takes several months for your menstrual periods to return to a regular pattern. Until this happens, it's more difficult to pinpoint when ovulation occurs or to estimate a due date if pregnancy occurs.

Once a month, a woman's ovaries release an egg, which enters her fallopian tube and begins traveling toward her uterus in a process called ovulation. Fertilization (when the sperm and egg unite) takes place in the fallopian tube. Once the fertilized egg reaches the uterus, it implants itself within the uterine wall and begins to grow into a baby. An egg that isn't fertilized is shed along with the lining of the uterus during menstruation.

To result in pregnancy, intercourse must take place within the 72 hours before the egg released at ovulation enters the fallopian tube.

A sperm is capable of fertilizing an egg for many hours after ejaculation, but an egg is fertile for only a very brief time. Your best chance of becoming pregnant is generally 12 to 14 days before the date your period is due.

When the Wait Seems Too Long

Among couples who have frequent sexual intercourse without using any contraception, three out of four will become pregnant within six months. About 10 percent don't become pregnant within a year. If you're unable to become pregnant after one year of unprotected sexual intercourse, you, your partner, or both of you may have a fertility problem. Your gynecologist, your partner's urologist, or your family physician can determine whether you should visit a specialist or clinic that treats infertility problems.

Chapter 4

Adoption: Where Do I Start?

Adopting a child can be one of the most rewarding experiences of your life. However, for adoption beginners, the adoption process can seem overwhelmingly complicated, time consuming, and frustrating—especially if you are eager to get started. This chapter provides some basic information about possible adoption alternatives and is designed to give you an understanding of the adoption process.

Adoption at the end of the 1990s is very different from what it was even ten years ago. Prospective adoptive families can feel vulnerable as they attempt to learn as much as possible in the shortest period of time to become informed consumers of adoption services.

The first step is to read and to educate yourself about adoption in general, the types of children available to adopt, and the various avenues to adoption. There are many informational resources available—guidebooks are listed at the end of this chapter along with an annotated list of national adoption organizations. Adoptive parent support groups throughout the United States have members willing to assist those who are considering adoption. State adoption specialists in each state can send you information to help get you started. As you learn more, you will become better prepared to make the choices that are best for you.

National Adoption Information Clearinghouse, fact sheet, revised 1999; available at http://www.calib.com/naic/factsheets/start.htm.

What Kinds of Children Are Available for Adoption?

Families of all kinds adopt children of all kinds, from newborns to teenagers, of every race and ethnicity, and from many countries around the world.

U.S.-born Infants

Many prospective parents seek to adopt healthy infants, often of a background similar to their own. In the United States, a relatively small percentage of healthy, Caucasian infants are placed for adoption. Most Caucasian infants are placed through agencies and independent adoptions.

African-American, Hispanic, and mixed-race infants are available through both public and private adoption agencies. The adoption of American Indian children (of all ages) by non-Indians is strictly limited by the Federal Indian Child Welfare Act (P.L.95-608). Fees and waiting times for infants vary tremendously, depending on the type of adoption involved.

Children with Special Needs

Many children with special needs are available for adoption. These children may be older (grade school through teens); may have physical, emotional, or mental disabilities; or may be brothers and sisters who should be adopted together. Usually, these children are in the care of a state foster care system. Both public agencies and some private agencies place children with special needs.

In addition, national, regional, and state adoption exchanges will assist in linking prospective parents with these children. Adoption exchanges and agencies usually have photolistings and descriptions of available children, and many now provide information about waiting children on the Internet. In many cases, financial assistance in the form of adoption subsidies is available to help parents with the legal, medical, and living costs associated with caring for a child with special needs.

Intercountry Adoption

Many children from other countries are available for adoption. Russia, China, Korea, India, and countries in Eastern Europe, Central America, and South America are the source countries for most foreign-born children adopted by Americans. More than 700 U.S. private agencies place children from foreign countries, and a few countries allow families to work with attorneys rather than agencies.

There are strict immigration requirements for adopting children from other countries, as well as substantial agency fees and transportation, legal, and medical costs. It is important that you choose a licensed, knowledgeable organization, because the intercountry adoption process is lengthy and complex.

As a prospective parent, you should carefully consider the emotional and social implications of adopting a child of a different nationality. Just as in transracial adoption of a U.S. child, you are adopting a culture as well as a child. Agencies seek families who will help a child learn about and appreciate his or her native culture because it is part of who he or she is.

What Options Are Available?

People considering adoption have a range of options:

- Agency adoptions (permissible in many states)
  - through the local public agency
  - through licensed private agencies (includes both domestic and intercountry programs)
- Independent agencies
  - identified adoptions (allowed in most states)
  - using attorneys or other intermediaries defined by state law
  - using adoption facilitators (allowed in only a few states)

Since adoption laws in the state where you live govern your options, it is essential that you know what types of placements are allowed or not allowed by your state's laws. If you pursue an adoption across states lines, you must comply with the laws in both states before the child can join your family. All 50 states, the District of Columbia, and the U.S. Virgin Islands have enacted legislation (called the Interstate Compact on the Placement of Children) that governs how children can be placed across state lines.

In weighing your options, you should evaluate your ability to tolerate risk. Of the options outlined above, agency adoptions provide the greatest assurance of monitoring and oversight since agencies are required to adhere to licensing and procedural standards. Independent adoptions by attorneys at least provide assurance that attorneys must adhere to the standards of the Bar Association and some attorneys who specialize in adoption are members of the American Academy of Adoption Attorneys, a professional membership organization with standards of ethical practice.

Adoptive placements by facilitators offer the least amount of supervision and oversight. This does not mean that there are not ethical professionals with good standards of practice; it simply means there are few or no oversight mechanisms in place at this time.

Who Can Adopt?

Adoptive parents may be married or single, childless or already parenting other children. Having a disability does not automatically disqualify you from adopting a child; rather, agencies will want to ensure that you can care for a child and meet his or her needs throughout his or her childhood. Divorce or a history of marital or personal counseling does not automatically eliminate you as a candidate. You are not required to own your own home or to have a high income in order to give children what they need—permanence, stability, a lifetime commitment, and a chance to be part of a family. Children do not need "perfect" parents—they need one or more caring and committed individuals willing to meet their needs and to incorporate them into a nurturing family environment.

Increasing numbers of agencies and some foreign countries are now placing children with single applicants. Follow-up research studies of successful single parent adoptions have shown single adoptive parents as mature, independent, and having a wide and supportive network of family and friends. In fact, single adoptive parents are often the placement of choice for children who have trouble dealing with two parents due to a history of abuse or neglect.

For many infant adoptions in the United States, however, agency criteria for applicants are more restrictive. Often agencies will only consider couples married at least one to three years, between the ages of 25 and 40, and with stable employment income. Some agencies accept applicants who are older than 40. Some agencies require that the couple have no other children and be unable to bear children. Some agencies require that one parent not work outside the home for at least six months after the adoption. Agencies placing infants will discuss their specific eligibility regulations and placement options with you.

Steps in Agency Adoption

There are several steps you must complete for any type of adoption through an agency. In addition to the four basic procedures described below, other procedures may be necessary, depending upon your particular needs and those of the child and the birth parents.

(1) Select an Adoption Agency

There are both private and public adoption agencies. A private adoption agency is supported by private funds and should be licensed or approved by the state in which it operates. A public agency is the local branch of your state social service agency. Most public agencies handle only special needs adoptions—not infant or intercountry adoptions. Below are descriptions of both types of agencies.

Using a Private Agency

To obtain the names of local private agencies, look under "Adoption Agencies" or "Social Services" in the Yellow Pages. You can obtain a free copy of your state's agency listing from the National Adoption Information Clearinghouse (NAIC). If you have Internet access, you can visit the NAIC website at http://www.calib.com/naic/databases/nadd/naddatabase.htm to access the *National Adoption Directory* online. You should check with your state adoption specialist, the Better Business Bureau local to the agency, and the state Attorney General's office regarding any complaints that might have been lodged by other adoptive families. You may also wish to check with local adoptive parent support groups for their recommendations of reputable agencies.

Private agencies handle both domestic and intercountry adoptions. You will need to decide which kind of child you want to join your family. Fees charged by private adoption agencies range from $5,000 to more than $30,000 for both domestic and intercountry adoptions. Make sure you ask any agency you might work with what its fees are and what the schedule is for paying them. You should also ask what services are and are not covered by the fees. Most will allow you to pay fees in installments due at particular points during the adoption process. If the fee policy is clear from the beginning, any misunderstandings about payment will be less likely.

Using a Public Agency

You can find an appropriate agency listed in your telephone book in the government section under a name such as "Department of Social Services" or "Department of Public Welfare." Each state organizes its agencies somewhat differently. They may be organized regionally or by county. To begin, call your county office and ask to speak to the adoption specialist. If the county office cannot help you, ask to be referred to the regional or state office.

In general, public agencies will accept adoption applications from families wanting to adopt older children, sibling groups, or children with special physical or psychological needs. Many of the children awaiting placement from public agencies are children of color.

Adoption services through a public agency are usually free or available for a modest fee, since the services are funded through state and federal taxes. As mentioned earlier, federal or state subsidies are sometimes available to assist families adopting a child with special needs. If a child has no special needs, adoptive parents may only be asked to pay legal fees, which are often quite reasonable. In some cases, subsidies may even be available for the legal fees, too.

Children in the custody of a public agency were either abused, neglected, or abandoned by their birth parents. Abuse and neglect can leave physical and emotional scars. It is important to discuss all aspects of a child's history with the agency social workers and to discuss the availability of counseling or other services, just in case they might be needed, before deciding to adopt a child with a traumatic history.

Another parenting option available through public agencies is foster parenting. Children are placed with foster parents to give birth parents a chance to improve their situations. Birth parents are offered counseling and services during this time. Foster parents receive a monthly stipend for a child's living expenses. In general, the goal of the foster care program is to reunite the child with his or her birth parents if at all possible. However, there is a growing trend toward freeing children for adoption (that is, terminating the parental rights of the birth parents) as quickly as possible to prevent years of drifting in foster care. Recent federal legislation (Adoption and Safe Families Act of 1997—P.L. 105-89) has mandated courts to seek termination of parental rights when a child has been in foster care for 15 out of the past 22 months unless there are extenuating circumstances.

More and more foster parents are adopting their foster children. This is particularly true for foster children of color or those with special needs. In almost all states, the vast majority of children adopted from the public foster care system were adopted by their foster parents or by their relatives.

Recently some states have changed the way they perceive their parenting programs. They consider foster parenting and adoption to be a continuum of service, rather than two discrete functions. As a result, agency personnel may ask you at the time of application if you want to be only foster parents, only adoptive parents, or foster/adoptive parents. Foster/adoptive parents are willing to be foster parents while that is the child's need and understand that the agency will make all efforts to reunite the child with the birth parents. However, if the child is freed for adoption, the foster/adoptive parents may be given priority consideration as his or her potential adoptive parents.

It will take some soul searching on your part to decide whether foster parenting is an appropriate option for you. If you can stand some uncertainty, it is a viable option, especially if you have your heart set on a young child and you do not have the funds for a private agency or independent adoption. You must be able to maturely face the prospect of a child being reunited with birth parents, feel sincerely that reunification is indeed in the best interest of the child at that time, and be prepared to handle the grief that would accompany such a loss.

If you are considering this option, discuss becoming a foster/adoptive parent with the agency social workers and other foster parents who have adopted their former foster children.

(2) Complete the Application and Preplacement Inquiry

When you contact an agency, you may be invited to attend an agency-sponsored orientation session. Here you and other applicants will learn about the agency's procedures and available children and receive the application forms. The agency will review your completed application to determine whether to accept you as a client. If accepted by a private agency, you will probably have to pay a registration fee at this point.

The next step is the preplacement inquiry known as the "home study" or the "family assessment." The home study is an evaluation (required by state law) of you as a prospective adoptive family and of the physical and emotional environment into which the child would be placed. It is also a preparation for adoptive parenthood. It consists of a series of interviews with a social worker, including at least one interview in your home. During this process, you will, with the social worker's assistance, consider all aspects of adoptive parenthood and identify the type of child you wish to adopt. Some agencies use a group approach to the educational part of the adoption preparation process because it creates a built-in support group among adoptive families.

Many of the questions asked in the home study are personal and may seem intrusive if you are not expecting them. These questions are necessary for the social worker's evaluation of you as a prospective parent. Some of the questions are about your income, assets, and health and the stability of the marriage (if married) and/or family relationships. Physical exams to ensure that you are healthy are usually required. Some states require that prospective adoptive parents undergo a fingerprint and background check to ensure that you do not have a felony conviction for domestic violence or child abuse. A home study is usually completed in a few months, depending upon the agency's requirements and the number of other clients.

(3) Be Prepared to Wait

Adopting a child always requires a waiting period. If you want to adopt a Caucasian infant, be prepared to wait at least one year from the time the home study is completed, and more frequently two to five years. It is difficult to estimate the waiting period more specifically because birth parents usually select and interview the family they wish to parent their child. Applicants wishing to adopt African-American infants may have a shorter wait, probably less than six months. If you want to adopt a child with special needs, you can begin now to review photolistings to learn more about waiting children and to look for children who might be right for your family. Intercountry adoptions, on the other hand, may take a year or more but the wait and the process will be somewhat more predictable. For any type of adoption, even after a child is found, you may have to wait weeks or months while final arrangements are made.

(4) Complete the Legal Procedures

After a child is placed with you, you must fulfill the legal requirements for adoption. Hiring an attorney may be necessary at this time, if you have not already retained one.

Usually a child lives with the adoptive family for at least six months before the adoption is finalized legally, although this period varies according to state law—unlike some intercountry adoptions, however, where the adoption is completed before the child leaves his or her country. During this time before the adoption is finalized, the agency will provide supportive services. The social worker may visit several times to ensure that the child is well cared for and to write up the required court reports. After this period, the agency will submit a written recommendation of approval of the adoption to the court, and you or your attorney can then file with the court to complete the adoption.

For intercountry adoptions, finalization of the adoption depends on the type of visa the child has, and the laws in your state. The actual adoption procedure is just one of a series of legal processes required for intercountry adoption. You must also fulfill the U.S. Immigration and Naturalization Service's requirements and then proceed to naturalize your child as a citizen of the United States.

Independent Adoptions

Adoptions can sometimes be arranged without an agency. Initial contacts can be made directly between a pregnant woman and adoptive parents or by the pregnant woman and an attorney, depending on state law. Independent adoption is legal in all but a few states, but there are significant variations regarding specific aspects of adoption laws of which you should be aware.

If you pursue this approach, retain an experienced adoption attorney to explain the adoption laws in your state. Talk to other adoptive parents. Become familiar with the Interstate Compact on the Placement of Children (ICPC), because in interstate adoptions you will be required to comply with the adoption laws of both states. You certainly do not want your adoption to be challenged because of failing to comply with the relevant adoption laws.

To initiate an independent adoption, you must first locate a birth mother interested in relinquishing her child. In the states where it is legal, advertising in the classified section of local newspapers has proven to be a successful method for bringing birth parents and adoptive parents together. You can advertise on your own or use a national adoption advertising consultant. Another way to locate a birth mother is to send an introductory letter, photo, and resume describing your family life, home, jobs, hobbies, and interests to crisis pregnancy centers, obstetricians, and all of your friends and colleagues who might possibly lead you to the right person. Some families have even advertised on the Internet.

Simply locating a birth mother is only the first step. You also need to know about the birth father. States have recognized the rights of birth fathers to be involved in decisions about their children, including adoptions. Many states have established registries (putative father registries) as a way for birth fathers to register their intention to support and be involved in their child's life. Several high-profile lawsuits have involved contested adoptions where birth fathers were not notified of, and subsequently objected to, the adoptive placement of the child.

Expenses involved in an independent adoption vary. It is customary for adoptive parents to pay for the birth mother's medical and legal expenses, in addition to their own. Some states also require the adoptive parents to pay for counseling for the birth parents so that the court can be satisfied that they both fully comprehend what they are planning to do. A home study, for which there is a fee, conducted by a certified social worker or a licensed child-placing agency is usually required. In some states, the adoptive parents may also help out with the birth mother's living or clothing expenses. Again, with each of these issues, you must know your state adoption laws and what they allow or prohibit in an adoption

A few states permit adoption facilitators to act as "matchmakers" who recruit and counsel birth parents and then make introductions to prospective adoptive families. The facilitators charge families for their services and allow the birth parents and the adoptive family to make the rest of the placement arrangements.

Each potential independent adoption situation is different, and this method can be expensive. It is not uncommon for the expenses in an independent adoption to equal those of a private agency adoption, unless the birth mother has health insurance or is covered by medical assistance. Since many birth parents change their minds after the child is born, prospective adoptive families must often deal with the loss of funds paid for birth parent expenses in addition to the loss of the anticipated baby. Some adoptive parents purchase adoption insurance as a way to guard against such financial risks; insurance underwriters require that families work with pre-approved agencies or attorneys in order to purchase this insurance.

Identified adoption is a form of independent adoption in which a birth mother and adoptive parents locate one another, but then go together to a licensed adoption agency—in a few states, this is the only type of independent adoption allowed. The agency conducts the home study for the adoptive parents and counsels the birth mother. All the parties know that the birth mother's baby will be placed with that couple. This process combines some of the positive elements of all types of adoption: the birth mother can feel confident that her child will have a future with an approved, loving family, and the adoptive parents can feel confident that the birth mother has thought through her decision carefully. As in any adoption, however, a birth mother may still change her mind about placing the child.

Many couples who have adopted infants independently found it was the right solution for them. It may be the solution for you; however, it is not for everyone. Some adoptive parents who have adopted independently say later that it might have been nice to have had the emotional support and thoughtful preparation for adoption that an adoption agency provides. Most parents want to be well-prepared to help their children deal with adoption issues they will face at different points in their lives. Some parents seek support before and after adopting independently by joining adoptive parent support groups.

Openness in Adoption

An increasing number of adoption professionals feel that openness between the birth parents and adoptive parents benefits the child. Information about both parties can be exchanged directly. The birth parents can do some anticipatory grieving for their loss, while the adoptive parents can prepare to bond immediately with their baby. In this approach, it has even been known for a birth mother to use the adoptive mother as her labor coach when delivering the baby.

Follow-up research on families who have open adoption placements suggests that there are several important benefits to openness. Adoptive families generally report that they do not fear the birth parents (who know them and the child) will return to claim the child. In addition, parents report that their children do not display confusion about who is the parent. Children can ask the difficult questions directly about the reasons they were placed for adoption. Birth parents report a confidence in the rightness of their very difficult decision when they have the security of knowing the adoptive parents and knowing how the child is doing.

Researchers plan to continue their follow-up studies of open adoption placements and to continue to report their findings to professionals and families alike.

How You Can Learn More About Adoption

This chapter gives a basic overview of the steps and issues involved with becoming an adoptive parent. For more in-depth information, you should read adoption guidebooks that are available at your public library or bookstore. Some of these publications are listed on the following page. If you have Internet access (most public libraries are connected), you can find adoption resources online but verify their credibility by cross checking.

Various organizations offer educational programs on adoption. Community colleges, adoption agencies, hospitals, religious groups, local YMCAs, and other organizations may offer adoption preparation programs in your community. You can also call a local private or public adoption agency to find out about their parent preparation programs or to obtain informative publications produced by the agency.

Related Clearinghouse Factsheets

The Clearinghouse factsheets identified in the text are as follows:
- Adopting Children with Developmental Disabilities
- Adopting a Child with Special Needs
- Creating a Family by Birth and Adoption
- The Sibling Bond: Its Importance in Foster Care and Adoptive Placement
- Intercountry Adoption
- Single Parent Adoption: What You Need to Know
- Subsidized Adoption: A Source of Help for Children with Special Needs and Their Families
- Providing Background Information to Adoptive Parents
- Parenting the Sexually Abused Child
- Foster Parent Adoption: What Parents Should Know
- The Adoption Home Study Process
- Open Adoption
- The Value of Adoptive Parent Groups

Clearinghouse Services Online

Factsheets: If you have Internet access, you can find the factsheets listed above online at http://www.calib.com/naic/factsheets/index.htm

State Adoption Law Summaries: Summaries of several elements of state adoption laws are found online at http://www.calib.com/naic/laws/index.htm

Agency & Adoptive Parent Support Group Listings: Find state-specific listings of agencies, attorney referral organizations, and adoptive parent support groups at http://www.calib.com/naic/databases/nadd/naddatabase.htm

Guidebooks

AFA's Guide to Adoption. St. Paul, MN: Adoptive Families of America, annually updated.

Alexander-Roberts, Colleen. *The Essential Adoption Handbook.* Dallas, TX: Taylor Publishing, 1993.

Beauvais-Godwin, Laura, and Raymond Godwin. *The Independent Adoption Manual, From Beginning to Baby.* Lakewood, NJ: The Advocate Press, 1993.

_____. *The Complete Adoption Book.* Holbrook, MA: Adams Media Corporation, 2000.

Bolles, Edmund Blair. *The Penguin Adoption Handbook.* New York: Viking Penguin, 1993.

Craig-Oldsen, Heather L. *From Foster Parent to Adoptive Parent: Helping Foster Parents Make an Informed Decision About Adoption.* Atlanta: Child Welfare Institute, 1988.

Gilman, Lois. *The Adoption Resource Book.* New York: Harper and Row, 1998.

Johnston, Patricia. *Launching a Baby's Adoption: Practical Strategies for Parents and Professionals.* Indianapolis, IN: Perspective Press, 1997.

Marindin, Hope. *Handbook for Single Adoptive Parents.* Chevy Chase, MD: Committee for Single Adoptive Parents, 1998.

Rosenthal, James A., and Victor K. Groze. *Special-Needs Adoption: A Study of Intact Families.* New York: Praeger, 1992.

Schooler, Jayne E. *The Whole Life Adoption Book*. Colorado Springs, CO: Pifion Press, 1993.

Sifferman, K. A. *Adoption: A Legal Guide for Birth and Adoptive Parents*. Hawthorne, NJ: Career Press, Inc., 1994.

Walker, Elaine L., and Teresa Walsh, illustrator. *Loving Journeys: Guide to Adoption*. Peterborough, NH: Loving Journeys, 1992.

Wirth, Eileen M., and Joan Worden. *How to Adopt a Child from Another Country*. Nashville, TN: Abingdon Press, 1993.

Directory

National Adoption Directory. National Adoption Information Clearinghouse. Updated annually. Cost is $25.00, including postage. Prepayment is required. The directory is available online on the NAIC website at http://www.calib.com/naic/databases/

Adoptive Organizations

Adoptive Families of America
Adoptive Families Magazine
(212) 877-1839
Fax (212) 382-8910
(800) 372-3300 (order information)
Website: http://www.adoptivefam.org

American Academy of Adoption Attorneys
PO Box 33053
Washington, DC 20033-0053
(202) 832-2222
Website: http://www.adoptionattorneys.org
(membership organization for adoption attorneys)

Children Awaiting Parents, Inc.
700 Exchange St.
Rochester, NY 14608
(716) 232-5110
Website: http://www.GGW.org/adopt/cap
(publishes *CAP Book* photolisting of waiting children)

Child Welfare League of America
440 First St., NW, Ste. 310
Washington, DC 20001
(202) 638-2952
Website: http://www.cwla.org

National Adoption Center
1500 Walnut St., Ste. 701
Philadelphia, PA 19102
(215) 735-9988 or (800) TO-ADOPT
Website: http://www.adopt.org
(family recruitment & online photolisting of waiting children)

National Adoption Foundation
100 Mill Plain Rd.
Danbury, CT 06811
(203) 791-3811
(revolving adoption bank loan & grants to adoptive families)

National Adoption Information Clearinghouse
330 C St., SW
Washington, DC 20447
(703) 352-3488 or (888) 251-0075
Website: http://www.calib.com/naic
(information service of US DHHS Children's Bureau)

National Council for Adoption
1930 17th St., NW
Washington, DC 20009-6207
(202) 328-1200
Website: http://www.ncfa-usa.org

National Resource Center for Special Needs Adoption
16250 Northland Dr., Ste. 120
Southfield, MI 48075
(248) 443-7080
Website: http://www.spaulding.org/adoption/NRC-adoption.html
(training & technical assistance on special needs adoption)

North American Council on Adoptable Children
970 Raymond Ave., Ste. 106
St. Paul, MN 55114-1149
(651) 644-3036
Website: http://www.nacac.org
(advocacy & information on subsidy)

One Church, One Child
1000 16th St., NW
Suite 702
Washington, D.C. 20036
(202) 789-4333
(church-based recruitment of & support to families of color)

Resolve, Inc.
1310 Broadway
Somerville, MA 02144-1731
(617) 623-1156
Website: http://www.resolve.org
(info & support to families dealing with infertility)

Part Two:

Special Family Planning Issues

Chapter 5

Infertility

Chapter Contents

Section 5.1

Overcoming Infertility

FDA Consumer, January-February 1997; revised February 1997; available at http://www.fda.gov/fdac/features/1997/197_fert.html.

—by Tamar Nordenberg; illustrations by Renée Gordon

Myth or fact: If a couple is having trouble conceiving a child, the man should try wearing loose underwear? That's a fact, according to a study on "Tight-fitting Underwear and Sperm Quality" published June 29, 1996, in the scientific journal *The Lancet*. Tight-fitting underwear—as well as hot tubs and saunas—is not recommended for men trying to father a child because it may raise testes temperature to a point where it interferes with sperm production.

But couples having difficulty getting pregnant can tell you the solution is almost never as simple as wearing boxers instead of briefs. Lisa (who asked that her last name not be used) tried for more than two years to get pregnant without success. "Everyone gave me advice," she says. "My mother said I should just go to church and pray more. My friends said, 'Try to relax and not think about it' or 'You're just overstressed. You work too much.'"

Actually, psychological stress is more likely a result of infertility than the cause, according to Resolve, a nonprofit consumer organization specializing in infertility.

"Fertility problems are a huge psychological stressor, a huge relationship stressor," says Lisa Rarick, M.D., director of the Food and Drug Administration's division of reproductive and urologic drug products.

So, while going on a relaxing vacation may temporarily relieve the stress that comes with fertility problems, a solution may require treatment by a health-care professional. Treatment with drugs such as Clomid or Serophene (both clomiphene citrate) or Pergonal, Humegon, Metrodin, or Fertinex (all menotropins) are used in some cases to correct a woman's hormone imbalance. Surgery is sometimes used to repair damaged reproductive organs. And in about 10 percent of cases, less conventional, high-tech options like in vitro fertilization are used.

Will the therapies work? "Talking about the success rate for fertility treatments is like saying, 'What's the chance of curing a headache?'" according to Benjamin Younger, M.D., executive director of the American Society for Reproductive Medicine. "It depends on many things, including the cause of the problem and the severity." Overall, Younger says, about half of couples that seek fertility treatment will be able to have babies.

A Year without Pregnancy

Infertility is defined as the inability to conceive a child despite trying for one year. The condition affects about 5.3 million Americans, or 9 percent of the reproductive age population, according to the American Society for Reproductive Medicine.

Ironically, the best protection against infertility is to use a condom while you are not trying to get pregnant. Condoms prevent sexually transmitted diseases, a primary cause of infertility.

Even a completely healthy couple can't expect to get pregnant at the drop of a hat. Only 20 percent of women who want to conceive become pregnant in the first ovulation cycle they try, according to Younger.

To become pregnant, a couple must have intercourse during the woman's fertile time of the month, which is right before and during ovulation. Because it's tough to pinpoint the exact day of ovulation, having intercourse often during the approximate time maximizes the chances of conception.

After a year of frequent intercourse without contraception that doesn't result in pregnancy, a couple should go to a health-care professional for an evaluation. In some cases, it makes sense to seek help for fertility problems even before a year is up.

A woman over 30 may wish to get an earlier evaluation. "At age 30, a woman begins a slow decline in her ability to get pregnant," says Younger. "The older she gets, the greater her chance of miscarriage, too." But a woman's fertility doesn't take a big drop until around age 40.

"A man's age affects fertility to a much smaller degree and 20 or 30 years later than in a woman," Younger says. Despite a decrease in sperm production that begins after age 25, some men remain fertile into their 60s and 70s.

A couple may also seek earlier evaluation if:

- The woman isn't menstruating regularly, which may indicate an absence of ovulation that would make it impossible for her to conceive without medical help.

- The woman has had three or more miscarriages (or the man had a previous partner who had had three or more miscarriages).

- The woman or man has had certain infections that sometimes affect fertility (for example, pelvic infection in a woman, or mumps or prostate infection in a man).

- The woman or man suspects there may be a fertility problem (if, for example, attempts at pregnancy failed in a previous relationship).

The Man or the Woman?

Impairment in any step of the intricate process of conception can cause infertility. For a woman to become pregnant, her partner's sperm must be healthy so that at least one can swim into her fallopian tubes. An egg, released by the woman's ovaries, must be in the fallopian tube ready to be fertilized. Next, the fertilized egg, called an embryo, must make its way through an open-ended fallopian tube into the uterus, implant in the uterine lining, and be sustained there while it grows. (See diagram.)

It is a myth that infertility is always a "woman's problem." Of the 80 percent of cases with a diagnosed cause, about half are based at least partially on male problems (referred to as male factors)—usually that the man produces no sperm, a condition called azoospermia, or that he produces too few sperm, called oligospermia.

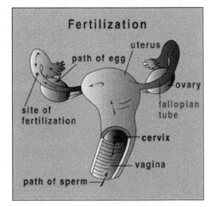

Lifestyle can influence the number and quality of a man's sperm. Alcohol and drugs—including marijuana, nicotine, and certain medications—can temporarily reduce sperm quality. Also, environmental toxins, including pesticides and lead, may be to blame for some cases of infertility.

The causes of sperm production problems can exist from birth or develop later as a result of severe medical illnesses, including mumps and some sexually transmitted diseases, or from a severe testicle injury, tumor, or other problem. Inability to ejaculate normally can prevent conception, too, and can be caused by many factors, including diabetes, surgery of the prostate gland or urethra, blood pressure medication, or impotence.

The other half of explained infertility cases are linked to female problems (called female factors), most commonly ovulation disorders. Without ovulation, eggs are not available for fertilization. Problems with ovulation are signaled by irregular menstrual periods or a lack of periods altogether (called amenorrhea). Simple lifestyle factors—including stress, diet, or athletic training—can affect a woman's hormonal balance. Much less often, a hormonal imbalance can result from a serious medical problem such as a pituitary gland tumor.

Other problems can also lead to female infertility. If the fallopian tubes are blocked at one or both ends, the egg can't travel through the tubes into the uterus. Such blockage may result from pelvic inflammatory disease, surgery for an ectopic pregnancy (when the embryo implants in the fallopian tube rather than in the uterus), or other problems, including endometriosis (the abnormal presence of uterine lining cells in other pelvic organs).

A medical evaluation may determine whether a couple's infertility is due to these or other causes. If a medical and sexual history doesn't reveal an obvious problem, like improperly timed intercourse or absence of ovulation, specific tests may be needed.

Tests for Both

The man's evaluation focuses on the number and health of his sperm. The laboratory first examines a sperm sample under a microscope to check sperm number, shape, and movement. Further tests may be needed to look for infection, hormonal imbalance, or other problems.

Male tests include:

- **X-ray:** If damage to one or both of the vas deferens (the ducts in the male that transport the sperm to the penis) is known or suspected, an x-ray is taken to examine the organs.

- **Mucus penetrance test:** Test of whether the man's sperm are able to swim through a drop of the woman's fertile vaginal mucus on a slide (also used to test the quality of the woman's mucus).

- **Hamster-egg penetrance assay:** Test of whether the man's sperm will penetrate hamster egg cells with their outer cells removed, indicating somewhat their ability to fertilize human eggs.

For the woman, the first step in testing is to determine if she is ovulating each month. This can be done by charting changes in morning body temperature, by using an FDA-approved home ovulation test kit (which is available over the counter), or by examining cervical mucus, which undergoes a series of hormone-induced changes throughout the menstrual cycle.

Checks of ovulation can also be done in the physician's office with simple blood tests for hormone levels or ultrasound tests of the ovaries. If the woman is ovulating, further testing will need to be done.

Common female tests include:

- **Hysterosalpingogram:** An x-ray of the fallopian tubes and uterus after they are injected with dye, to show if the tubes are open and to show the shape of the uterus.

- **Laparoscopy:** An examination of the tubes and other female organs for disease, using a miniature light-transmitting tube called a laparoscope. The tube is inserted into the abdomen through a one-inch incision below the navel, usually while the woman is under general anesthesia.

- **Endometrial biopsy:** An examination of a small shred of uterine lining to see if the monthly changes in the lining are normal.

Some tests require participation of both partners. Samples of cervical mucus taken after intercourse can show whether sperm and mucus have properly interacted. Also, a variety of tests can show if the man or woman is forming antibodies that are attacking the sperm.

Drugs and Surgery

Depending on what the tests turn up, different treatments are recommended. Eighty to 90 percent of infertility cases are treated with drugs or surgery.

Therapy with the fertility drug Clomid or with a more potent hormone stimulator—Pergonal, Metrodin, Humegon, or Fertinex—is often recommended for women with ovulation problems. The benefits of each drug and the side effects, which can be minor or serious but rare, should be discussed with the doctor. Multiple births occur in 10 to 20 percent of births resulting from fertility drug use.

Other drugs, used under very limited circumstances, include Parlodel (bromocriptine mesylate), for women with elevated levels of a hormone called prolactin, and a hormone pump that releases gonadotropins necessary for ovulation.

If drugs aren't the answer, surgery may be. Because major surgery is involved, operations to repair damage to the woman's ovaries, fallopian tubes, or uterus are recommended only if there is a good chance of restoring fertility.

In the man, one infertility problem often treated surgically is damage to the vas deferens, commonly caused by a sexually transmitted disease, other infection, or vasectomy (male sterilization).

Other important tools in the battle against infertility include artificial insemination and the so-called assisted reproductive technologies. (See "Science and ART.")

Fulfillment Regardless

Lisa became pregnant without assisted reproductive technologies, after taking ovulation-promoting medication and undergoing surgery to repair her damaged fallopian tubes. Her daughter is now 4 years old.

"It was definitely worth it. I really appreciate having my daughter because of what I went through," she says. But Lisa and her husband won't try to have a second child just yet. "At some point you have to stop trying to have a baby, stop obsessing over what might be an unreachable goal," she says.

When having a genetically related baby seems unachievable, a couple may decide to stop treatment and proceed with the rest of their lives. Some may choose to lead an enriched life without children. Others may choose to adopt.

And no, according to Resolve, you're not more likely to get pregnant if you adopt a baby.

Science and ART

Sometimes it may be necessary or preferable to get pregnant without intercourse. A woman may choose to get pregnant with the sperm of someone who is not her partner.

In some cases, a woman may not be able to become pregnant with her partner because his sexual problems make it impossible for him to ejaculate normally during sex, or because the sperm have to bypass the vagina if the vaginal mucus cannot support them, or for other reasons. In these cases, through artificial insemination, the semen is placed into the woman's uterus or vaginal canal using a hollow, flexible tube called a catheter.

New, more complex assisted reproductive technologies, or ART, procedures, including in vitro fertilization (IVF), have been available since the birth in 1978 of Louise Brown, the world's first "test tube baby." IVF makes it possible to combine sperm and eggs in a laboratory for a baby that is genetically related to one or both partners.

IVF (illustrated in the diagram at right) is often used when a woman's fallopian tubes are blocked. First, medication is given to stimulate the ovaries to produce multiple eggs. Once mature, the eggs are suctioned from the ovaries (1) and placed in a laboratory culture dish with the man's sperm for fertilization (2). The dish is then placed in an incubator (3). About two days later, three to five embryos are transferred to the woman's uterus (4). If the woman does not become pregnant, she may try again in the next cycle.

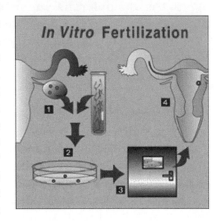

In Vitro Fertilization

Other ART procedures, based on many of the same principles, include:

- **Gamete intrafallopian transfer, or GIFT:** Similar to IVF, but used when the woman has at least one normal fallopian tube. Three to five eggs are placed in the fallopian tube, along with the man's sperm, for fertilization inside the woman's body.

- **Zygote intrafallopian transfer, or ZIFT (also called tubal embryo transfer):** A hybrid of IVF and GIFT. The eggs retrieved from the woman's ovaries are fertilized in the lab and replaced in the fallopian tubes rather than the uterus.

- **Donor egg IVF:** For women who, for example, have impaired ovaries or carry a genetic disease that can be transferred to the offspring. Eggs are donated by another healthy woman and fertilized in the lab with the male partner's sperm before being transferred to the female partner's uterus.

- **Frozen embryos:** Excess embryos are frozen, to be thawed in the future if the woman doesn't get pregnant on the first cycle or wants another baby in the future.

New treatments for male factors are fast-evolving. Intracytoplasmic sperm injection is one of the most exciting new procedures, according to Benjamin Younger, M.D., executive director of the American

Society for Reproductive Medicine. A single egg is injected with a single sperm to produce an embryo that can implant and grow in the uterus.

About two-thirds of births from ART procedures are single births. Of the rest, almost all are twins, with about 6 percent resulting in the birth of triplets or more.

To get more information about infertility, send a self-addressed stamped envelope to: Resolve, 1310 Broadway, Somerville, MA 02144-1731, or call their National Helpline at (617) 623-0744.

Tamar Nordenberg is a staff writer for *FDA Consumer.*

Section 5.2

Facts about Infertility

"Fact Sheet: Infertility," © 1998 ASRM (American Society for Reproductive Medicine); available at http://www.asrm.org/fact/infertility.html; reprinted with permission.

- Infertility affects 61 million American women and their partners, about 10% of the reproductive age population.
- Infertility is a disease of the reproductive system that affects the male or female with almost equal frequency.
- Recent improvements in medication, microsurgery, and in vitro fertilization (IVF) techniques make pregnancy possible for more than half of the couples pursuing treatments.
- 25% of infertile couples have more than one factor that contributes to their infertility.
- In approximately 40% of infertile couples, the male partner is either the sole cause or a contributing cause of infertility.
- Tubal blockage and/or peritoneal factors account for approximately 35% of all female infertility problems.
- Irregular or abnormal ovulation accounts for approximately 25% of all female infertility cases.

- Endometriosis is found in about 35% of infertile women who have laparoscopy as part of their infertility work-up.

- Approximately 20% of couples who have a complete work-up are diagnosed with unexplained infertility because no specific cause is identified.

- IVF is a method of assisted reproduction in which a man's sperm and the woman's egg are combined in a laboratory dish, where fertilization occurs. The resulting embryo is then transferred to the uterus to develop naturally. Usually, two to four embryos are transferred with each cycle.

- Other techniques of assisted reproduction include gamete intrafallopian transfer (GIFT), zygote intrafallopian transfer (ZIFT), IVF with donor eggs, donor sperm, and donor embryos, and micromanipulation of eggs and embryos.

- There are more than 70,000 babies born in the United States as a result of all assisted reproductive technologies (ART), including 45,000 as a result of IVF.

- According to the most recent statistics (1995), the success rate of ART procedures are as follows:

  IVF—22.3% live birth per egg retrieval

  GIFT—26.8% live birth per egg retrieval

  ZIFT—27.7% live birth per egg retrieval

Chapter 6

When Pregnancy Is Unplanned

Chapter Contents

Section 6.1

What If I'm Pregnant?

Text adapted from *What If I'm Pregnant?*, © revised version April 1998
Planned Parenthood® Federation of America, Inc., original copyright 1993
PPFA, PPFA Web Site © 1998, Planned Parenthood® Federation of America,
Inc.; available at http://plannedparenthood.org/WOMENSHEALTH/
whatifpregnant.htm; reprinted with permission.

Women may ask this question at many times in their lives—especially when their periods are late. Most women want to become mothers when they are ready and can plan for it. Adult and teenage women often face difficult decisions when pregnancy is unplanned. If you think you're pregnant, you may be asking yourself lots of other questions, too:

- "Is having a baby the best choice for me?"
- "Is raising a child by myself the best choice for me?"
- "Is raising a child with a partner the best choice for me?"
- "Is placing the baby for adoption the best choice for me?"
- "Is having an abortion the best choice for me?"

You want to choose what's right for you. But first, be sure you are pregnant.

How Can I Be Sure I'm Pregnant?

A urine or blood test performed by medical professionals is the surest way to find out.

You can get home pregnancy tests at most drugstores. They are simple to use. But they are not accurate unless you very carefully read and follow the instructions in the package. To be sure, have your pregnancy test done at your clinician's office or at a Planned Parenthood center or other family planning clinic.

If your test is "positive," you will need a pelvic exam. The clinician will feel the size of your uterus to estimate how long you have been pregnant. Then you will need to decide what you want to do.

What Are My Choices?

You have three choices if you are pregnant.
- You can choose to have a baby and raise the child.
- You can choose to have a baby and place your child for adoption.
- You can choose to end the pregnancy.

There is no right or wrong choice for everyone. Only you can decide which choice is right for you.

How Can I Decide which Choice Is Best for Me?

Consider each of your choices carefully. Ask yourself:
- Which choice(s) could I live with?
- Which choice(s) would be impossible for me?
- How would each choice affect my everyday life?
- What would each choice mean to the people closest to me?

It may help to take time and ask yourself:
- What is going on in my life?
- What are my plans for the future?
- What are my spiritual and moral beliefs?
- What do I believe is best for me in the long run?
- What can I afford?

Talk about your feelings with your partner, someone in your family, or a trusted friend. All family planning clinics have specially trained counselors. These counselors can talk with you about your options. Your counselor will try to make sure that you are not being pressured into any decision against your will. You may bring your partner, your parents, or someone else if you wish.

Find out as much as you can about all your choices. Here is some information to consider.

How Soon Do I Have to Decide?

If there is a chance that you will continue the pregnancy— you should begin prenatal care as soon as possible. You should have a medical exam early in your pregnancy to make sure that you are healthy and the pregnancy is normal.

If you are considering abortion—you should make your decision as soon as possible. Abortion is very safe, but the risks increase the longer a pregnancy goes on.

While you are deciding what to do, take good care of yourself. If you do decide to have a child, you will want it to be healthy and well.

- Get enough good food—fruits, vegetables, cereals, breads, beans, rice, and dairy products as well as fish, meat, and poultry.
- Keep your body in good shape. Stay active and get regular exercise.
- Get plenty of sleep.
- Do not smoke.
- Do not drink alcohol or drinks with caffeine, like coffee and cola.
- Do not eat junk food.
- Don't take any drugs or medications—not even aspirin—without checking with your clinic doctor.

You can get complete information about prenatal care and how to pay for it from your family doctor, your local Planned Parenthood center, other family planning clinics, women's health centers, and your state's department of family services. Good prenatal care is very important for a baby's health.

To make an appointment with the Planned Parenthood nearest you about your pregnancy options and prenatal care call toll-free 1-800-230-PLAN.

What about Raising a Child?

One of your choices is to continue your pregnancy and raise a child. Being a parent is exciting, rewarding, and demanding. It can help you grow, understand yourself better, and enhance your life.

There are two ways to raise a child.

- You might want to raise the child with a partner.
- You might want to raise the child without a partner.

Parenting with a Partner

Most of us look forward to finding a life partner—someone with whom we can share the pleasures, responsibilities, and difficulties of family life. You may want to consider marriage if you intend to parent with a partner.

Marriage is a serious legal contract binding both partners. Each one accepts legal as well as moral and emotional obligations to the other. Every state has its own laws about marriage. If you are under 18, contact your local marriage license bureau or consult your religious adviser to find out about the laws in your state.

Consider premarital counseling if marriage is one of your choices. Taking the time to talk about marriage with a counselor can make a big difference. See a private counselor or get counseling through your church, temple, mosque, or some other community service. Family counseling is also beneficial for all couples, married or not—whenever they consider beginning or expanding a family.

With or without marriage, a life partnership can succeed if both people:

- are deeply committed to make it work
- understand what each expects from the relationship.

Here are some things to consider if you are thinking about parenting with a partner:

		True	False
1.	I'll get what I want in life if I start a family now.	___	___
2.	My/his parents are pushing us into marriage.	___	___
3.	We're both financially and emotionally ready.	___	___
4.	We get upset when we talk about a long-term, committed relationship.	___	___
5.	I know what to expect of my partner.	___	___
6.	My partner knows what to expect of me.	___	___
7.	Marriage will make us feel less guilty about sex.	___	___
8.	He knows that he's responsible for child care and housework, too.	___	___
9.	We'd stay together even if I weren't pregnant.	___	___
10.	I'm prepared to be a single parent if things don't work out between us.	___	___

REMEMBER: A child can bring joy and many other rewards to a relationship. A child can also strain the best relationship. If your commitment is not solid, the relationship may fail.

Think about what your answers mean to you. You may want to discuss your answers with your partner, someone in your family, a friend, a trusted religious advisor, your counselor.

Parenting without a Partner

The challenge of raising a child alone can also be exciting and rewarding. It is easier if you find and use all the support you can. Be sure to let family and friends know that you hope for their support before you decide to become a single parent.

Even with the help of your family and friends, being a single parent is not easy. It is often complicated and frustrating. Your child's needs will constantly change and so will your ability to meet those needs. You may want to consider counseling to help you through these changes. You may find out about counseling from your local department of children's services.

Your child will look to you for love and care—all day, every day. And you can take great pleasure helping your child grow into a happy, independent, and responsible adult. But there will be no breaks. It takes years for children to become responsible for themselves. And convenient, affordable childcare is difficult to find.

It takes a lot of money to raise a child. Earning a living for you and your child will be a real challenge—even if you have finished school and can get a good job. Your own parent(s) may find it hard to help you out with all the bills. Welfare payments barely cover the basics.

Because your child will need you so much, you may become more dependent on your own family and friends—for help with the child, for money, and for emotional support. You may have to give up a lot of freedom to be a good single parent. On the other hand, because you will not have to make compromises with a partner, you can raise the child as you wish—with your values, principles, and beliefs.

Parenting requires lots of love and unlimited energy and patience. There will be times when you may feel that you are not doing a good job at it. To feel good about being a single parent, it must be what you want to do—for a long time. You already know what that means if you have other children. If you don't, talk with a single mother or with a counselor who works with single mothers.

Here are some things to consider if you are thinking about parenting without a partner:

		True	False
1.	Loving my baby will get me through hard times.	——	——
2.	I'm being pressured to keep the baby.	——	——
3.	I'm willing to put school and career on hold.	——	——
4.	I'll be more dependent on other people.	——	——
5.	Money won't be a problem.	——	——
6.	My baby will give me all the love I need.	——	——
7.	I know someone who is always available and who I can trust to take care of the child when I'm at work or school or when I'm sick.	——	——
8.	Having another child will strengthen my family.	——	——
9.	I'll find a life partner more easily with a child.	——	——
10.	My family and friends will be supportive.	——	——

Think about what your answers mean to you. You may want to discuss your answers with someone in your family, a friend, a trusted religious advisor, or your counselor.

To make an appointment with the Planned Parenthood nearest you for referrals to couples-counseling professionals and family-service organizations call toll-free 1-800-230-PLAN.

What about Placing the Baby for Adoption?

One of your choices is to complete your pregnancy and let someone else raise your child. Many women who make this choice are happy knowing that their children are loved and living in good homes. But some women find that the pain of being separated from their children is deeper and longer lasting than they expected.

There are two kinds of adoption:

- **Closed Adoption**—the names of the birth mother and the adoptive parents are kept secret from one another.

- **Open Adoption**—the birth mother may select the adoptive parents for her child. She and the adoptive parents may choose to get to know one another. They may also choose to have an on-going relationship.

Adoption is legal and binding whether it is open or closed. Few adoptions are reversed by the courts. You will have to sign "relinquishment papers" some time after your baby is born. After signing, you may be given a limited period of time during which you may change your mind. In most states, minors do not need a parent's consent to choose adoption. However, the child's father can demand custody of the child unless he has already signed release papers for the adoption.

Adoption laws are different in every state. Find out in advance what they are in your state. Talk with an adoption counselor or lawyer before deciding on any arrangement. Be sure to read everything very carefully before you sign. It is always best to have a lawyer review all documents first.

There are thousands of women and men waiting to adopt newborn children. However, there is no guarantee that homes will be found for all children waiting to be adopted. This is especially true of children of color and children with disabilities.

Adoption is arranged in three ways:

- **Agency (licensed) adoption:** the birth parents "relinquish" their child to the agency. The agent places the child into the adoptive home.
- **Independent (unlicensed) adoption:** the birth parents relinquish their child directly into the adoptive home.
- **Adoption by relatives:** the court grants legal adoption to relatives.

All adoptions must be approved by a judge in a family or surrogate court.

Agency Adoption

You could place your child through a public or private agency that is licensed by the government. These agencies:

- provide counseling
- handle legal matters
- make hospital arrangements for your child's birth
- select a home for your child
- refer you to agencies that may help you financially

Sometimes an agency is able to help find a home for you during your pregnancy. In agency adoption, your name and the adoptive parents' names are usually kept secret. However, some licensed agencies also offer various open adoption options.

Most religious organizations can help you locate a licensed adoption agency. You can also look in the Yellow Pages® under "Adoption Agencies" and "Social Service Organizations." You can also contact your state, county, or local department of family or child services, or your local Planned Parenthood.

The National Council for Adoption hotline can refer you to licensed agencies in your area Call: 1-202-328-8072. If you are pregnant you can call collect. Or you can write to the National Council for Adoption, 1930 17th Street, N.W., Washington, DC, 20009. The general phone number is 202-328-1200. The website address is http://www.ncfa-usa.org.

Independent Adoption

You can arrange an independent adoption through a doctor or lawyer or someone else who knows a couple that wants to adopt. Some states have private, independent adoption centers that provide counseling. These centers are run by women and men who want to adopt. Independent adoptions are not legal in some states because there is a risk that birth mothers and adoptive parents may be exploited.

An independent adoption is usually an open adoption. The adoptive parents will often agree to pay for your hospital and medical bills until the child is born. They may even pay for your living expenses during that time. Usually the adoptive parents hire one lawyer to represent them and you. If you choose independent adoption, you should consider having a lawyer of your own. To find one, contact your local state bar association, Family Court, local family service organization, or the Legal Aid Society. A social worker can also help you find a lawyer.

You will be asked to sign a "take into care" form after you give birth. This allows the adoptive parents to take the child home while the state studies their family life and home environment. The study takes six to eight weeks. During this time, both you and the prospective parents can change your minds. When the study is over, you will be asked to sign "relinquishment papers."

For information and referrals about independent adoption, call the Independent Adoption Center hotline: 1-800-877-OPEN. Or write to the Independent Adoption Center, 391 Taylor Boulevard, Suite 100, Pleasant Hill, California 94523. The website address is http://www.adoptionhelp.org/nfediac. Planned Parenthood and other family planning centers can also provide information about independent adoption.

Adoption by Relatives

You may want your child to stay in your own family. However, independent adoptions with a relative must also be approved by a family- or surrogate-court judge. Your relatives will have to be studied by a state agency before the adoption can be finalized. And you will have no more right to the child than if you placed it with strangers.

Think about what your answers mean to you. You may want to discuss your answers with your partner, someone in your family, a friend, a trusted religious advisor, or your counselor.

Foster Care

In some cities and counties, temporary foster care may be available for the children of mothers who need more time to decide between adoption and parenting.

Here are some things to consider if you are thinking about adoption:

		True	False
1.	I can accept my child living with someone else.	____	____
2.	Going through pregnancy and delivery won't change my mind.	____	____
3.	I'm willing to get good prenatal care.	____	____
4.	I'm choosing adoption because abortion scares me.	____	____
5.	The child's father will approve of adoption.	____	____
6.	No one is pressuring me to choose adoption.	____	____
7.	I'll know my child will be treated well.	____	____
8.	I won't be jealous of the adoptive parents.	____	____
9.	I care what other people will think.	____	____
10.	I respect women who place their children for adoption.	____	____

You and the child's father must both sign a legal foster care agreement to have another family care for your child. It's a good idea to consider a legal contract even if someone in your family provides the foster care. Legal contracts can help prevent misunderstandings.

Foster care agreements include:

- how often you agree to visit your child
- how long your child will stay with the foster care family
- how much money you may have to pay for the child's care
- how often you must see the social worker

You could lose your child if you don't keep your part of the agreement. It is important to remember that foster care is only temporary and is not a good substitute for a permanent home.

Laws about foster care vary from state to state. To find out more about foster care, consult your state's Department of Child Welfare or talk to someone at your local Planned Parenthood.

To make an appointment with the Planned Parenthood nearest you to discuss adoption and your other pregnancy options, call toll-free 1-800-230-PLAN.

What about Abortion?

One of your choices is abortion. Abortion is a legal and safe procedure. More than 90 percent of abortions occur during the first 12 weeks of pregnancy.

Vacuum aspiration is the usual method of early abortion. First, the cervix is numbed. Then the embryo or fetus is removed through a narrow tube with vacuum suction. The surgery takes about five minutes.

Early medical abortion is available in a small number of clinics that are participating in clinical trials. This method uses the medication mifepristone or methotrexate. Medical abortion is not yet widely available.

Early abortion is usually done in a clinic, doctor's office, or hospital. You don't need to stay overnight. Most likely, you can return to your normal activities the next day. Abortions performed later in pregnancy may be more complicated but are still safer than having a baby.

Abortion is one of the safest operations available. Serious complications are rare. But the risk of complications increases the longer a pregnancy continues.

Most women say that early abortion feels like menstrual cramps. Other women say it feels very uncomfortable. Still others feel very little.

You will need to sign a form that says you:

- have been **informed** about all your options
- have been **counseled** about the procedure, its risks, and how to care for yourself afterward
- have **chosen** abortion of your own free will

Most teenagers consult their parents before an abortion. But telling a parent is not required in all states. Many states do require a woman under 18 to tell a parent or get a parent's permission. If she cannot talk with her parents, or chooses not to, she can speak with a judge. The judge will decide whether she is mature enough to make her own decision about abortion. If she is not mature enough, the judge will decide if abortion is in her best interest. Find out about the law in your state. Your local Planned Parenthood can help you with this process.

Most women feel relieved after an abortion. Some experience anger, regret, guilt, or sadness for a short time. These feelings may be complicated by the abrupt hormonal changes that take place after abortion. Serious, long-term emotional problems after abortion are rare. They are more likely after childbirth.

You are more likely to experience serious regrets after abortion if you have strong religious feelings against it. Be sure to examine your moral concerns before choosing abortion. Counseling is available before and after abortion.

Uncomplicated abortion should not affect future pregnancies.

Abortions during the first 12 weeks of pregnancy can be performed in a clinician's office. Abortions are also available in many Planned Parenthood clinics, in many other reproductive health clinics, and in some hospitals. Most large cities and many smaller communities have abortion providers. Look in the Yellow Pages under "abortion."

Ask beforehand about payment. Some places want to be paid in advance. Some accept credit cards. Sometimes payment plans can be worked out. Some insurance plans cover part or all of the cost. In all states, Medicaid will pay for abortion if the woman's life is in danger. In some states, Medicaid will pay for abortion for other reasons, too. Check with your local Planned Parenthood or your state or local health or welfare department for the kind of Medicaid coverage in your state.

Think about what your answers mean to you. You may want to discuss your answers with your partner, someone in your family, a friend, a trusted religious advisor, or your counselor.

You can get abortion information and assistance at Planned Parenthood and other family planning centers, women's health centers,

---

Here are some things to consider if you are thinking about abortion:

		True	False
1.	No one is pressuring me to choose abortion.		
2.	I have strong religious beliefs against abortion.		
3.	I look down on women who have abortions.		
4.	I'd rather have a child at another time.		
5.	I can afford to have another child.		
6.	I can afford to have an abortion.		
7.	I care about what other people will think.		
8.	I can handle the abortion experience.		
9.	I'll go before a judge if necessary.		
10.	I would do anything to end this pregnancy.		

---

youth centers, and departments of health or social services. Or you can call the National Abortion Federation hotline: 1-800-772-9100.

To make an appointment with the Planned Parenthood nearest you for counseling about abortion and your other pregnancy options, call toll-free 1-800-230-PLAN.

Section 6.2

Are You Pregnant and Thinking about Adoption?

National Adoption Information Clearinghouse, fact sheet, 1992; available at http://www.calib.com/naic/factsheets/pregnant.htm.

—by Debra G. Smith

If you are pregnant and not sure that you want to keep the baby, you might be thinking about adoption.

Pregnancy causes many changes, both physical and emotional. It can be a very confusing time for a woman, even in the best of circumstances. Talking to a counselor about your options might help. But how do you start?

This section gives you, the birth mother, information about counseling and adoption. It addresses many questions you might have:

- Who can I talk to about my options?
- Should I place my child for adoption?
- What are the different types of adoption?
- How do I arrange an adoption through an agency?
- How do I arrange a private adoption?
- What if my baby is a child of color?
- How do I arrange for future contact with my child if I want it?

If you want more information on these adoption issues, or any others, please contact the National Adoption Information Clearinghouse at (703) 352-3488 or 1 (888) 251-0075, 330 C Street, SW, Washington, D.C. 20447.

Who Can I Talk to about My Options?

If you want to talk to a professional about your options, there are different places you can go. Counseling at the places listed on the next page will be free or cost very little.

- *Crisis pregnancy center*—This is a place where they talk only to pregnant women. It might even have a maternity center attached where you could live until the baby is born.
- *Family planning clinic*—This is a place where women get birth control information or pregnancy tests.
- *Adoption agency*—This choice is good if you are already leaning strongly in the direction of adoption.
- *Health Department or Social Services*—A food stamps or welfare worker can tell you which clinic or department is the right one.
- *Mental health center or family service agency*—Counselors at these places help all kinds of people in all kinds of situations.

No matter where you go for counseling, a counselor should always treat you with respect and make you feel good about yourself. A counselor may have strong feelings about adoption, abortion, and parenting a child. In order to make up your own mind, it is important for you to get clear answers from your counselor to your questions that will help you choose the best option.

If you are not happy with the answers you get, you may wish to find a counselor at another place. The Clearinghouse can tell you about crisis pregnancy centers and adoption agencies in each state, and can also help you find other counseling agencies in your area.

Should I Place My Child for Adoption?

The decision to place a child for adoption is a difficult one. It is an act of great courage and much love. Remember, adoption is permanent. The adoptive parents will raise your child and have legal authority for his or her welfare. You need to think about these questions as you make your decision.

Have I Explored All Possibilities?

Pregnancy can affect your feelings and emotions. Are you only thinking about adoption because you have money problems, or because your living situation is difficult? These problems might be temporary. Have you called Social Services to see what they can do, or asked friends and family if they can help? If you have done these things and still want adoption, you will feel more content with your decision.

Will the Adoptive Parents Take Good Care of My Child?

Prospective adoptive parents are carefully screened and give a great deal of information about themselves. They are visited in their home several times by a social worker and must provide personal references. They are taught about the special nature of adoptive parenting before an adoption takes place. By the time an agency has approved adoptive parents for placement, they have gotten to know them very well, and feel confident they would make good parents. This does not promise that they will be perfect parents, but usually decent people who really want to care for children.

Will My Child Wonder Why I Placed Him (or Her)for Adoption?

Probably. But adoption in the year 2000 is probably a lot different from what it was when you were growing up. Most adopted adults realize that their birth parents placed them for adoption out of love, and because it was the best they knew how to do. Hopefully your child will come to realize that a lot of his or her wonderful traits come from you. And if you have an open adoption, it is likely that you will be able to explain to the child why you chose adoption.

Why Am I Placing My Child for Adoption?

If your answer is because it is what you, or you and your partner, think is best, then it is a good decision. Now it is time to move forward, and not feel guilty.

What Are the Different Types of Adoption?

There are two types of adoptions, confidential and open.

Confidential: The birth parents and the adoptive parents never know each other. Adoptive parents are given background information about you and the birth father that they would need to help them take care of the child, such as medical information.

Open: The birth parents and the adoptive parents know something about each other. There are different levels of openness:

- **Least open**—You will read about several possible adoptive families and pick the one that sounds best for your baby. You will not know each other's names.

- **More open**—You and the possible adoptive family will speak on the telephone and exchange first names.

- **Even more open**—You can meet the possible adoptive family. Your social worker or attorney will arrange the meeting at the adoption agency or attorney's office.

- **Most open**—You and the adoptive parents share your full names, addresses, and telephone numbers. You stay in contact with the family and your child over the years, by visiting, calling, or writing each other.

Talk to your counselor about the type of adoption that is best for you. Do you want to help decide who adopts your child? Would you mind if a single person adopted your child, or a couple of a different race than you? Would you like to be able to share medical information with your child's family that may only become known in the future?

If you have strong feelings about these things, work with an agency or attorney who you feel will listen to what you want.

If you do not have strong feelings about these things, the adoption agency or attorney will decide who adopts your child based on who they think can best care for the child.

How Do I Arrange an Adoption through an Agency?

In all states, you can work with a licensed child placing (adoption) agency. In all but four states, you can also work directly with an adopting couple or their attorney without using an agency (see next page).

Private adoption agencies arrange most infant adoptions. To find private adoption agencies in your area, either contact the Clearinghouse or look in the yellow pages of your local phone book under "Adoption Agencies."

There are several types of private adoption agencies. Some are for profit and some are nonprofit. Some work with prospective adoptive parents of a particular religious group, though they work with birth parents of all religions.

When you contact adoption agencies, ask the social workers as many questions as you need to ask so that you understand the agencies' rules.

The agency social worker will ask you questions to find out some information about you and the baby's father, such as your medical histories, age, race, physical characteristics, whether you have been to see a doctor since you became pregnant, whether you have been pregnant or given birth before, and whether you smoked cigarettes, took any drugs, or drank any alcohol since you became pregnant. The social worker asks these questions so that the baby can be placed with parents who will be fully able to care for and love the baby, not so that she can turn you down.

How Do I Arrange a Private Adoption?

An adoption arranged without an adoption agency is called an independent or private adoption. It is legal in all states except Connecticut, Delaware, Massachusetts, and Minnesota. With a private adoption, you need to find an attorney to represent you. Look for an attorney who will not charge you a fee if you decide not to place your baby for adoption. You also need to find adoptive parents. Here's how you find both of these.

To Find an Attorney

Legal Aid—This is a service available in most communities for people who cannot afford a private attorney, Sometimes it is located at a university law school. Note: Some states allow the adopting parents to pay your legal fees, so going to Legal Aid may not be necessary.

State Attorney Association or the American Academy of Adoption Attorneys—These groups can refer you to an attorney who handles adoptions in your area. Contact the Clearinghouse for the address and telephone number of your state attorney association. You can contact the American Academy of Adoption Attorneys at P.O. Box 33053, Washington, DC 20033-0053.

To Find Adoptive Parents

Personal Ads—Some newspapers carry personal ads from people seeking to adopt. You call the number in the ad and get to know each other over the telephone. If you think you want to work with the couple, have your attorney call their attorney. The attorneys will work out all the arrangements according to what you and the adoptive parents want and the laws of your state.

Your Doctor—He or she may know about couples who are seeking a child, and be able to help arrange the adoption.

Adoptive Parent Support Groups—Parents who have already adopted may know other people seeking to adopt. You can find out more about these groups from the Clearinghouse.

National Matching Services—These services help birth parents and adoptive parents find one another. Contact the Clearinghouse for more information.

Of course, personal referrals are always good. Ask friends and family if they know any attorneys or possible adoptive parents.

What If My Baby Is a Child of Color?

There are some special considerations if your baby is a child of color, such as African American, Hispanic, Native American, or biracial.

Some adoption agency workers try almost always to place children of color with a family where at least one of the adoptive parents is the same race as the child. Some believe that a loving family, period, is more important, and that as long as the adoptive parents honor the heritage of the child, that family is okay with them.

If you want to, you can choose which kind of agency you work with and what kind of family your child goes to. Sometimes not a lot of families of color are waiting to adopt. This is because people of color sometimes do not know that there are babies available for adoption, or they may feel uncomfortable about the formal adoption process.

Unfortunately, this means that some agencies may not be as welcoming to you as they could be. They are afraid that they will not find a family for your child right away. Your child might have to be placed in a foster home until a permanent family can be found.

There are some adoption agencies that specialize in finding families for children of color. They work very hard to let people know that children of color are available for adoption. They also try to make the adoption process less confusing and complicated.

Contact the Clearinghouse for the names, addresses, and telephone numbers of adoption agencies that specialize in working with families of color, or for all the adoption agencies in your state. This information is free.

How Do I Arrange for Future Contact with My Child If I Want It?

If you decide on a confidential adoption, you may still wish to make sure that your child can contact you in the future. There are things you can do now to make that happen.

Many people who are adopted as children later want to meet their birth parents. They have to figure out a way to get around state laws that will not allow them to see their own original birth certificates. Because of these problems, many states, and some private national organizations, have set up adoption registries to help people find one another.

A registry works like this: You leave the information about the birth of the child and your address and telephone number. You must keep your address and telephone number current. You can register at any time, even years after the child is born.

When your child is an adult, he or she can call or write this registry. If what the child knows about his or her birth matches what the registry has, the registry will release your current address and telephone number to the child, and you could be contacted.

There is another way to ensure that your child can contact you if he or she wishes. Some adoption agencies and attorneys who arrange private adoptions will hold a letter in their file in which you say why you chose adoption and how to get in touch with you if the child ever wants to. If the agency or attorney that you are working with will not agree to do this, you may wish to work with somebody else.

There are several national organizations that offer ongoing advice and support to birth parents, information about contact and reunion with their children, and many other things. People in these organizations have already gone through what you are going through. They will be very helpful and understanding if you need someone to talk to. These organizations or the staff of the Clearinghouse can refer you to a group near you.

Chapter 7

Teens and Sex

Chapter Contents

Section 7.1

Facts in Brief: Teen Sex and Pregnancy

Sexual Activity

- Most very young teens have not had intercourse: 8 in 10 girls and 7 in 10 boys are sexually inexperienced at age 15.

- The likelihood of teenagers' having intercourse increases steadily with age; however, about 1 in 5 young people do not have intercourse while teenagers.

- Most young people begin having sex in their mid-to-late teens, about 8 years before they marry; more than half of 17-year-olds have had intercourse.

- While 93% of teenage women report that their first intercourse was voluntary, one-quarter of these young women report that it was unwanted.

- The younger women are when they first have intercourse, the more likely they are to have had unwanted or nonvoluntary first sex—7 in 10 of those who had sex before age 13, for example.

- Nearly two-thirds (64%) of sexually active 15–17-year-old women have partners who are within two years of their age; 29% have sexual partners who are 3–5 years older, and 7% have partners who are six or more years older.

- Most sexually active young men have female partners close to their age: 76% of the partners of 19-year-old men are either 17 (33%) or 18 (43%); 13% are 16, and 11% are aged 13–15.

Contraceptive Use

- A sexually active teenager who does not use contraceptives has a 90% chance of becoming pregnant within one year.

Sex is rare among very young teenagers, but common in the later teenage years.

% who have had sexual intercourse at different ages, 1995

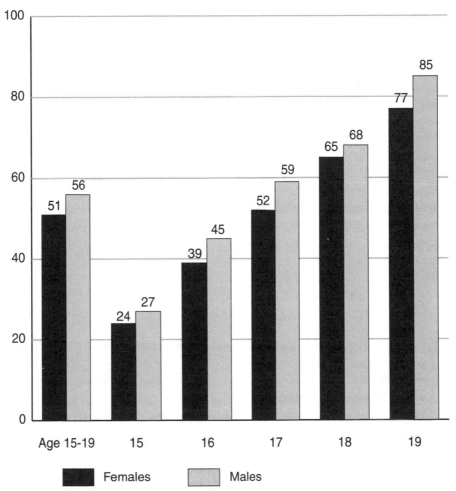

Sources: 1995 National Survey of Family Growth and 1995 National Survey of Adolescent Males.

- Teenage women's contraceptive use at first intercourse rose from 48% to 65% during the 1980s, almost entirely because of a doubling in condom use. By 1995, use at first intercourse reached 78%, with 2/3 of it condom use.

- 9 in 10 sexually active women and their partners use a contraceptive method, although not always consistently or correctly.

- About 1 in 6 teenage women practicing contraception combine two methods, primarily the condom and another method.

- The method teenage women most frequently use is the pill (44%), followed by the condom (38%). About 10% rely on the injectable, 4% on withdrawal, and 3% on the implant.

- Teenagers are less likely than older women to practice contraception without interruption over the course of a year, and more likely to practice contraception sporadically or not at all.

Sexually Transmitted Diseases (STDs)

- Every year 3 million teens—about 1 in 4 sexually experienced teens—acquire an STD.

- In a single act of unprotected sex with an infected partner, a teenage woman has a 1% risk of acquiring HIV, a 30% risk of getting genital herpes, and a 50% chance of contracting gonorrhea.

- Chlamydia is more common among teens than among older men and women; in some settings, 10–29% of sexually active teenage women and 10% of teenage men tested for STDs have been found to have chlamydia.

- Teens have higher rates of gonorrhea than do sexually active men and women aged 20–44.

- In some studies, up to 15% of sexually active teenage women have been found to be infected with the human papillomavirus, many with a strain of the virus linked to cervical cancer.

- Teenage women have a higher hospitalization rate than older women for acute pelvic inflammatory disease (PID), which is most often caused by untreated gonorrhea or chlamydia. PID can lead to infertility and ectopic pregnancy.

Teen Pregnancy

- Each year, almost 1 million teenage women—10% of all women aged 15–19 and 19% of those who have had sexual intercourse—become pregnant.

- The overall U.S. teenage pregnancy rate declined 17% between 1990 and 1996, from 117 pregnancies per 1,000 women aged 15–19 to 97 per 1,000.

- 78% of teen pregnancies are unplanned, accounting for about 1/4 of all accidental pregnancies annually.

- 6 in 10 teen pregnancies occur among 18–19-year-olds.

- Teen pregnancy rates are much higher in the United States than in many other developed countries—twice as high as in

Teen Pregnancy Outcomes

More than half (56%) of the 905,000 teenage pregnancies in 1996 ended in births (2/3 of which were unplanned).

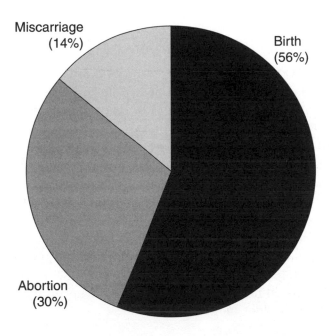

England and Wales or Canada, and nine times as high as in the Netherlands or Japan.

- Steep decreases in the pregnancy rate among sexually experienced teenagers accounted for most of the drop in the overall teenage pregnancy rate in the early-to-mid 1990s. While 20% of the decline is because of decreased sexual activity, 80% is due to more effective contraceptive practice.

Childbearing

- 13% of all U.S. births are to teens.
- The fathers of babies born to teenage mothers are likely to be older than the women: About 1 in 5 infants born to unmarried minors are fathered by men 5 or more years older than the mother.
- 78% of births to teens occur outside of marriage.
- Teens now account for 31% of all nonmarital births, down from 50% in 1970.
- 1/4 of teenage mothers have a second child within 2 years of their first.

Teen Mothers and Their Children

- Teens who give birth are much more likely to come from poor or low-income families (83%) than are teens who have abortions (61%) or teens in general (38%).
- 7 in 10 teen mothers complete high school, but they are less likely than women who delay childbearing to go on to college.
- In part because most teen mothers come from disadvantaged backgrounds, 28% of them are poor while in their 20s and early 30s; only 7% of women who first give birth after adolescence are poor at those ages.
- 1/3 of pregnant teens receive inadequate prenatal care; babies born to young mothers are more likely to be low-birth-weight, to have childhood health problems, and to be hospitalized than are those born to older mothers.

Abortion

- Nearly 4 in 10 teen pregnancies (excluding those ending in miscarriages) are terminated by abortion. There were about 274,000 abortions among teens in 1996.

- Since 1980, abortion rates among sexually experienced teens have declined steadily, because fewer teens are becoming pregnant, and in recent years, fewer pregnant teens have chosen to have an abortion.

- The reasons most often given by teens for choosing to have an abortion are being concerned about how having a baby would change their lives, feeling that they are not mature enough to have a child and having financial problems.

- 29 states currently have mandatory parental involvement laws in effect for a minor seeking an abortion: AL, AR, DE, GA, ID, IN, IO, KS, KY, LA, MD, MA, MI, MN, MS, MO, NE, NC, ND, OH, PA, RI, SC, SD, UT, VA, WV, WI, and WY.

- 61% of minors who have abortions do so with at least one parent's knowledge; 45% of parents are told by their daughter. The great majority of parents support their daughter's decision to have an abortion.

Sources

The data in this fact sheet are the most current available. Most of the data are from research conducted by The Alan Guttmacher Institute (AGI) or published in the peer-reviewed journal *Family Planning Perspectives* and the 1994 AGI report *Sex and America's Teenagers*. Additional sources include the Centers for Disease Control and Prevention and the National Center for Health Statistics.

Section 7.2

Birth Control Choices for Teens

Text adapted from *Birth Control Choices for Teens*, © revised version December 1997 Planned Parenthood® Federation of America, Inc., copyright PPFA 1997, PPFA Web Site © 1998, Planned Parenthood® Federation of America, Inc.; available at http://www.plannedparenthood.org/TEENISSUES/BCCHOICES/BCCHOICES.HTML; reprinted with permission.

To choose which birth control method to use, you need to consider how well each one will work for you:

- How well will it fit into your lifestyle?
- How effective will it be?
- How safe will it be?
- How affordable will it be?
- How reversible will it be?
- Will it help protect against sexually transmitted infections?

Having Sex Is about Making Choices

- We choose when we are ready and when we want to wait.
- We choose our partners.
- We choose what we want to do and what we don't want to do with our partners.
- We can choose to do it in the safest way.

Teens who have vaginal intercourse need to make choices about birth control. One of the great joys of life can be having a baby—when we are ready and are able to provide all the love and care a child needs. One of the great setbacks in life can be an unintended pregnancy—especially for a young woman.

Sex partners should:

- Have each other's consent.
- Be honest with each other.

- Treat each other as equals.
- Be attentive to each other's pleasure.
- Protect each other against physical and emotional harm, unintended pregnancy, and sexually transmitted infections.
- Accept responsibility for their actions.
- Have access to safe and effective means to prevent unintended pregnancy and sexually transmitted infections.

If You Choose Continuous Abstinence...

...you will not have sex play with a partner. This will keep sperm from joining egg.

Effectiveness
- 100%
- Prevents sexually transmitted infections.

Advantages
- No medical or hormonal side effects.
- Many religions endorse abstinence for unmarried people.

Possible Problems
- Difficult for many people to abstain from sex play for long periods.
- People often forget to protect themselves against pregnancy or sexually transmitted infections when they stop abstaining.

Cost
- None.

Advantage for Teens

Sexual relationships present physical and emotional risks. Abstinence is a very good way to postpone taking those risks until women and men are mature enough to handle them.

Women who postpone vaginal intercourse until their 20s have certain health advantages. They are less likely to suffer from sexually transmitted infections, infertility, and cancer of the cervix than women who have vaginal intercourse at younger ages.

If You Choose Outercourse...

...you will enjoy sex play without vaginal intercourse. This will keep sperm from joining egg. Outercourse includes:

- Masturbation—Masturbation is the most common way we enjoy sex. Partners can enjoy it together while hugging and kissing or watching one another. Masturbating together can deepen a couple's intimacy.
- Erotic Massage—Many couples enjoy arousing one another with body massage. They stimulate each other's sex organs with their hands, bodies, or mouths. They take turns bringing each other to orgasm.
- Body Rubbing—Many couples rub their bodies together, especially their sex organs, for intense sexual pleasure and orgasm.

Effectiveness
- Nearly 100%.
- Pregnancy is possible if semen or pre-ejaculate is spilled near the opening of the vagina.
- Effective against HIV and other serious sexually transmitted infections, unless body fluids are exchanged through oral or anal intercourse.

Advantages
- No medical or hormonal side effects.
- Can be used as safer sex if no body fluids are exchanged.
- May prolong sex play and enhance orgasm.
- Can be fully satisfying without the risks of sexual intercourse.

Possible Problems

- Difficult for many people to abstain from vaginal intercourse for long periods.

Cost

- None.

Advantage for Teens

Outercourse can give complete satisfaction for both partners and take a lot of pressure off young women and men.

Many teen women get little or no pleasure from sexual intercourse because their partners do not know how to give them pleasure. Outercourse helps partners learn about their bodies and how to give themselves and each other sexual pleasure.

Women have very different sexual response cycles than men. Men usually have one orgasm, and it is usually some time before they can have another. Women can have frequent and multiple orgasms. But most women don't have orgasms from vaginal stimulation. Most of them get orgasms when the clitoris is stimulated—whether or not they are having vaginal intercourse. Sex play without intercourse can help women learn how to have orgasms.

Men also enjoy outercourse—even if they're shy about it in front of their partners. Outercourse allows men to be truly erotic without worrying about how well they perform.

Caution:

Outercourse is almost the same as foreplay. Both add to sexual excitement and pleasure. The difference is that foreplay is meant to lead to intercourse. Outercourse may also add to a couple's desire to take a risk and have intercourse. Couples who use outercourse for birth control must not give in to that impulse. Be careful, don't turn outercourse into foreplay unless you are ready to use another form of birth control.

If You Choose Norplant®...

...your clinician will put six small capsules under the skin of your upper arm. Capsules constantly release small amounts of progestin, a hormone that:

- prevents release of egg
- thickens cervical mucus to keep sperm from joining egg.

Removal can be done at any time. Must be done by clinician.

Effectiveness
- 99.96%
- Not effective against sexually transmitted infections. Use a condom for good protection against infection.

Advantages
- Protects against pregnancy for five years.
- No daily pill.
- Nothing to put in place before intercourse.
- Can use while breastfeeding (six weeks after delivery).
- Can be used by some women who cannot take the Pill.

Possible Problems
- Side effects include irregular, late, and absent periods as well as other discomforts, including: headaches, nausea, depression, nervousness, dizziness, and weight gain.
- Medical procedure needed for insertion and removal.
- Possible scarring at insertion site.
- Rarely, infection at insertion site.
- Rarely, difficult removal.

Cost
- $500–$600: exam, implants, insertion.
- $100–$200: removal.
- Some health centers charge according to income.

Advantage for Teens

Many teen women lead active and unpredictable life styles. They some-times forget to take the Pill or to make an appointment for an injection. With Norplant®, women can have long-term, reliable protection against pregnancy for five years—without having to remember anything—except to use a condom for protection against sexually transmitted infections.

Caution:

Although it has not been proven, some scientists believe that prolonged use of Norplant® and other progestin-only implants or injections may de-crease bone mass in young women.

If You Choose Depo-Provera®...

...your clinician will give you a shot of the hormone progestin in your arm or buttock every 12 weeks to:
- prevent release of egg
- thicken cervical mucus to keep sperm from joining egg
- prevent fertilized egg from implanting in uterus.

Effectiveness
- 99.7% Not effective against sexually transmitted infections. Use a condom for good protection against infection.

Advantages
- Protects against pregnancy for 12 weeks.
- No daily pill.
- Nothing to put in place before intercourse.
- Can be used while breastfeeding (starting six weeks after delivery).
- Can be used by some women who cannot take the Pill.
- Protects against: cancer of the lining of the uterus, iron defi-ciency anemia.

Possible Problems

- Side effects include irregular, late, and absent periods as well as other discomforts, including: weight gain, headaches, depression, and abdominal pain.
- Side effects cannot be reversed until medication wears off (up to 12 weeks).
- May cause delay in getting pregnant after shots are stopped.

Cost

- $30–$75 per injection. May be less at clinics.
- $35–$125: exam. Some family planning clinics charge according to income.

Advantage for Teens

Injection is one of the most private prescription methods of birth control. No one can tell you're using it. There is no packaging or other evidence of use that might embarrass some users.

Caution:

Although it has not been proven, some scientists believe that prolonged use of Depo-Provera® or other progestin-only implants or injections may decrease bone mass in young women.

If You Choose the Pill...

...your clinician will prescribe the right Pill for you. Take one Pill once a day. Complete one pill-pack every month. Combination pills contain estrogen and progestin. Mini-pills contain only progestin. Pills contain hormones that work in different ways.

- Combination pills prevent release of egg.
- Both types thicken cervical mucus to keep sperm from joining egg.
- Both types also may prevent fertilized egg from implanting in uterus.

Effectiveness

- 97%–99.9% Not effective against sexually transmitted infections. Use a condom for good protection against infection.

Advantages

- Nothing to put in place before intercourse.
- More regular periods.
- Less: menstrual cramping, acne, iron deficiency anemia, and premenstrual tension.
- Protects against: ovarian and endometrial cancers, pelvic inflammatory disease, and non-cancerous breast tumors.
- Fewer tubal pregnancies.

Possible Problems

- Must be taken daily.
- Rare but serious health risks, including: blood clots, heart attack, and stroke. Women over 35 who smoke and those who are greatly overweight are at greater risk.
- Possible side effects include temporary irregular bleeding, depression, nausea, and other discomforts.

Cost

- $15–$25: monthly pill-pack at drugstores. Often less at clinics.
- $35–$125: exam.
- Some health centers charge according to income

Advantage for Teens

The Pill is often appropriate for teens, even if they are not having intercourse, because teen women are more likely than older women to have cramps and irregular periods. Women who remember to take the Pill at the same time every day have fewer cramps and more regular periods than women who don't take the Pill.

Caution:

Don't smoke while you take the Pill.
Doing so will increase your risk of heart attack, blood clots, and stroke.

Don't forget to take your pill.
About one out of three users often forget to take the Pill. The Pill won't work for anyone who forgets to take it every day.

- If you choose the Pill, schedule taking it with something else you do every day—like brushing your teeth.

- If you forget ONE active combination pill, take it as soon as you remember. This means you may take two pills in one day. If you forget two or more pills, call your clinician immediately.

- Remember to take your pill whether or not you're having sex.

Don't share your pills.
Prescription methods like the Pill, diaphragm, and cervical cap are personalized for each woman's use. They should not be shared.

If You Choose the Condom...

...you will cover the penis before intercourse with a sheath made of thin latex, plastic, or animal tissue to keep sperm from joining egg. Lubricate condoms with spermicide to immobilize sperm.

Effectiveness
- 88%–98%
- Latex condoms are effective against sexually transmitted infections, including HIV, the virus that can cause AIDS.
- Plastic condoms are still being tested for effectiveness against infection. Animal tissue condoms may not protect against viruses such as HIV and hepatitis B.
- Increase your protection:
  — Also use spermicides.

— Do not use oil-based lubricants, like Vaseline®, on latex condoms.

— Use correctly: Place rolled condom on tip of hard penis. Squeeze air out of half-inch space at tip. Pull back foreskin and roll condom down over penis. Smooth out any air bubbles. Lubricate with water-based lubricant, like K-Y® jelly.

— Hold condom against penis to withdraw.

Advantages

• Inexpensive and easy to buy in drugstores, supermarkets, etc.

• Can help relieve premature ejaculation.

• Can be put on as part of sex play.

• Can be used with other methods of birth control to prevent sexually transmitted infections.

Possible Problems

• Allergies to latex or spermicide.

• Decreased sensation.

• Breakage.

Cost

• 25¢ and up: dry.

• 50¢ and up: lubricated.

• $2.50 and up: plastic, animal tissue, textured.

• Some health centers give them away or charge very little.

Advantage for Teens

One out of four teens has a sexually transmitted infection. Teens are also likely to have more than one partner during their adolescence, which increases the likelihood of their getting an infection. Latex condoms are the best protection against infection for women and men of all ages who have sexual intercourse. They are also cheap and widely available.

Caution:

The cervix in pregnant women, young girls, and teen women is especially vulnerable to infection. Even as mature adults, women's sexual anatomy makes them 10 to 20 times more likely than men to become infected with sexually transmitted infections.

No matter how old you are, it is very important to use condoms with your other method of birth control whenever you are at risk for getting a sexually transmitted infection.

If You Choose the Diaphragm or Cervical Cap...

...your clinician will fit you with a shallow latex cup (diaphragm) or a thimble-shaped latex cap (cervical cap). Clinician also will show you how to coat diaphragm or cap with spermicide and put it in your vagina to keep sperm from joining egg.

Effectiveness
- 82%–94%: diaphragm
- 82%–91%: cervical cap for women who have not had a child
- 64%–74%: cervical cap for women who have had a child
- Not effective against sexually transmitted infections. Use a condom for good protection against infection.

Advantages
- No medicinal or hormonal side effects.
- Inexpensive.

Possible Problems
- Can be messy.
- Allergies to latex or spermicide.
- Cannot use during vaginal bleeding or infection.
- May interrupt sex play.
- Diaphragm:
  — Increased risk of bladder infection.

- Cervical Cap:
  - Difficult for some women to use.
  - Only four sizes. Difficult to fit some women.

Cost

- $13–$25: diaphragm or cap.
- $50–$125: examination.
- $8: supplies of spermicide jelly or cream.
- Some health centers charge according to income.

Advantage for Teens

Many teen women have vaginal intercourse only now and then. Many of them prefer to use the diaphragm or cap on those occasions. That way they avoid the possible, ongoing side effects of other prescription methods.

Caution:

Prescription methods like the diaphragm, cervical cap, and the Pill are personalized for each woman's use. Do not share them with friends. The *diaphragm* should be checked to see if it's the right size after a weight change of 10 or more pounds, childbirth, or abortion. The *cervical cap* should be checked for size after childbirth.

If You Choose Over-the-Counter Birth Control for Women...

...you will follow package instructions and insert vaginal pouch (female condom) or spermicides—contraceptive foam, cream, jelly, film, or suppository—deep into your vagina shortly before intercourse to keep sperm from joining egg. Spermicides immobilize sperm.

Follow package instructions to remove pouch. Spermicides in other methods dissolve in vagina.

Effectiveness

- 72%–97% contraceptive foam, creams, jelly, film, or suppository

- 79%–95% pouch
- Pouch provides some protection against sexually transmitted infection, including HIV. Use condoms with all other birth control methods for protection against infection.

Advantages

- Easy to buy in drugstores, supermarkets, etc.
- Insertion may be part of sex play.
- Erection unnecessary to keep pouch in place.

Possible Problems

- Can be messy.
- Allergies; may irritate vagina or penis.
- Outer ring of pouch may slip into vagina during intercourse.
- Difficulty inserting pouch.

Cost

- $2.50: pouch.
- $8–$18: applicator kits of foam and gel.
- $4–$8: refills, films, and suppositories.
- Some health centers charge according to income.

Advantage for Teens

Many teen women have vaginal intercourse only now and then. Many of them prefer to use over-the-counter methods on those occasions. That way they avoid the possible, ongoing side effects of prescription methods.

Four Methods NOT Usually Recommended for Teens

1. Sterilization
2. The IUD (Intrauterine Device)
3. Withdrawal
4. Periodic Abstinence or Fertility Awareness Methods (FAMs)

1. Sterilization

an operation to keep sperm from joining egg.

- **Tubal sterilization:** Intended to permanently block a woman's tubes where sperm join egg.
- **Vasectomy:** Intended to permanently block a man's tubes that carry sperm.

Effectiveness

- 99.6%–99.8%. Not effective against sexually transmitted infections.

Reason Not Recommended for Teens

This method is intended to be permanent. It is not appropriate for anyone who may want to have a child in the future. Because people so often change their minds about having families, sterilization is usually discouraged for people under 30 who have not had children.

2. The IUD (Intrauterine Device)

a small plastic device inserted into the uterus. The IUD contains copper or hormones that:

- keep sperm from joining egg
- prevent fertilized egg from implanting in uterus.

Effectiveness

- 97.4%–99.2%. Not effective against sexually transmitted infections.

Reason Not Recommended for Teens

- Unless she has had a child, a young woman's uterus may be too small to hold an IUD.

- IUD users who get certain sexually transmitted infections can develop pelvic inflammatory disease and become unable to have children. Teenagers are at very high risk for these infections. One out of four teenagers has at least one of these infections.

Withdrawal

the man pulls his penis out of the vagina before he ejaculates (comes) to keep sperm from joining egg.

Effectiveness

- 81%–96%. Not effective against sexually transmitted infections.

Reason Not Recommended for Teens

- Some men lack the experience and self-control to pull out in time.

- Some men have been known to say they will pull out, and then they get so excited and carried away that they don't.

- Some men cannot tell when they are going to ejaculate.

- Some men ejaculate very quickly, before they realize it.

- Before ejaculation, almost all penises leak fluid that can cause pregnancy.

Periodic Abstinence or Fertility Awareness Methods (FAMs)

a professional teaches a woman how to chart her menstrual cycle and to detect certain physical signs that help her predict "unsafe" days. She must abstain from intercourse (periodic abstinence) or use barrier contraceptives during nine or more "unsafe" days of her cycle (Famous).

The physical signs that are charted include:

- daily basal body temperature
- daily texture of cervical mucus
- occurrence of menstrual cycles.

Effectiveness

- 80%–99%. Not effective against sexually transmitted infections.

Reason Not Recommended for Teens

- These methods work best for women with very regular periods.

- Teen women often have irregular periods.

- Their partners may not wish to cooperate in using this method.

- A teen's relationship may not be as stable or as committed as is necessary for developing the trust and cooperation necessary for effective use of this method.

Emergency Contraception:

- can help prevent pregnancy after unprotected vaginal intercourse.
- is available from health care providers, Planned Parenthood health centers, and other women's health and family planning centers.
- is provided in two ways:
  - emergency hormonal contraception—doses of certain birth control pills that are started within three days of unprotected intercourse
  - insertion of an IUD within 5–7 days of unprotected intercourse.
- is for use only if a woman is sure she is not already pregnant. It keeps the egg from joining with the sperm or prevents the egg from implanting in the uterus. It will not cause an abortion.

Effectiveness

- A woman's risk of pregnancy varies from day to day during her menstrual cycle. Emergency contraception can reduce that risk:
- **Emergency "morning-after" pills**—Treatment initiated within 72 hours of unprotected intercourse reduces the risk of pregnancy by at least 75%.
- **Emergency IUD insertion**—Insertion within 5–7 days of unprotected intercourse reduces the risk of pregnancy by 99.9%.

Possible Problems

Emergency hormonal contraception:

- nausea
- vomiting
- breast tenderness, irregular bleeding, fluid retention, and headaches.

Emergency IUD insertion:

- cramps.

You May Want Emergency Contraception If:

- His condom broke or slipped off, and he ejaculated inside your vagina.

- Your diaphragm or cervical cap slipped out of place, and he ejaculated inside your vagina.

- He forced you to have unprotected vaginal intercourse.

- You miscalculated your "safe" days for periodic abstinence or fertility awareness methods.

- You forgot to take your birth control pill more than two days in a row.

- You weren't using any birth control.

- He didn't pull out in time.

Contact your health care provider immediately if you have unprotected intercourse when you think you might become pregnant.

For a confidential appointment with the Planned Parenthood health center nearest you, call 1-800-230-PLAN.

To reach the Emergency Contraception Hot Line for information and referrals call 1-888-NOT-2-LATE.

Section 7.3

On the Teen Scene: Preventing STDs

FDA Consumer, June 1993, with revisions made in February 1995 and
April 1998, Pub. No. (FDA) 98-1210; available at http://www.fda.gov/opacom/
catalog/ots_stds.html.

—by Judith Levine Willis

You don't have to be a genius to figure out that the only sure way to
avoid getting sexually transmitted diseases (STDs) is to not have sex.

But in today's age of AIDS, it's smart to also know ways to lower
the risk of getting STDs, including HIV, the virus that causes AIDS.

Infection with HIV, which stands for human immunodeficiency virus, is spreading among teenagers. According to the Centers for Disease Control and Prevention (CDC), as of June 30, 1997, 2953 people
had been diagnosed with HIV or AIDS when they were in their teens
and 107,281 when in their twenties. Because it can be many years from
the time a person becomes infected to when the person develops symptoms and is diagnosed with HIV infection, many people diagnosed in
their twenties likely contracted HIV in their teens.

You may have heard that birth control can also help prevent AIDS
and other STDs. This is only partly true. The whole story is that only
one form of birth control currently on the market—latex condoms (thin
rubber sheaths used to cover the penis)—is highly effective in reducing the transmission (spread) of HIV and many other STDs.

The Food and Drug Administration (FDA) has approved the marketing of male condoms made of polyurethane for people allergic to
latex. (See "New Information on Labels.") Reality Female Condom, another form of birth control made of polyurethane, may give limited protection against STDs, but it is not as effective as male latex condoms.

So people who use other kinds of birth control, such as the pill, diaphragm, Norplant®, Depo-Provera®, cervical cap, or IUD, also need
to use condoms to help prevent STDs.

Here's why: Latex condoms work against STDs by keeping blood,
a man's semen, and a woman' s vaginal fluids—all of which can carry
bacteria and viruses—from passing from one person to another. For
many years, scientists have known that male condoms (also called
safes, rubbers, or prophylactics) can help prevent STDs transmitted
by bacteria, such as syphilis and gonorrhea, because the bacteria can't

get through the condom. More recently, researchers discovered that latex condoms can also reduce the risk of getting STDs caused by viruses, such as HIV, herpes, and hepatitis B, even though viruses are much smaller than bacteria or sperm.

After this discovery, FDA, which regulates condoms as medical devices, worked with manufacturers to develop labeling for latex condoms. The labeling tells consumers that although latex condoms cannot entirely eliminate the risk of STDs, when used properly and consistently they are highly effective in preventing STDs. FDA also provided a sample set of instructions and requested that all condoms include adequate instructions.

Make the Right Choice

Male condoms now sold in the United States are made either of latex (rubber), polyurethane, or natural membrane (called "lambskin," but actually made of sheep intestine). Scientists found that natural skin condoms are not as effective as latex condoms in reducing the risk of STDs because natural skin condoms have naturally occurring tiny holes or pores that viruses may be able to get through. Only latex condoms labeled for protection against STDs should be used for disease protection, unless one of the partners is allergic to latex. In that case, a polyurethane condom can be used.

Some condoms have lubricants added and some have spermicide (a chemical that kills sperm) added. The package labeling tells whether either of these has been added to the condom.

Lubricants may help prevent condoms from breaking and may help prevent irritation. But lubricants do not give any added disease protection. If an unlubricated condom is used, a water-based lubricant (such as K-Y Jelly), available over-the-counter (without prescription) in drugstores, can be used but is not required for the proper use of the condom. Do not use petroleum-based jelly (such as Vaseline), baby oil, lotions, cooking oils, or cold creams because these products can weaken latex and cause the condom to tear easily.

Some condoms have added spermicide—an active chemical in spermicides, nonoxynol-9, kills sperm. But spermicides alone (as sold in creams and jellies over-the-counter in drugstores) and spermicides used with the diaphragm or cervical cap do not give adequate protection against HIV and other STDs. For the best disease protection, a latex condom should be used from start to finish every time a person has sex.

FDA requires condoms to be labeled with an expiration date. Condoms should be stored in a cool, dry place out of direct sunlight. Closets and drawers usually make good storage places. Because of possible exposure to extreme heat and cold, glove compartments of cars are not a good place to store condoms. For the same reason, condoms shouldn't be kept in a pocket, wallet, or purse for more than a few hours at a time. Condoms should not be used after the expiration date, usually abbreviated EXP and followed by the date.

Condoms are available in almost all drugstores, many supermarkets, and other stores. They are also available from vending machines. When purchasing condoms from vending machines, as from any source, be sure they are latex, labeled for disease prevention, and are not past their expiration date. Don't buy a condom from a vending machine located where it may be exposed to extreme heat or cold or to direct sunlight.

How to Use a Condom

- Use a new condom for every act of vaginal, anal, and oral (penis-mouth contact) sex. Do not unroll the condom before placing it on the penis.

- Put the condom on after the penis is erect and before any contact is made between the penis and any part of the partner's body.

- If the condom does not have a reservoir top, pinch the tip enough to leave a half-inch space for semen to collect. Always make sure to eliminate any air in the tip to help keep the condom from breaking.

- Holding the condom rim (and pinching a half-inch space if necessary), place the condom on the top of the penis. Then, continuing to hold it by the rim, unroll it all the way to the base of the penis. If you are also using water-based lubricant, you can put more on the outside of the condom.

- If you feel the condom break, stop immediately, withdraw, and put on a new condom.

- After ejaculation and before the penis gets soft, grip the rim of the condom and carefully withdraw.

- To remove the condom, gently pull it off the penis, being careful that semen doesn't spill out.

• Wrap the condom in a tissue and throw it in the trash where others won't handle it. (Don't flush condoms down the toilet because they may cause sewer problems.) Afterwards, wash your hands with soap and water.

Latex condoms are the only form of contraception now available that human studies have shown to be highly effective in protecting against the transmission of HIV and other STDs. They give good disease protection for vaginal sex and should also reduce the risk of disease transmission in oral and anal sex. But latex condoms may not be 100 percent effective, and a lot depends on knowing the right way to buy, store and use them.

Judith Levine Willis is a member of FDA's Public Affairs Staff.

New Information on Labels

Information about whether a birth control product also helps protect against sexually transmitted diseases (STDs), including HIV infection, is emphasized on the labeling of these products, because a product that is highly effective in preventing pregnancy will not necessarily protect against sexually transmitted diseases.

Labels on birth control pills, implants such as Norplant®, injectable contraceptives such as Depo-Provera®, intrauterine devices (IUDs), and natural skin condoms will state that the products are intended to prevent pregnancy and do not protect against STDs, including HIV infection (which leads to AIDS). Labeling of natural skin condoms will also state that consumers should use a latex condom to help reduce risk of many STDs, including HIV infection.

Laboratory tests show that organisms as small as sperm and the HIV virus cannot pass through polyurethane condoms. But the risks of STDs, including HIV infection, have not been well studied in actual use with polyurethane condoms. So unless one or both partners is allergic to latex, latex condoms should be used.

Labeling for latex condoms states that if used properly, latex condoms help reduce risk of HIV transmission and many other STDs. This statement, a modification from previous labeling, now appears on individual condom wrappers, on the box, and in consumer information.

Besides highlighting statements concerning sexually transmitted diseases and AIDS on the consumer packaging, manufacturers will add a similar statement to patient and physician leaflets provided with the products.

FDA may take action against any products that don't carry the new information.

FDA is currently reviewing whether similar action is necessary for the labeling of spermicide, cervical caps, and diaphragms.

Looking at a Condom Label

Like other drugs and medical devices, FDA requires condom packages to contain certain labeling information. When buying condoms, look on the package label to make sure the condoms are:

- made of latex
- labeled for disease prevention
- not past their expiration date (EXP followed by the date).

STD Facts

- Sexually transmitted diseases affect more than 12 million Americans each year, many of whom are teenagers or young adults.
- Using drugs and alcohol increases your chances of getting STDs because these substances can interfere with your judgment and your ability to use a condom properly.
- Intravenous drug use puts a person at higher risk for HIV and hepatitis B because IV drug users usually share needles.
- The more partners you have, the higher your chance of being exposed to HIV or other STDs. This is because it is difficult to know whether a person is infected, or has had sex with people who are more likely to be infected due to intravenous drug use or other risk factors.
- Sometimes, early in infection, there may be no symptoms, or symptoms may be confused with other illnesses.
- You cannot tell by looking at someone whether he or she is infected with HIV or another STD.

STDs can cause:

- pelvic inflammatory disease (PID), which can damage a woman's fallopian tubes and result in pelvic pain and sterility
- tubal pregnancies (where the fetus grows in the fallopian tube instead of the womb), sometimes fatal to the mother and always fatal to the fetus
- cancer of the cervix in women
- sterility—the inability to have children—in both men and women
- damage to major organs, such as the heart, kidney, and brain, if STDs go untreated
- death, especially with HIV infection.

See a doctor if you have any of these STD symptoms:

- discharge from vagina, penis, or rectum
- pain or burning during urination or intercourse
- pain in the abdomen (women), testicles (men), or buttocks and legs (both)
- blisters, open sores, warts, rash, or swelling in the genital or anal areas or mouth
- persistent flu-like symptoms—including fever, headache, aching muscles, or swollen glands—which may precede STD symptoms.

Chapter 8

Pregnancy and Contraception after the Age of 35

Chapter Contents

Section 8.1

Later-age Pregnancy

"Later-age Pregnancy: Preparing for the Happy, Healthy Event after 40,"
Mayo Clinic Health Oasis; originally published in *Mayo Clinic Women's Health
Source*, September 1997; © 2000 Mayo Foundation for Medical Education and
Research; available at http://www.mayohealth.org/mayo/9708/htm/aged_p.htm;
reprinted with permission.

Preparing for the Happy, Healthy Event after 40

You read about the 63-year-old California woman who just had a
baby. And now you're wondering if you could fit a baby in before you
qualify for Social Security. Maybe.

If you're in your 40s, your chances of getting pregnant are around
50 percent. If you've had no luck getting pregnant naturally, you can
increase your odds of carrying and delivering a baby to about 10 percent with infertility treatment. But the whole issue of infertility treatment is another story. Before you check into the possibilities of getting
pregnant, check out your health.

Although most older mothers (older than age 40) have uncomplicated pregnancies and healthy babies, you're at higher risk than
younger women for complications.

Facing Chromosome Abnormalities

One of the biggest issues for older mothers is the risk of having a
child with chromosome abnormalities. The most common is Down syndrome, a condition that causes mental retardation and defects of the
heart and other organs. While your risk of having a child with Down
syndrome is relatively low—only about 1 percent at age 40—it's still
greater than when you were 20 (see "Putting Your Risks into Perspective").

There are, however, two prenatal tests—amniocentesis and chorionic villus sampling (CVS)—that detect chromosome disorders. Both
tests carry a slight risk of miscarriage. If your test findings are abnormal, you'll be faced with the difficult decision of whether to continue or terminate the pregnancy.

Taking Care of You

Diabetes and high blood pressure are more common in women in their 40s. Diabetic mothers are at greater risk for pre-eclampsia, preterm delivery, placental problems, or stillbirth. Women with diabetes are also more likely to have a child with poor fetal growth or birth defects. Blood pressure also normally rises during pregnancy, which can worsen an existing condition, putting you at risk of seizures or stroke.

Even if you don't have diabetes or high blood pressure, you have an increased chance of developing pregnancy-related diabetes (gestational diabetes) as well as pregnancy-induced hypertension (PIH). Both gestational diabetes and PIH increase the chances of eclampsia, a complication characterized by high blood pressure, swelling of your face and hands, and protein in your urine. Eclampsia can impair your nervous system function, leading to seizures, stroke, or other serious complications.

Both conditions occur infrequently and complications are rare. Gestational diabetes is controlled with diet and exercise (and insulin injections for about 15 percent of women). PIH is treated with bed rest and close monitoring of your condition as well as the baby's, both during pregnancy and delivery.

Other Concerns

Your chances of having twins or triplets also goes up as you age, even without infertility treatment. As an older mother, the possibility of multiple births is riskier to your health as well as the babies'.

Your chances of cesarean delivery are also about 40 percent higher than a younger woman's. Although a cesarean delivery is riskier than a vaginal delivery, most are uncomplicated and require only a slightly longer hospital stay and recovery time.

Planning Ahead

Here's what you can do to improve the health odds for you and your baby:

- Control existing health problems such as high blood pressure or diabetes.

- Lose weight if you're overweight. Women who are overweight when they get pregnant are more likely to develop problems during pregnancy.

- Take prenatal vitamins containing folic acid before getting pregnant to help prevent neural tube defects such as spina bifida, a condition in which the tissue over the baby's spinal cord doesn't close.

- Learn about your health risks and the diagnostic tests you may want to have to detect chromosome abnormalities.

The Benefits of Waiting

Although later-age pregnancy can put you at higher risk for a number of health complications, there's an upside. As a potential older mother, you may be more mature, realistic, and dedicated to the idea of having a baby than a woman in her 20s. You've probably also given a lot of thought to the changes a new baby will bring.

Putting Your Risks into Perspective

This chart shows you the odds of having a child with a chromosome abnormality. Down syndrome is in a category by itself because it's the most common chromosome abnormality in infants. It does, however, also fall within the category of all chromosome abnormalities.

Age	Down syndrome	All chromosome abnormalities
20	1 in 1,667	1 in 526
35	1 in 378	1 in 192
40	1 in 106	1 in 66
45	1 in 30	1 in 21

Section 8.2

Perimenopause: Pathways to Change

—by Arthur F. Haney, M.D.; Kirtly Parker Jones, M.D.; Leon Speroff, M.D.; and Susan Wysocki, R.N.C., N.P.

Your body goes through many physical changes during your lifetime. The perimenopause—the six- to eight-year period of transition for women around the menopause—is one of those times of change.

The purpose of this section is to help you understand the peri-menopause, the kinds of frequently encountered changes you can expect, and what this period of transition can mean for you.

What Is the Perimenopause?

The perimenopause is a time of change experienced by most women. During this transition period you will experience a decrease in your ability to become pregnant and an increase in irregular menstrual cycles.

The perimenopause is a normal life transition and each woman's experience is different. It can give you an opportunity to positively influence all areas of your life—physical, personal, social, and professional. The perimenopause serves as a signal to make health commitments for your future.

When Does the Perimenopause Occur?

Menopause—the ending of the active functioning of your ovaries—usually occurs between the ages of 45 and 55, but every woman follows her own biologic clock. The perimenopause is the time of change around the menopause, and usually lasts about eight years.

How Will I Recognize It?

During the perimenopause you may experience changes in your menstrual cycle and breasts. So-called "hot flashes" and vaginal dryness usually occur after the menopause because of a decrease in female hormones.

It is important to see your health care provider—physician, nurse clinician, or physician assistant—yearly during these times of change.

Changes in Menstrual Cycle

- The most common sign of perimenopause is a change in your menstrual cycle. There is a wide variation in the length of menstrual cycles in women. As you enter the perimenopause your own cycles may become more irregular.

- You should talk to your health care provider if you are experiencing heavy vaginal bleeding, long intervals of spotting, or have gone more than two months without a period. These symptoms can be signs of abnormalities of the uterine lining which are easily treated.

Breast Changes

- Variations in breast tenderness or fullness are common with the menstrual cycle and pregnancy. You may be unable to predict breast tenderness or fullness as your cycle changes. Any lumps in your breast should be evaluated by your health care provider. Your provider may suggest mammography based on your personal and family history.

Will I Experience Emotional Changes?

Most women do not find the perimenopause to be difficult. In fact, for most, it is a normal transition in their lives.

During this period emotional swings can occur in both men and women. They generally concern issues such as children leaving home, parents growing older, or a career change. They aren't usually due to the perimenopause itself.

Menopause is not believed to cause depression. If you are feeling depressed, talk to your health care provider about treatment for depression—not for perimenopause.

Will My Sex Life Change?

Most women do not experience major changes in their sex lives after the perimenopause. Your sex life will probably be the same after the perimenopause as before.

You may notice more vaginal dryness during the perimenopause. This is your body's normal response to a decreased level of the hormone estrogen which occurs after menopause. Your health care provider can discuss the options available to deal with vaginal dryness, such as the use of lubricants that you can by in any drug store.

Should I Still Use Birth Control?

It is possible to become pregnant during the perimenopause, though it is less likely than in your twenties or thirties. To avoid unintended pregnancy, contraception remains an important part of health planning.

Birth control methods can have additional health benefits. Low-dose birth control pills, for example, can correct irregular bleeding and reduce the risk of ovarian and uterine cancer. Implants or "the shot" can have similar benefits. The IUD can be a good method during this time. Male and female condoms, cervical caps, and the diaphragm can also be useful.

No one method is perfect for every person, so talk to your provider to find out what is best for you.

What about Sexually Transmitted Diseases?

You're just as likely now as ever to contract a sexually transmitted disease (STD) such as herpes and HIV/AIDS. Condoms (both male and female) help reduce the risk of contracting an STD. Discuss your concerns with your provider to find out what your risks might be.

Are There Other Types of Therapy?

You may want to consider hormone therapy. Some health benefits include protection against osteoporosis and cardiovascular disease, and prevention of hot flashes. Consult your provider for advice.

What about Diet and Exercise?

The perimenopause is a good time to plan for a vigorous, healthy second half of your life. That means establishing good habits such as regular exercise, a healthy diet, and stopping smoking. Preventive health care is important throughout your life. If you aren't already maintaining a healthy lifestyle, now is a good time to start.

How Can I Find Out More?

For more information about the perimenopause please contact your health care provider or write:

ARHP
2401 Pennsylvania Avenue, NW, Suite 350
Washington, DC 20037-1718
(202) 466-3825

Section 8.3

Oral Contraceptives vs. HRT

Mayo Clinic Health Oasis, August 13, 1998; originally published in *Mayo Clinic Women's Health Source*, August 1998; © 2000 Mayo Foundation for Medical Education and Research; available at http://www.mayohealth.org/mayo/9808/htm/thepillsb.htm; reprinted with permission.

If your doctor recommends the pill for your perimenopausal symptoms, you can safely stay on that regimen until you go through menopause. At that time, you can switch to hormone replacement therapy (HRT).

What's the difference between the pill and HRT? Dosage. HRT has only one-quarter to one-eighth the amount of estrogen and progesterone as the birth control pill. The lower the dosage of these hormones, the fewer the side effects.

"As long as you have even occasional periods, it's better to take the pill than hormone replacement therapy," says Lynne Shuster, M.D., Mayo Clinic internist. "That's because the amount of hormones in HRT isn't enough to stop ovulation. You'd still get periods, but they'd be irregular and the flow unpredictable. Plus you'd be at risk of pregnancy. Once you go through menopause, HRT is a better option. You can determine the best time to make the switch from the pill to HRT by using one of three options," says Dr. Shuster.

- **Option #1**—You can stop the pill for a few months. If your period resumes on its own, you haven't gone through menopause.

- **Option #2**—Your doctor can check your level of follicle stimulating hormone (FSH) and estrogen (estradiol) with a blood test. FSH levels increase as menopause approaches and estradiol decreases. If your FSH level is above 30 and your estradiol is less than 20, you've probably gone through menopause. The test needs to be done at the end of your hormone-free week.

- **Option #3**—You can stay on the pill until it's very likely you've gone through menopause—usually around age 52—and then just switch to HRT, if pregnancy prevention isn't an issue. Even if you stay on the pill 1 or 2 years past menopause, there's no danger to your health. Taking oral contraceptives won't delay menopause, but they can conceal it because you wouldn't have hot flashes.

Section 8.4

Contraception and the Late Premenopause

Progress in Human Reproduction Research, World Health Organization, no. 40, 1996; available at http://www.who.int/hrp/progress/40/04.html.

The late premenopause begins at 35–40 years of age and ends with the menopause. It is a period when childbearing is associated with greater risks than previously and when there are distinctive contraceptive requirements. In most parts of the world, childbearing by women in this age group is not desired, and may be actively discouraged, although a trend towards late childbearing has been noted in some developed countries.

Although sexual intercourse becomes less frequent as couples grow older, and fecundity also declines, the probability of pregnancy still exists if contraceptive methods are not used. Research has shown that half of all women in their early forties are still fertile. Without contraception, the annual risk of pregnancy is around 10 percent for women aged 40–44 and 2–3 percent for women aged 45–49, and the risk may not be zero for women over 50. In women over 45 years who have not menstruated for one year the probability of subsequent menstruation (which could be ovulatory) is estimated to be 2–10 percent. There is a clearly established need for contraception until the menopause is established.

As the number of ovarian follicles declines and hormonal changes occur, the number of menstrual cycles without ovulation increases and the oocytes that are released are less capable of being fertilized. Attempts at assisted reproduction confirm the reduction of fertility after the age of 35. A study of nulliparous women undergoing artificial insemination showed that the probability of success was 74 percent in women under 30 years but fell to 54 percent above 35 years. Smoking may exacerbate these trends.

Pregnancy in women over the age of 35 is usually unwanted and many women opt for abortion where it is legal. For example, in the United Kingdom official statistics show that 45 percent of the pregnancies among women over 40 are terminated by legal abortion. Pregnancy over the age of 35 also carries increased health risks for both mother and fetus. The maternal mortality rate in women in their forties is four times higher than among women in their twenties. Rates of spontaneous abortion are double (26 percent for women in their forties) as are perinatal mortality rates. The risk of chromosomal anomalies in the fetus increases with the age of the mother, and where tests are available for these anomalies women carrying an abnormal fetus often choose to have an abortion if this is legal. There may also be social pressure against late pregnancy; in some cultures it is unacceptable for a woman to become pregnant after the arrival of her first grandchild.

The ratio of risk to benefit of contraceptive use in the late premenopause has to be seen in the light of the prevailing risk of maternal mortality. In countries where maternal mortality rates are high, the effectiveness of contraceptives in preventing pregnancy will be of utmost importance. In developing countries contraception protects women against the morbidity and mortality that is associated with a high number of pregnancies and deliveries.

Combined Oral Contraceptives

The dosage of hormones in combined oral contraceptives was reduced after studies in the 1970s and 1980s showed that high-dose preparations had adverse health effects, most notably on the cardiovascular system. The products currently on the market contain 4–5 times less estrogen than in the 1960s, and similarly reduced amounts of progestogen.

In 1986 the Programme began a large study to evaluate the safety of low-dose combined pills in different parts of the world. The study's findings, some of which were summarized in issue No. 39 of *Progress*, are based on research at 21 centres in 17 countries (12 developing and 5 developed). The study assessed the link between the risk of stroke and blood clots in the veins (venous thromboembolism) and the use of combined oral contraceptives in women aged 20–44 years.

The research showed that current use of combined oral contraceptives was associated with slightly increased risk of haemorrhagic and ischaemic stroke. In women under 35 years of age, use of oral contraceptives did not affect the risk of haerriorrhagic stroke in either developed or developing countries, and the risk of ischaemic stroke was low. In women aged over 35, however, there was a small but clear increase in risk. Factors such as smoking and high blood pressure increased this slight risk.

Stroke is rare in young women of reproductive age so the additional risk due to using oral contraceptives is very small. In European women, for instance, the extra risk of stroke due to low-dose oral contraceptives is around two cases per 100,000 users per year. Most of that extra risk is in women over 35 years of age.

With regard to venous thromboembolism, the study found a slight increase in risk, especially in women with high body weight or with a history of high blood pressure during pregnancy. The increased risk of venous thromboembolism becomes apparent within the first few months of starting to use the pill and disappears within a few months of stopping. There was no evidence of a higher risk with age.

Another disease that is extremely rare among younger women, and therefore among most users of combined oral contraceptives, is breast cancer. However, the chance of a woman developing breast cancer increases during and after the menopause so any long-term additional risk from oral contraceptive use would be a significant problem.

An analysis of studies on hormonal contraception and breast cancer that was reported in issue No. 39 of *Progress* showed that there is a small increase in risk for current users of the pill (relative risk 1.24) and that this risk reduces gradually during the 10 years after discontinuing use. Ten years after a woman stops using the pill, therefore, her risk of breast cancer is the same as that of a woman who has never used oral contraceptives.

The incidence of breast cancer goes up steeply between the ages of 35 and 50. Consequently, since oral contraceptives increase risk slightly and since this risk decreases only gradually over a number of years, the age at which a woman last uses oral contraceptives is a major factor in determining the excess risk to which she is exposed. On average, the incidence of breast cancer in developing countries is less than half of that in developed countries.

In developed countries, oral contraceptives are used mainly by young women. Use declines sharply in those over 25. For women who discontinue use of the pill at age 25, the additional risk of breast cancer declines by the time they reach the age at which their natural risk increases. For women who use oral contraceptives at older ages, the additional risk is higher. In developed countries, among women who continue using oral contraceptives until the age of 40 the cumulative incidence of breast cancer at age 50 is estimated at 199 per 10,000 and at age 60 is 394 per 10,000 (compared with 180 per 10,000 at age 50 and 380 per 10,000 at age 60 among women in the general population). Among women in developing countries who continue using the pill until age 40, the cumulative incidence of breast cancer at age 50 is estimated at 80 per 10,000, and at age 60 is estimated at 155 per

10,000 (compared with 72 per 10,000 at age 50 and 150 per 10,000 at age 60 among the general population).

Progestogen-Only Contraceptives

Contraceptive progestogens can be administered in several forms: progestogen-only pills, levonorgestrel implants such as Norplant®, injectable depot forms such as DMPA (depot medroxyprogesterone acetate), and levonorgestrel-releasing intrauterine devices (IUDs). In general, women who are at risk of cardiovascular complications and for whom combined oral contraceptives are not recommended may decide to use progestogen-only preparations. These preparations have lower doses of progestogen than combined oral contraceptives though their efficacy may be lower.

One disadvantage of all forms of progestogen-only contraceptives is their tendency to disrupt the menstrual cycle and cause irregular bleeding. This could be a concern for women over the age of 40 who are more prone to irregular bleeding anyway, although the irregularity is more of a problem during the first few months of progestogen use and declines over time. Enlargement of the ovarian follicles may also occur.

Intrauterine Devices (IUDs)

Copper-bearing IUDs are used in many parts of the world. Their efficacy is long-lasting and is likely to suit the needs of women over the age of 35 who are usually more interested in having no more children than in spacing pregnancies. The use of IUDs may be extended until the menopause is established.

Studies of the use of IUDs by European women aged over 35 have shown a low incidence of side-effects, including bleeding, and a low infection rate. One European study found that, in women who were aged over 35 when the IUD was inserted, there were fewer IUD removals during nine years of observation and fewer side-effects than in women who were under 35 at the time of insertion.

The chief problem with the use of the IUD by women over 35 years is that it accentuates the already increased incidence of uterine bleeding. Removal of the IUD is advised in cases of bleeding or pain in order to protect women from anaemia or infection and to speed up diagnosis of organic causes of bleeding.

The levonorgestrel-releasing IUD combines high efficacy with a reduction of the amount and duration of menstrual bleeding. This latter effect is due to a local suppressive action on the endometrium resulting from the release of constant low levels of progestogen. A multicentre European study showed that, after five years of IUD use, women using the levonorgestrel-releasing IUD had significantly fewer IUD removals because of bleeding than did women using the copper-bearing IUD. According to a WHO Scientific Group on the Menopause, which met in Geneva in 1994, the levonorgestrel-releasing IUD "appears to be a suitable contraceptive for the late premenopausal years, because it has a high acceptability and causes minimal bleeding problems." This IUD can also be used to treat menorrhagia. There is one problem, however. Hormone-releasing IUDs are expensive and may not be affordable in developing countries.

Barrier Methods

The most common contraceptive barrier methods are diaphragms and condoms. Their efficacy is less than that of IUDs and oral contraceptives. Reported pregnancy rates among women aged 35–39 years using barriers methods are at best 1.1 per 100 woman-years. The condom has the advantage of giving protection against sexually transmitted diseases.

Coitus-related methods of contraception are preferred by some couples because they allow user control. This may, however, create some difficulty for men around age 50 who are the likely partners of late premenopausal women. If their sexual potency is reduced, self-administered contraceptive methods may make the problem worse.

Diaphragms and condoms are suitable methods for women nearing the menopause when both fecundity and the frequency of coitus are low. However, contraceptive failures may occur and these methods will be more useful if emergency contraception and abortion back-up services are available.

Sterilization

The various methods for female sterilization include tubal resection, cautery, and occlusion of the tube using bands or clips. When a couple has a family of the size they desire, male or female sterilization is a good contraceptive option because there should be little need for a reversible method. In the United Kingdom, more than 40 percent of couples over 40 years of age have selected sterilization as their method of family planning, and a similar situation exists in many developed countries. Recent research suggests that female sterilization may have the added benefit of a protective effect against ovarian cancer. Surgical sterilization requires, of course, adequate health care to minimize the risk of infection and other possible complications.

Natural Family Planning

There are few data on the appropriateness of natural methods of fertility regulation in the years of the late premenopause. However, the irregular menstrual cycles that occur in a large proportion of women make the use of safe periods impractical.

Key Conclusions

1. Combined oral contraceptives containing low doses of an estrogen and a progestogen are suitable for healthy, non-smoking women over the age of 35.

2. Progestogen-only contraceptives may be suitable for late premenopausal women.

3. Both copper-bearing and progestogen-releasing IUDs are effective, long-lasting, and safe contraceptives for late premenopausal women.

4. Barrier methods may be the method of choice for late premenopausal women whose fertility and frequency of coitus are low.

5. Male or female sterilization is an excellent contraceptive option for women approaching the menopause.

Chapter 9

Equity in Prescription Insurance and Contraceptive Coverage

Nearly half of all pregnancies in the United States are unintended, and more than half of all unintended pregnancies end in abortion (Henshaw, 1998). Contraceptives have a proven track record of enhancing the health of women and children, preventing unintended pregnancy, and reducing the need for abortion. However, although contraception is part of basic health care for women, far too many insurance policies exclude this vital coverage.

In fact, while most employment-related insurance policies in the United States cover prescription drugs in general, the vast majority does not include equitable coverage for prescription contraceptive drugs and devices (Alan Guttmacher Institute [AGI, 1994). Similarly, while most policies cover outpatient medical services in general, they often exclude outpatient contraceptive services from that coverage (AGI, 1994). This failure is costly, both for insurers who may have to pay for either maternity care or abortion, and the families whose physical and financial well-being is threatened by unintended pregnancy and lack of access to equitable coverage for contraceptives.

Efforts were already underway to address the inequity in prescription coverage for women when Viagra®, a drug to treat erectile dysfunction, was introduced on the U.S. market in the spring of 1998. Within two months of its entrance into the U.S. market, more than

"Fact Sheet: Equity in Prescription Insurance and Contraceptive Coverage," PPFA Web Site © 1999, Planned Parenthood® Federation of America, Inc.; available at http://www.plannedparenthood.org/library/ BIRTHCONTROL/EPICC_facts.html; reprinted with permission.

113

one half of the prescriptions for Viagra received insurance coverage. Such coverage has yet to be extended to intrauterine devices (IUDs) or diaphragms (Goldstein, 1998), prompting national organizations such as the American College of Obstetricians and Gynecologists and Planned Parenthood Federation of America (PPFA) to condemn the gender bias in prescription coverage.

In Congress:

In 1998, PPFA won a major legislative victory with the enactment of a contraceptive coverage requirement in the Federal Employees Health Benefits Plan (FEHBP). This provision is based on amendments to the Treasury-Postal Service appropriations bill (H.R. 4104), sponsored by Representative Nita Lowey (D-NY) in the House and Senators Olympia Snowe (R-ME) and Harry Reid (D-NV) in the Senate. The provision guarantees coverage of prescription contraceptive drugs and devices for federal employees by all plans participating in the FEHBP that cover other prescription drugs and devices. Contraceptive coverage for federal employees was again included in the FY 2000 Treasury and General Government Appropriations Act signed into law by President Clinton on September 29, 1999 (PL 106-58).

In 1999, Senators Olympia Snowe (R-ME) and Harry Reid (D-NV) and Representatives James Greenwood (R-PA) and Nita Lowey (D-NY) reintroduced the Equity in Prescription Insurance and Contraceptive Coverage Act to provide equity in insurance coverage for contraception in the private market. The bill simply seeks to establish parity for contraceptive prescriptions and related medical services within the context of coverage already guaranteed by each insurance plan.

Under this legislation, plans already covering prescription drugs and devices would include equal coverage for prescription contraceptive drugs and devices. Also, plans that include coverage for outpatient medical services would include outpatient contraceptive services in that coverage. The bill defines contraceptive services as "consultations, examinations, procedures, and medical services, provided on an outpatient basis and related to the use of contraceptive methods (including natural family planning) to prevent an unintended pregnancy." (S. 1200, 1999; H.R. 2120, 1999)

In the States:

In 1998, Maryland became the first state to enact a law requiring health insurers to provide comprehensive coverage of all contraceptives approved by the U.S. Food and Drug Administration (Mantius, 1999). A total of 22 states considered bills to improve insurance coverage of contraception in 1998. These bills generally required that insurers that cover prescription drugs include coverage for FDA-approved prescription contraceptive drugs and devices—along with associated medical services such as exams, insertion, and removal.

In April 1999, Georgia Governor Roy E. Barnes signed into law this year's first contraceptive equity provision, making Georgia the second state to enact a law requiring health insurers to provide comprehensive coverage of all FDA-approved contraceptives (Mantius, 1999). Since then, Vermont, Maine, Nevada, Connecticut, North Carolina, Hawaii, New Hampshire, and California have also enacted contraceptive equity laws. In total, contraceptive equity legislation has been introduced in 21 states.

While plans routinely cover other prescriptions and outpatient medical services, contraceptive coverage is meager or nonexistent in many insurance policies.

- Half of indemnity plans and Preferred Provider Organizations (PPOs), 20 percent of Point of Service (POS) networks, and 7 percent of Health Maintenance Organizations (HMOs) cover no reversible contraception (AGI, 1994).

- In 1998, less than two months after Viagra entered the U.S. market, more than half of all prescriptions received some insurance reimbursement. Overall coverage for oral contraceptives did not reach this level until they had been on the market for almost 40 years—coverage for diaphragms and IUDs still lags far behind (Goldstein, 1998).

- Even plans that do provide some coverage typically do not cover all of the five most commonly used reversible contraceptive methods (oral contraceptives, the IUD, diaphragm, Norplant® and Depo-Provera®). Less than 20 percent of traditional indemnity plans and PPOs, and less than 40 percent of POS networks or HMOs, routinely allow women to choose among these five contraceptive methods (AGI, 1994).

- Coverage of prescription drugs usually does not even include coverage for oral contraceptives, the most commonly used reversible contraceptive method in the United States. Although 97 percent of typical indemnity policies cover prescription drugs in general, only 33 percent include oral contraceptives in that coverage. This leaves two-thirds of typical indemnity plans covering "prescription drugs" but not the prescription so many women need access to—oral contraceptives (AGI, 1994).

Contraception is basic health care for women, and a critical contributor to improved maternal and child health.

- Ready access to contraceptive-related health services increases the likelihood that the estimated 15 million Americans who contract sexually transmitted infections each year will be diagnosed and treated (Kaiser Family Foundation, 1998).

- As they help women avoid unplanned pregnancies, contraceptive services help women plan pregnancies. A study of 45,000 women suggests that women who used family planning services in the two years before conception were more likely than women who had not used such services to receive early and adequate prenatal care (Jamieson & Buescher, 1992).

- The National Commission to Prevent Infant Mortality estimated that 10 percent of infant deaths could be prevented if all pregnancies were planned—in 1989 alone, 4,000 infant lives could have been saved (1990).

Insurers have relied on women and their families paying out of pocket for contraceptive services and supplies, forcing financial decisions that may result in the use of less effective or less medically appropriate contraceptive methods.

- Women of reproductive age currently spend 68 percent more in out-of-pocket health care costs than men (Women's Research and Education Institute, 1994). Much of the gender gap in expenses is due to reproductive health-related supplies and services.

- The more effective forms of contraception are generally also the most expensive, often costing hundreds of dollars at the onset of patient use (AGI, 1994). Women and their families who must pay out of pocket may well opt for less expensive and sometimes less effective methods, increasing their risk for unintended pregnancies.

- Cost analyses have shown that if health insurance policies were to include coverage for these contraceptive supplies, costs to employers would be minimal—as little as $1.43 per employee per month (Darroch, 1998).

The correlation is clear. Contraception prevents unintended pregnancy, helps women plan their pregnancies, and reduces the need for abortion.

- In any single year, 85 of 100 sexually active women of reproductive age not using a contraceptive method become pregnant. In contrast, of 100 oral contraceptive users, only between 0.1 and 5 percent become pregnant during the first year of use (Trussell, et al., 1998).

- Because the likelihood of pregnancy is so great when contraception is not used, 53 percent of all unintended pregnancies in the U.S. occur among the 10 percent of fertile women who use no method and leave pregnancy to chance (Harlap, et al., 1991).

- Reducing unintended pregnancy is key to reducing the number of abortions—more than half of unintended pregnancies end in abortion (Henshaw, 1998).

Part Three:

An Overview of Contraception

Chapter 10

Protecting Against Unintended Pregnancy: A Guide to Contraceptive Choices

—by Tamar Nordenberg

I am 20 and have never gone to see a doctor about birth control. My boyfriend and I have been going together for a couple of years and have been using condoms. So far, everything is fine. Are condoms alone safe enough, or is something else safe besides the Pill? I do not want to go on the Pill.
—Letter to the Kinsey Institute for Research in Sex, Gender, and Reproduction

This young woman is not alone in her uncertainty about contraceptive options. A 1995 report by the National Academy of Sciences' Institute of Medicine, *The Best Intentions: Unintended Pregnancy and the Well-being of Children and Families,* attributed the high rate of unintended pregnancies in the United States, in part, to Americans' lack of knowledge about contraception. About 6 of every 10 pregnancies in the United States are unplanned, according to the report.

Being informed about the pros and cons of various contraceptives is important not only for preventing unintended pregnancies but also for reducing the risk of illness or death from sexually transmitted diseases (STDs), including AIDS. (See "Preventing HIV and Other STDs.")

FDA Consumer, April 1997; revised June 1997; available at http://www.pueblo.gsa.gov/cic_text/health/contracept/397_baby.html.

The Food and Drug Administration (FDA) has approved a number of birth control methods, ranging from over-the-counter male and female condoms and vaginal spermicides to doctor-prescribed birth control pills, diaphragms, intrauterine devices (IUDs), injected hormones, and hormonal implants. Other contraceptive options include fertility awareness and voluntary surgical sterilization.

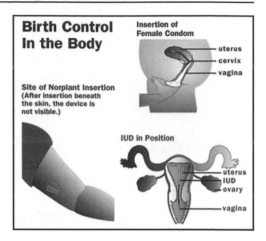

"On the whole, the contraceptive choices that Americans have are very safe and effective," says Dennis Barbour, president of the Association of Reproductive Health Professionals, "but a method that is very good for one woman may be lousy for another."

The choice of birth control depends on factors such as a person's health, frequency of sexual activity, number of partners, and desire to have children in the future. Effectiveness rates, based on statistical estimates, are another key consideration. FDA has developed a more consumer-friendly effectiveness table, which the agency will encourage all contraceptives marketers to add to their products' labeling. A copy of the table can be obtained by sending a request to FDA's Office of Women's Health, 5600 Fishers Lane (HF-8), Room 15-61, Rockville, MD 20857.

Barrier Methods

Male Condom

The male condom is a sheath placed over the erect penis before penetration, preventing pregnancy by blocking the passage of sperm.

A condom can be used only once. Some have spermicide added, usually nonoxynol-9 in the United States, to kill sperm. Spermicide has not been scientifically shown to provide additional contraceptive protection over the condom alone. Because they act as a mechanical barrier, condoms prevent direct vaginal contact with semen, infectious genital secretions, and genital lesions and discharges.

Most condoms are made from latex rubber, while a small percentage are made from lamb intestines (sometimes called "lambskin" condoms). Condoms made from polyurethane have been marketed in the United States since 1994.

Except for abstinence, latex condoms are the most effective method for reducing the risk of infection from the viruses that cause AIDS, other HIV-related illnesses, and other STDs.

Some condoms are prelubricated. These lubricants don't provide more birth control or STD protection. Non-oil-based lubricants, such as water or K-Y jelly, can be used with latex or lambskin condoms, but oil-based lubricants, such as petroleum jelly (Vaseline), lotions, or massage or baby oil, should not be used because they can weaken the material.

Female Condom

The Reality Female Condom, approved by FDA in April 1993, consists of a lubricated polyurethane sheath shaped similarly to the male condom. The closed end, which has a flexible ring, is inserted into the vagina, while the open end remains outside, partially covering the labia.

The female condom, like the male condom, is available without a prescription and is intended for one-time use. It should not be used together with a male condom because they may not both stay in place.

Diaphragm

Available by prescription only and sized by a health professional to achieve a proper fit, the diaphragm has a dual mechanism to prevent pregnancy. A dome-shaped rubber disk with a flexible rim covers the cervix so sperm can't reach the uterus, while a spermicide applied to the diaphragm before insertion kills sperm.

The diaphragm protects for six hours. For intercourse after the six-hour period, or for repeated intercourse within this period, fresh spermicide should be placed in the vagina with the diaphragm still in place. The diaphragm should be left in place for at least six hours after the last intercourse but not for longer than a total of 24 hours because of the risk of toxic shock syndrome (TSS), a rare but potentially fatal infection. Symptoms of TSS include sudden fever, stomach upset, sunburn-like rash, and a drop in blood pressure.

Cervical Cap

The cap is a soft rubber cup with a round rim, sized by a health professional to fit snugly around the cervix. It is available by prescription only and, like the diaphragm, is used with spermicide.

It protects for 48 hours and for multiple acts of intercourse within this time. Wearing it for more than 48 hours is not recommended because of the risk, though low, of TSS. Also, with prolonged use of two or more days, the cap may cause an unpleasant vaginal odor or discharge in some women.

Sponge

The vaginal contraceptive sponge has not been available since the sole manufacturer, Whitehall Laboratories of Madison, N.J., voluntarily stopped selling it in 1995. It remains an approved product and could be marketed again.

The sponge, a donut-shaped polyurethane device containing the spermicide nonoxynol-9, is inserted into the vagina to cover the cervix. A woven polyester loop is designed to ease removal.

The sponge protects for up to 24 hours and for multiple acts of intercourse within this time. It should be left in place for at least six hours after intercourse but should be removed no more than 30 hours after insertion because of the risk, though low, of TSS.

Vaginal Spermicides Alone

Vaginal spermicides are available in foam, cream, jelly, film, suppository, or tablet forms. All types contain a sperm-killing chemical.

Studies have not produced definitive data on the efficacy of spermicides alone, but according to the authors of *Contraceptive Technology*, a leading resource for contraceptive information, the failure rate for typical users may be 21 percent per year.

Package instructions must be carefully followed because some spermicide products require the couple to wait 10 minutes or more after inserting the spermicide before having sex. One dose of spermicide is usually effective for one hour. For repeated intercourse, additional spermicide must be applied. And after intercourse, the spermicide has to remain in place for at least six to eight hours to ensure that all sperm are killed. The woman should not douche or rinse the vagina during this time.

Hormonal Methods

Combined Oral Contraceptives

Typically called "the pill," combined oral contraceptives have been on the market for more than 35 years and are the most popular form of reversible birth control in the United States. This form of birth control suppresses ovulation (the monthly release of an egg from the ovaries) by the combined actions of the hormones estrogen and progestin.

If a woman remembers to take the pill every day as directed, she has an extremely low chance of becoming pregnant in a year. But the pill's effectiveness may be reduced if the woman is taking some medications, such as certain antibiotics.

Besides preventing pregnancy, the pill offers additional benefits. As stated in the labeling, the pill can make periods more regular. It also has a protective effect against pelvic inflammatory disease, an infection of the fallopian tubes or uterus that is a major cause of infertility in women, and against ovarian and endometrial cancers.

The decision whether to take the pill should be made in consultation with a health professional. Birth control pills are safe for most women—safer even than delivering a baby—but they carry some risks.

Current low-dose pills have fewer risks associated with them than earlier versions. But women who smoke—especially those over 35—and women with certain medical conditions, such as a history of blood clots or breast or endometrial cancer, may be advised against taking the pill. The pill may contribute to cardiovascular disease, including high blood pressure, blood clots, and blockage of the arteries.

One of the biggest questions has been whether the pill increases the risk of breast cancer in past and current pill users. An international study published in the September 1996 journal *Contraception* concluded that women's risk of breast cancer 10 years after going off birth control pills was no higher than that of women who had never used the pill. During pill use and for the first 10 years after stopping the pill, women's risk of breast cancer was only slightly higher in pill users than non-pill users.

Side effects of the pill, which often subside after a few months' use, include nausea, headache, breast tenderness, weight gain, irregular bleeding, and depression.

Doctors sometimes prescribe higher doses of combined oral contraceptives for use as "morning after" pills to be taken within 72 hours of unprotected intercourse to prevent the possibly fertilized egg from reaching the uterus. On June 28, 1996, FDA's Advisory Committee for Reproductive Health Drugs concluded that certain oral contraceptives are safe and effective for this use. At press time in January 1997, no drug firm had submitted an application to FDA to label its pills for this use, and the agency had not yet acted on the committee's recommendation. [In September 1998, the FDA approved the PREVEN™ Emergency Contraceptive Kit produced by Gynetics Inc., which to date is the only product packaged and marketed exclusively for use as an emergency contraceptive.]

Mini-pills

Although taken daily like combined oral contraceptives, minipills contain only the hormone progestin and no estrogen. They work by reducing and thickening cervical mucus to prevent sperm from reaching the egg. They also keep the uterine lining from thickening, which prevents a fertilized egg from implanting in the uterus. These pills are slightly less effective than combined oral contraceptives.

Mini-pills can decrease menstrual bleeding and cramps, as well as the risk of endometrial and ovarian cancer and pelvic inflammatory disease. Because they contain no estrogen, minipills don't present the risk of blood clots associated with estrogen in combined pills. They are a good option for women who can't take estrogen because they are breast-feeding or because estrogen-containing products cause them to have severe headaches or high blood pressure.

Side effects of mini-pills include menstrual cycle changes, weight gain, and breast tenderness.

Injectable Progestins

Depo-Provera®, approved by FDA in 1992, is injected by a health professional into the buttocks or arm muscle every three months. Depo-Provera prevents pregnancy in three ways: It inhibits ovulation, changes the cervical mucus to help prevent sperm from reaching the egg, and changes the uterine lining to prevent the fertilized egg from implanting in the uterus. The progestin injection is extremely effective in preventing pregnancy, in large part because it requires little effort for the woman to comply: She simply has to get an injection by a doctor once every three months.

The benefits are similar to those of the minipill and another progestin-only contraceptive, Norplant®. Side effects are also similar and can include irregular or missed periods, weight gain, and breast tenderness.

(See "Depo-Provera: The Quarterly Contraceptive" in the March 1993 *FDA Consumer*.)

Implantable Progestins

Norplant®, approved by FDA in 1990, and the newer Norplant® 2, approved in 1996, are the third type of progestin-only contraceptive. Made up of matchstick-sized rubber rods, this contraceptive is surgically implanted under the skin of the upper arm, where it steadily releases the contraceptive steroid levonorgestrel.

The six-rod Norplant provides protection for up to five years (or until it is removed), while the two-rod Norplant 2 protects for up to three years. Norplant failures are rare, but are higher with increased body weight.

Some women may experience inflammation or infection at the site of the implant. Other side effects include menstrual cycle changes, weight gain, and breast tenderness.

Intrauterine Devices

An IUD is a t-shaped device inserted into the uterus by a health-care professional. Two types of IUDs are available in the United States: the ParaGard CopperT 380A and the Progestasert Progesterone T. The ParaGard IUD can remain in place for 10 years, while the Progestasert IUD must be replaced every year.

It's not entirely clear how IUDs prevent pregnancy. They seem to prevent sperm and eggs from meeting by either immobilizing the sperm on their way to the fallopian tubes or changing the uterine lining so the fertilized egg cannot implant in it.

IUDs have one of the lowest failure rates of any contraceptive method. "In the population for which the IUD is appropriate—for those in a mutually monogamous, stable relationship who aren't at a high risk of infection—the IUD is a very safe and very effective method of contraception," says Lisa Rarick, M.D., director of FDA's division of reproductive and urologic drug products.

The IUD's image suffered when the Dalkon Shield IUD was taken off the market in 1975. This IUD was associated with a high incidence of pelvic infections and infertility, and some deaths. Today, serious complications from IUDs are rare, although IUD users may be at in-creased risk of developing pelvic inflammatory disease. Other side effects can include perforation of the uterus, abnormal bleeding, and cramps. Complications occur most often during and immediately af-ter insertion.

Traditional Methods

Fertility Awareness

Also known as natural family planning or periodic abstinence, fer-tility awareness entails not having sexual intercourse on the days of a woman's menstrual cycle when she could become pregnant or using a barrier method of birth control on those days.

Because a sperm may live in the female's reproductive tract for up to seven days and the egg remains fertile for about 24 hours, a woman can get pregnant within a substantial window of time—from seven days before ovulation to three days after. Methods to approximate when a woman is fertile are usually based on the menstrual cycle, changes in cervical mucus, or changes in body temperature.

"Natural family planning can work," Rarick says, "but it takes an extremely motivated couple to use the method effectively."

Withdrawal

In this method, also called coitus interruptus, the man withdraws his penis from the vagina before ejaculation. Fertilization is prevented because the sperm don't enter the vagina.

Effectiveness depends on the male's ability to withdraw before ejaculation. Also, withdrawal doesn't provide protection from STDs, including HIV. Infectious diseases can be transmitted by direct con-tact with surface lesions and by pre-ejaculatory fluid.

Surgical Sterilization

Surgical sterilization is a contraceptive option intended for people who don't want children in the future. It is considered permanent be-cause reversal requires major surgery that is often unsuccessful.

Female Sterilization

Female sterilization blocks the fallopian tubes so the egg can't travel to the uterus. Sterilization is done by various surgical techniques, usually under general anesthesia.

Complications from these operations are rare and can include infection, hemorrhage, and problems related to the use of general anesthesia.

Male Sterilization

This procedure, called a vasectomy, involves sealing, tying, or cutting a man's vas deferens, which otherwise would carry the sperm from the testicle to the penis.

Vasectomy involves a quick operation, usually under 30 minutes, with possible minor postsurgical complications, such as bleeding or infection.

Contraceptive Research

Research continues on effective contraceptives that minimize side effects. One important research focus, according to FDA's Rarick, is the development of birth control methods that are both spermicidal and microbicidal to prevent not only pregnancy but also transmission of HIV and other STDs.

Preventing HIV and Other STDs

Some people mistakenly believe that by protecting themselves against pregnancy, they are automatically protecting themselves from HIV, the virus that causes AIDS, and other sexually transmitted diseases (STDs). But the male latex condom is the only contraceptive method considered highly effective in reducing the risk of STDs.

Unlike latex condoms, lambskin condoms are not recommended for STD prevention because they are porous and may permit passage of viruses like HIV, hepatitis B, and herpes. Polyurethane condoms are an alternative method of STD protection for those who are latex-sensitive.

Because it is a barrier method that works in much the same way as the male condom, the female condom may provide some protection against STDs. Both condoms should not be used together, however, because they may not both stay in place.

According to an FDA advisory committee panel that met November 22, 1996, it appears, based on several published scientific studies, that some vaginal spermicides containing nonoxynol-9 may reduce the risk of gonorrhea and chlamydia transmission. However, use of nonoxynol-9 may cause tissue irritation, raising the possibility of an increased susceptibility to some STDs, including HIV.

As stated in their labeling, birth control pills, Norplant®, Depo-Provera®, IUDs, and lambskin condoms do not protect against STD infection. For STD protection, a male latex condom can be used in combination with non-condom methods. The relationship of the vaginal barrier methods—the diaphragm, cap and sponge—to STD prevention is not yet clear.

Tamar Nordenberg is a staff writer for *FDA Consumer*.

Chapter 11

Consumer-Friendly Birth Control Information

Pregnancy Rates for Birth Control Methods
(For One Year of Use)

The following table provides estimates of the percent of women likely to become pregnant while using a particular contraceptive method for one year. These estimates are based on a variety of studies.

"Typical Use" rates mean that the method either was not always used correctly or was not used with every act of sexual intercourse (e.g., sometimes forgot to take a birth control pill as directed and became pregnant), or was used correctly but failed anyway.

"Lowest Expected" rates mean that the method was always used correctly with every act of sexual intercourse but failed anyway (e.g., always took a birth control pill as directed but still became pregnant).

U.S. Food and Drug Administration (FDA), May 13, 1997. Data adapted from R. A. Hatcher, J. Trussell, F. Stewart, et al., *Contraceptive Technology*, 17th rev. ed., New York: Irvington Publishers Inc. (in press). Available at http://www.fda.gov/fdac/features/1997/conceptbl.html.

131

Method	Typical Use Rate of Pregnancy	Lowest Expected Rate of Pregnancy
Sterilization:		
Male Sterilization	0.15%	0.1%
Female Sterilization	0.5%	0.5%
Hormonal Methods:		
Implant (Norplant®)	0.09%	0.09%
Hormone Shot (Depo-Provera®)	0.3%	0.3%
Combined Pill (Estrogen/Progestin)	5%	0.1%
Mini-pill (Progestin only)	5%	0.5%
Intrauterine Devices (IUDs):		
Copper T	0.8%	0.6%
Progesterone T	2%	1.5%
Barrier Methods:		
Male Latex Condom[1]	14%	3%
Diaphragm[2]	20%	6%
Vaginal Sponge (no previous births)[3]	20%	9%
Vaginal Sponge (previous births)[3]	40%	20%
Cervical Cap (no previous births)[2]	20%	9%
Cervical Cap (previous births)[2]	40%	26%
Female Condom	21%	5%
Spermicide:		
(gel, foam, suppository, film)	26%	6%

MethodTypical Use	Lowest Expected Rate of Pregnancy	Rate of Pregnancy
Natural Methods:		
Withdrawal	19%	4%
Natural Family Planning (calendar, temperature, cervical mucus)	25%	1–9%
No Method:	85%	85%

[1] Used Without Spermicide
[2] Used With Spermicide
[3] Contains Spermicide

Chapter 12

Choosing a Birth Control Method

There are many kinds of birth control. And no one contraceptive is right for every person. That's why it's important to find what fits your needs.

The following table compares the five major reversible (non-permanent) types of birth control. This information can help you work with your doctor to choose a method that is right for you.

Each type of birth control discussed can help you prevent pregnancy, if you use it correctly. Using a combination of a latex condom and other methods can help protect you against both pregnancy and diseases, like AIDS, that are passed on through sexual contact.

In comparing your choices, you must decide what matters most to you in a birth control method. Share your concerns with your doctor, nurse practitioner, or other health care provider and don't hesitate to get more information if you need it.

To learn more about birth control methods, ask your doctor, nurse practitioner, or other health care provider. Make sure you have all the information you need to make the right choice, and be sure to use birth control correctly.

Excerpted from *Choosing a Birth Control Method*, an undated patient education booklet prepared by the Association of Reproductive Health Professionals under an educational grant from The Upjohn Company; available at http://www.arhp.org/cb.htm; reprinted with permission.

Key Factors	Barriers	IUDs	The Pill	Implants	Injections
Average success rate	low	moderately high	extremely high	extremely high	high
Length of protection	one sex act	8 years (copper)	continuous if taken daily	5 years	3 months
Average cost	$.50–$3.00/ use	$200–$300	$20–$25/ month	$450–$750/ insertion	$60–$75 (3 months)
Return to fertility after stopping use	immediate	immediate	immediate	immediate	6–18 months
Requires visit to clinicians to stop using	no	yes	no	yes	no
Privacy of use	no	usually (string may be felt by man)	requires supply of pills	some implants visible or felt in some women	yes
Protection against STDs/AIDS	yes	no	no	no	no
Provides other health benefits	no	no	yes	yes	yes

Chapter 13

Your Contraceptive Choices for Now, for Later

The Pill

(birth control pills; oral contraceptives)

What Is It?

- pills containing the hormones estrogen and progestin

How Does It Work?

- thickens cervical mucus, blocking sperm
- prevents ovulation
- prevents implantation of fertilized egg

How Is It Used?

- birth control pills are prescribed for women
- a pill must be taken by mouth every day for 21 or 28 days each cycle
- the pill should be taken at the same time each day
- pills must be taken on schedule, month after month

U.S. Department of Health and Human Services, Public Health Service, Office of Population Affairs, updated spring 1998. Source: Hatcher, R.A., J. Trussell, et al., *Contraceptive Technology*, 17th rev. ed., New York: Irvington Publishers, 1998.

How Well Does It Work?

- typical use: 95%
- perfect use: 99.9%
- failure rate increased with: some medications, missed pills, taking pills late
- use backup method for: first cycle, any missed pills, discontinuing pill, or if taking some medications

Does It Reduce the Risk for HIV/AIDS and STDs?

- does not reduce risk for HIV/AIDS or STDs
- may increase risk for chlamydia and cervicitis
- using a male, latex condom reduces the risk

What Are Its Main Advantages?

- reversible
- does not interfere with sex
- medically safe for most women
- regulates periods, lighter periods
- decreases menstrual pain and PMS
- may improve acne
- decreases risk for ovarian and endometrial cancer

What Are Some Possible Problems?

- side effects: nausea, weight gain, headaches, dizziness, breast tenderness, break-through bleeding (spotting between periods)
- more serious complications include depression, liver tumors
- may increase risk of stroke, heart attack, blood clots, and high blood pressure for some women (especially women over 35 who smoke)
- possible increased risk for breast cancer and cervical cancer

The Minipill

(progestin-only pill)

What Is It?

- pills containing the hormone progestin

How Does It Work?

- thickens cervical mucus, blocking sperm
- may or may not prevent ovulation
- prevents implantation of fertilized egg

How Is It Used?

- minipills are prescribed for women
- a pill must be taken by mouth every day
- the pill must be taken at the same time each day, without interruption

How Well Does It Work?

- typical use: 95%
- perfect use: 99.5%
- failure rate increased for women who take seizure medications
- use back-up method every time a pill is missed or taken late (even 3 hours late!)

Does It Reduce the Risk for HIV/AIDS and STDs?

- does not reduce risk for HIV/AIDS or STDs
- using a male, latex condom reduces the risk

What Are Its Main Advantages?

- reversible
- does not interfere with sex
- can be used by some women who cannot take regular birth control pills
- can be used while breastfeeding

What Are Some Possible Problems?

- progestin-only methods often cause changes in menstruation including: spotting, missed periods, irregular bleeding, heavy flow
- side effects: weight gain, headaches, breast tenderness, ovarian cysts

Norplant®

(progestin implant)

What Is It?

- a device placed under the skin ("implant") consisting of six, silicone tubes (capsules), each the size of a matchstick; releases low, constant level of hormone levonorgestrel (progestin) into the blood stream

How Does It Work?

- thickens cervical mucus, blocking sperm
- usually prevents ovulation
- prevents implantation of fertilized egg

How Is It Used?

- six capsules are placed under the woman's skin on inside of the upper arm
- capsules are inserted and removed by a clinician
- involves a minor surgical procedure using local anesthesia (numbing medicine)

How Well Does It Work?

- typical use: almost 100%
- perfect use: almost 100%
- effective immediately, if inserted within 7 days from the start of menstrual period
- effective for up to 5 years
- failure rate is high for women who take most seizure medications

Does It Reduce the Risk for HIV/AIDS and STDs?

- does not reduce risk for HIV/AIDS or STDs
- using a male, latex condom reduces the risk

What Are Its Main Advantages?

- reversible as soon as it is removed
- long lasting method
- nothing to remember
- does not interfere with sex
- can be used by women who cannot take estrogen
- may decrease menstrual cramps, pain, and blood loss
- can be used while breastfeeding

What Are Some Possible Problems?

- may have infection or pain in arm soon after insertion
- removal can be difficult
- some women have scarring at insertion site
- menstrual changes are common including: irregular bleeding, very light bleeding, heavy bleeding, missed periods or no periods
- side effects: weight gain, headaches, breast tenderness, hair loss, depression, ovarian cysts

Depo-Provera®

("the shot")

What Is It?

- a long-acting form of the hormone depo-medroxyprogesterone accetate (progestin) given by injection

How Does It Work?

- thickens cervical mucus, blocking sperm
- prevents ovulation
- prevents implantation of fertilized egg

How Is It Used?

- the woman is given an injection into the upper arm or buttocks every 3 months

How Well Does It Work?

- typical use: almost 100%
- perfect use: almost 100%
- works for 12 weeks
- failure rate increased if shot is not repeated every 12 weeks

Does It Reduce the Risk for HIV/AIDS and STDs?

- does not reduce risk for HIV/AIDS or STDs
- using a male, latex condom reduces the risk

What Are Its Main Advantages?

- lasts for 3 months
- does not interfere with sex
- can be used by women with a history of seizures (reduces seizures) or sickle cell anemia
- can be used while breastfeeding

What Are Some Possible Problems?

- need to return for shot every 3 months
- menstrual changes are common including: irregular bleeding, spotting, missed periods or no periods
- side effects: weight gain, depression, breast tenderness, headaches, allergic reaction
- side effects may last for up to 6 months after the last injection
- may cause delay in ability to get pregnant after discontinuation
- may cause bone density changes or bone loss; adverse effects on lipids

Emergency Contraceptive Pills
(ECPs)

What Is It?
- birth control pills taken in a specific way to prevent pregnancy after unprotected sex

How Does It Work?

Depending on when in the menstrual cycle ECPs are taken:
- prevents ovulation
- prevents implantation of fertilized egg

How Is It Used?
- first set of pills is taken within 72 hours after unprotected sex
- a second set of pills is taken exactly 12 hours later

How Well Does It Work?
- reduces the risk of pregnancy for a single act of unprotected sex by 75%

Does It Reduce the Risk for HIV/AIDS and STDs?
- does not reduce risk for HIV/AIDS or STDs

What Are Its Main Advantages?
- can be used after unplanned, unprotected sex
- can be used when usual method fails (for example, when a condom breaks)
- can be used after rape

What Are Some Possible Problems?
- frequently causes nausea and vomiting
- vomiting may reduce effectiveness
- should not be used if already pregnant
- may change time of next menstrual period (early or late)

143

- if period does not begin within 3 weeks of taking ECPs, get a pregnancy test

IUD

(intrauterine device)

What Is It?

- a medicated, plastic device that is placed into the uterus; a string attached to the IUD hangs down into the vagina
- the ParaGard® (CuT 380A) contains copper
- the Progestasert® release the hormone progesterone

How Does It Work?

- may inactivate sperm and/or egg, preventing fertilization
- creates an inflammatory condition in the uterus, preventing implantation of fertilized egg

How Is It Used?

- requires a simple medical procedure for insertion and removal
- the device is placed into the uterus, where it remains until it is removed
- the woman can check the correct placement of the device by feeling for the string

How Well Does It Work?

- the ParaGard® (CuT 380A) is effective for up to 10 years
  - typical use: 99.2%
  - perfect use: 99.4%
- the Progestasert® is effective for 1 year
  - typical use: 98%
  - perfect use: 98.5%

Does It Reduce the Risk for HIV/AIDS and STDs?

- does not reduce risk for HIV/AIDS or STDs
- may increase risk of HIV/STD transmission

- may increase risk of pelvic inflammatory disease (PID) soon after insertion
- using a male, latex condom reduces the risk
- should only be used by women at low risk for HIV/AIDS and STDs (only have sex with one uninfected partner)

What Are Its Main Advantages?
- reversible method
- does not interfere with sex
- nothing to remember (except checking the string)
- long-acting (up to 10 years with the CuT 380A)

What Are Some Possible Problems?
- up to 10% of women expel IUD during first year of use
- insertion requires a minor medical procedure which may be somewhat uncomfortable
- must be removed by a clinician
- possible uterine perforation at time of insertion
- may cause menstrual problems, including heavy bleeding and cramps
- increased risk for PID which may lead to infertility; may not be a good choice for women who have not had children
- should not be used by women who are at high risk for HIV/AIDS/STDs
- should not be used by women with diabetes, HIV infection, other impaired immune conditions, or anemia
- IUD may not stay in place (may fall out, move out of reach or become imbedded)
- partner may fell the string during sex

Abstinence

What Is It?
- a decision to not have sex (vaginal, oral, and anal)

How Does It Work?

- egg and sperm do not meet
- fertilization does not occur

How Is It Used?

- an individual makes a decision not to have sex and sticks to it
- a couple makes a decision not to have sex and sticks to it
- learning assertiveness, negotiation, and planning skills is helpful

How Well Does It Work?

- 100% effective as long as sex does not occur

Does It Reduce the Risk for HIV/AIDS and STDs?

- 100% reduced risk for sexual transmission of HIV/AIDS and STDs if abstaining from all forms of sex (vaginal, oral, and anal)
- does not reduce risk for HIV/AIDS and STDs if only abstaining from vaginal sex or if engaging in other risky behavior

What Are Its Main Advantages?

- eliminates the risk for sexually transmitting or contracting HIV/AIDS and STDs
- no health risks or side effects
- can be used at any time, regardless of prior sexual experience
- may be a strong value for some individuals, families, and religious groups
- allows users to focus on non-sexual aspects of relationship

What Are Some Possible Problems?

- may be hard to stick with
- requires learning and using decision-making, negotiation, and planning skills

Natural Family Planning

(Periodic Abstinence, Sympto-Thermal, Billings / Ovulation Method, Basal Body Temperature)

What Is It?

- a variety of methods that help to detect the fertile days of the menstrual cycle
- abstinence from sex during fertile days ("unsafe days")

How Does It Work?

- users abstain from sex on fertile days to prevent egg and sperm from meeting
- fertilization does not occur

How Is It Used?

- instruction from a qualified NFP instructor or clinician is recommended
- observing and charting daily signs of fertility or ovulation (release of the egg)
- basal body temperature (BBT) method: the temperature is taken and charted each day
- cervical mucus method: the cervical mucus is evaluated for signs of ovulation
- sympto-thermal method: combines BBT and cervical mucus methods, along with checking position of the cervix

How Well Does It Work?

- typical use: 81%
- perfect use: 91–99%

Does It Reduce the Risk for HIV/AIDS and STDs?

- does not reduce risk for HIV/AIDS or STDs
- using a male, latex condom reduces the risk

What Are Its Main Advantages?

- no health risks or side effects caused by method

- accepted by most religions
- can be used to determine fertile days when pregnancy is desired
- responsibility can be shared by couple

What Are Some Possible Problems?

- have to abstain from intercourse on fertile days (back-up method can be used on fertile days, if couple chooses not to abstain)
- temptation to take risks may occur
- care is needed to keep records and observe signs
- fertility signs and symptoms may be difficult for some women to identify

Calendar/Rhythm

What Is It?

- charting menstrual cycle to help detect fertile days
- abstinence from sex during fertile days ("unsafe days")

How Does It Work?

- users abstain from sex on fertile days to prevent egg and sperm from meeting
- fertilization does not occur

How Is It Used?

- woman charts menstrual cycle on a calendar
- fertile days are calculated based on the following assumptions: 1) ovulation occurs on day 14 (plus or minus 2 days) before the onset of the next menstrual period; 2) sperm live for 2–3 days; and 3) the egg lives for 24 hours

How Well Does It Work?

- typical use: 75%
- perfect use: 91%

Does It Reduce the Risk for HIV/AIDS and STDs?

- does not reduce risk for HIV/AIDS or STDs
- using a male, latex condom reduces the risk

What Are Its Main Advantages?

- no health risks or side effects caused by method
- accepted by most religions
- can also be used to determine fertile days when pregnancy is desired
- responsibility can be shared by couple

What Are Some Possible Problems?

- menstrual cycle can change due to stress, illness, or other factors making it difficult to predict ovulation and fertile days based on past cycles
- have to abstain from intercourse on fertile days (back-up method can be used on fertile days, if couple chooses not to abstain)
- temptation to take risks may occur
- care is needed to keep records

Withdrawal

What Is It?

- the practice of interrupting sex in order to ejaculate ("come") outside of the vagina

How Does It Work?

- egg and sperm do not meet
- fertilization does not occur

How Is It Used?

- the male withdraws his penis from the woman's vagina before ejaculation occurs
- male ejaculates outside of the vagina and away from the outer genital area

149

How Well Does It Work?

- typical use: 81%
- perfect use: may be as high as 96%
- effectiveness varies according to the skill and control of the male
- failure rate increases with repeated sex or inability to control ejaculation

Does It Reduce the Risk for HIV/AIDS and STDs?

- does not reduce risk for HIV/AIDS or STDs
- pre-ejaculate ("pre-come") may contain HIV and STDs
- using a male, latex condom reduces the risk

What Are Its Main Advantages?

- no health risks or side effects cause by method
- reversible
- no cost
- always available

What Are Some Possible Problems?

- requires good self control for the male
- may decrease pleasure and satisfaction
- some males may be unable to predict ejaculation and withdraw in time

Male Condom

("rubber")

What Is It?

- a sheath that covers the penis
- may be made of latex, plastic, or animal "skin"
- may be pre-lubricated and/or contain spermicide

How Does It Work?

- creates a barrier between the penis and the vagina
- collects and holds the semen

- egg and sperm do not meet
- fertilization does not occur

How Is It Used?

- condom is unrolled over the erect penis before sex
- male must hold the base of the condom to penis when withdrawing
- male must withdraw from vagina while penis is still erect
- condom is removed and discarded without spilling the semen near the vagina
- condoms cannot be reused

How Well Does It Work?

- typical use (condom alone): 84%
- perfect use (condom alone): 97%
- using a condom with spermicide increases the effectiveness up to 99%

Does It Reduce the Risk for HIV/AIDS and STDs?

- male, latex condoms reduce risk for HIV/AIDS and STDs
- animal "skin" condoms do not provide HIV/AIDS and STD protection

What Are Its Main Advantages?

- latex condoms reduce the risk for transmitting and contracting HIV/AIDS and STDs
- no prescription needed; can be purchased at most drugstores
- no health risks or side effects caused by method (except for those allergic to latex)
- delays premature ejaculation

What Are Some Possible Problems?

- condoms may slip off, or break
- proper use may interfere with spontaneity
- may affect sexual sensations

- may cause irritation or discomfort
- if allergic to latex can have a severe reaction; plastic condoms may be used
- latex condoms should not be used with oil-based lubricants

Female Condom

(vaginal pouch, Reality Female Condom®)

What Is It?

- a sheath made of polyurethane with rubber rings at each end
- covers the vagina, cervix, and vulva "from inside-out"

How Does It Work?

- creates a barrier between the penis and vagina
- collects and holds the semen
- egg and sperm do not meet
- fertilization does not occur

How Is It Used?

- must be inserted prior to contact between penis and vagina
- one ring is placed deep inside the vagina; the second ring remains outside of the vagina
- the condom is removed and discarded without spilling the semen
- used for one act of intercourse
- the condom cannot be reused

How Well Does It Work?

- typical use: 79%
- perfect use: 95%

Does It Reduce the Risk for HIV/AIDS and STDs?

- the female condom has not been well tested for HIV/AIDS and STD prevention
- in theory, all barrier methods provide some protection against HIV/AIDS and STDs

- female condom should not be used with a male latex condom
- if female is at high risk for HIV/AIDS or other STDs, using a male, latex condom **instead** reduces the risk

What Are Its Main Advantages?

- reversible
- can be bought at many drugstores
- can be placed in vagina up to 8 hours before use
- may not tear as easily as male condoms; polyurethane is stronger than latex

What Are Some Possible Problems?

- may slip out of place during sex
- may be difficult for some women to insert
- may affect sexual sensations
- may cause irritation or discomfort
- increased risk for toxic shock sydrome

Diaphragm with Spermicide

What Is It?

- dome-shaped, rubber cup with a flexible rim which covers the cervix

How Does It Work?

- cup acts as barrier to semen contact with the cervix
- spermicide kills sperm
- fertilization does not occur

How Is It Used?

- clinician fits woman with proper size and teaches correct use
- spermicide cream or gel/jelly is placed in the cup before insertion
- before sex, diaphragm is placed in the vagina, covering the cervix
- diaphragm is left in place for at least 6 hours after sex
- additional application of spermicide is needed for each act of intercourse

How Well Does It Work?

- typical use: 80%
- perfect use: 94%
- failure rate increases with increased sexual activity (more than 3 times a week)

Does It Reduce the Risk for HIV/AIDS and STDs?

- somewhat reduced risk for some STDs and PID
- uncertain protection against HIV/AIDS
- lowers risk for cancer of the cervix
- using a male, latex condom reduces the risk for HIV/AIDS and STDs

What Are Its Main Advantages?

- reversible
- can be used with or without partner cooperation
- can be placed in vagina up to 6 hours before sex

What Are Some Possible Problems?

- requires a prescription and clinic visit
- may be difficult for some women to insert
- some individuals are allergic to the rubber or the spermicide
- pelvic pressure, vaginal discharge, or vaginal irritation if left in too long
- increased risk for vaginal and urinary tract infections
- increased risk for toxic shock syndrome; must be removed within 24 hours
- cannot be used with oil-based lubricants or vaginal medications

Cervical Cap

What Is It?

- soft rubber cup with a firm rim that fits over the cervix
- similar to the diaphragm, but smaller

How Does It Work?

- covers and fits snugly around the cervix
- cup holds spermicide in contact with the cervix
- cup acts as barrier to semen contact with the cervix
- spermicide kills sperm
- fertilization does not occur

How Is It Used?

- clinician fits woman with cap and teaches correct use
- spermicide cream/gel/jelly is placed in the cap
- cap is placed deep inside the vagina covering the cervix
- must be left in place for at least 6 hours after sex
- can be left in place for up to 48 hours

How Well Does It Work?

- typical use in woman who has never had a baby: 80%
- perfect use in woman who has never had a baby: 91%

- typical use in woman who has already had a baby: 60%
- perfect use in woman who has already had a baby: 74%

Does It Reduce the Risk for HIV/AIDS and STDs?

- HIV/AIDS and STD protection has not been studied in the cap
- in theory, barrier methods provide some protection against HIV/AIDS and STDs
- using a male, latex condom reduces the risk

What Are Its Main Advantages?

- reversible
- can be used with or without partner cooperation
- can be used for repeated sex for up to 48 hours

What Are Some Possible Problems?

- few clinicians are trained to fit the cap

- some women have difficulty inserting and removing the cap
- should not be used during the menstrual period
- possible allergy to rubber or spermicide
- pelvic pressure, vaginal discharge, or vaginal irritation if left in too long
- increased risk for vaginal and urinary tract infections
- increased risk for toxic shock syndrome; must remove within 48 hours
- cannot be used with oil-based lubricants or vaginal medications

Vaginal Spermicides

What Is It?
- creams, gels/jellies, foams, films, suppositories that contain sperm-killing chemicals
- may be used alone or with barrier methods (condom, diaphragm, cap)

How Does It Work?
- kills sperm
- some forms block sperm from entering the cervix
- fertilization does not occur

How Is It Used?
- placed inside the vagina by hand or with an applicator before sex
- may be placed on condoms, or inside diaphragms or cervical cap

How Well Does It Work?
- typical use (spermicide only): 74%
- perfect use (spermicide only): 94%
- using a condom with spermicide increases effectiveness up to 99.9%
- some types are not effective until 10–15 minutes after placing in vagina; follow instructions
- only effective for about one hour when used alone
- additional application is needed for each act of intercourse

Does It Reduce the Risk for HIV/AIDS and STDs?

- somewhat reduced risk for some STDs
- uncertain action against HIV/AIDS
- using a male, latex condom reduces the risk

What Are Its Main Advantages?

- reversible
- no prescription needed
- available at most drugstores

What Are Some Possible Problems?

- may cause irritation or discomfort
- increased risk of vaginal and urinary tract infections
- some individuals are allergic to spermicides
- proper use may interrupt "sexual mood"
- may leak and feel messy

Female Sterilization

(tubal ligation)

What Is It?

- surgical procedure to block the fallopian tubes

How Does It Work?

- egg and sperm cannot meet
- fertilization does not occur

How Is It Used?

- local or general anesthesia is used
- a surgical procedure is performed in which the tubes are cut, clipped, or blocked
- the method is permanent

How Well Does It Work?

- typical use: 99.5%

- perfect use: 99.5%
- failure rate may be increased with some methods of tubal ligation

Does It Reduce the Risk for HIV/AIDS and STDs?

- does not reduce risk for HIV/AIDS or STDs
- using a male, latex condom reduces the risk
- reduces risk of ovarian cancer

What Are Its Main Advantages?

- permanent
- safe medical procedure (although male sterilization is easier and safer)
- does not interfere with sex
- nothing to remember

What Are Some Possible Problems?

- may require a 30-day waiting period; may have minimum age requirement
- risks of surgery, including: reaction to anesthetic, infection, and bleeding
- temporary pain at surgical site
- some individuals later regret decision
- if pregnancy occurs, risk of ectopic (tubal) pregnancy is high; any symptoms of pregnancy should be reported to health care provider immediately and evaluated
- reversal requires surgery, is very expensive, and may not be successful

Male Sterilization

(vasectomy)

What Is It?

- surgical procedure to block the vas deferens (male sperm tube)

How Does It Work?

- egg and sperm cannot meet

- fertilization does not occur

How Is It Used?

- a surgical procedure is performed in which the vas deferens are cut or blocked
- operation is performed under local anesthesia
- the method is permanent

How Well Does It Work?

- typical use: 99.8%
- perfect use: 99.9%
- vasectomy is not effective until sperm is cleared from the male system (takes about 15 ejaculations or 6 weeks)

Does It Reduce the Risk for HIV/AIDS and STDs?

- does not reduce risk for HIV/AIDS or STDs
- using a male, latex condom reduces the risk

What Are Its Main Advantages?

- permanent
- safe medical procedure
- easier and safer than female sterilization
- does not interfere with sex
- nothing to remember

What Are Some Possible Problems?

- risks of surgery, including: reaction to anesthetic, bleeding, and infection
- temporary bruising, swelling, tenderness of the scrotum
- some individuals later regret decision
- reversal requires surgery, is very expensive, and may not be successful

Chapter 14

Contraception at 20, 30, 40

—by Nancy Monson

The average woman is capable of bearing children for 36 years. Yet for 27 of those years, most women are actively trying to prevent pregnancy. Here's the latest on everything from the Pill to the female condom—and what works best when.

No one method of birth control can satisfy all women all the time—or even one woman in all her life stages. As she ages and her needs shift, every woman should reassess her method of contraception and consider these six factors:

- Her desire for children in the near or distant future;

- Her sexual behavior, which can put her at risk of unintended pregnancy and sexually transmitted diseases (STDs);

- Her personal—and family—health history, which may make some methods of birth control, such as the Pill, unsafe for her;

- Her habits, such as smoking;

- Her tolerance for certain side effects (say, the bleeding irregularities that accompany Norplant® use);

- Her (and her partner's) willingness and ability to use a particular method consistently and correctly.

The last issue is critical. "The effectiveness of some methods, like barrier contraceptives, are highly dependent on whether they are used consistently and correctly," says Herbert Peterson, M.D., chief of the Women' s Health and Fertility Branch at the Centers for Disease Control and Prevention in Atlanta. "Other methods like the intrauterine device, are less dependent on the user for effectiveness. In choosing a method of contraception, each woman will want to consider the extent to which she will actively participate in determining the method's effectiveness."

With birth control options expanding—three new methods have been approved by the Food and Drug Administration since 1990—a woman's chances of finding a workable method, no matter what her age, are better than ever.

Contraception in Your 20s

Many women in their twenties have a dual goal: to delay childbearing and to preserve fertility. Sexual encounters may be spontaneous and frequent: women 25 to 29 years old have typically had five male sexual partners, according to *Contraceptive Technology*, a comprehensive birth control manual. These behaviors put women at risk not only of pregnancy, but of acquiring STDs, which can compromise fertility. There are roughly 12 million cases of STDs each year, two-thirds of them in women and men under 25.

Among women 20 to 29, birth rates peak; today, half of all women who have had children started by age 26. Those who finish their families in their twenties often turn to sterilization, the second most popular contraceptive choice of this age group. There is no question, however, that half of all pregnancies in the twenties are unplanned or linked to failed contraceptives, according to the Alan Guttmacher Institute in New York City.

The Pill is the number-one contraceptive choice of women in their twenties. It is reliable, easy to use, and reversible, plus it allows for spur-of-the-moment encounters. It also offers a wealth of noncontraceptive health benefits, such as prevention of tubal pregnancy and pelvic inflammatory disease (PID), and long-term protection against uterine and ovarian cancer. But the Pill doesn't prevent STDs and may increase the risk of breast cancer in a small number of users.

And not every woman is a successful Pill taker. In a 1993 survey sponsored by the Upjohn Company (makers of Depo-Provera®) of 4,000 women aged 18 to 50, one of four Pill users forgot to take one or more of her pills during a three-month period. Inconsistent Pill use reduces pregnancy protection from almost 100 to 92 percent or lower. To be most effective oral contraceptives must be taken every day at the same time of day.

Women who are not good Pill takers or who wish to avoid dealing with their contraception on a daily basis can now opt for either of two virtually failsafe hormonal methods. Both Norplant, a five-year implantable contraceptive, and Depo-Provera, a three-month injectable, relieve women of the everyday responsibility of the Pill, though neither of these methods provides protection from STDs.

Of the nearly one million women who've chosen Norplant as their contraceptive, most are 18 to 29 years old and have already had at least one child. No statistical data are yet available regarding Depo-Provera, but it seems to appeal to a wide age range of women, including those in their twenties. Both methods, which rely on artificial progesterones, are convenient and dependable and Depo-Provera—unlike the Pill—doesn't cause nausea.

Like oral contraceptives, Depo-Provera helps protect against PID and uterine cancer. In theory, Norplant, which contains the same progestin found in many Pill formulations, should offer similar noncontraceptive advantages although that hasn't been proven in clinical trials. However, both Norplant and Depo-Provera can cause menstrual changes during the first year of use. Other side effects such as weight gain and breast tenderness have also been reported for both methods.

Though roughly 20 percent of women in their twenties use condoms, diaphragms, spermicides, or contraceptive sponges, these coitus-linked methods may not be ideal contraceptive choices for young women. That's because their degree of pregnancy protection depends on how carefully they're used. For a woman using a barrier method, the chance of getting pregnant over the course of a year ranges from 6 percent to 36 percent; if in the heat of passion you forget to use the barrier or insert it carelessly you'll be at the high end. Careless use also means you'll miss out on the protection afforded by barrier methods. Latex condoms, in particular, provide the best protection against STDs, including HIV, the virus that causes AIDS. For these reasons, doctors are now applauding a new "belt and suspenders" approach: using the condom and the Pill together.

In early studies of the newest prophylactic, the Reality female condom, women reportedly found it easy to use and were pleased that they could insert it long before intercourse. They also said it was softer than the male condom, transmitted heat, and felt good.

The least popular birth control method among women in their twenties is the intrauterine device, or IUD: Those under age 30 comprise roughly 10 percent of all IUD users. Some women in their twenties don't fit the profile of the ideal IUD user: a woman who is in a mutually monogamous long-term relationship and has had at least one child. In childless women the device may be expelled or it may cause PID, which can lead to infertility in a small number of women. The risk of an IUD causing PID is highest in women who are exposed to STDs, which is why the method isn't recommended for women with multiple partners. In general, women under age 24 and those who haven't had children are more vulnerable to infection than older women are.

One vitally important emergency option for women in their twenties is the morning-after, or postcoital, pill, which can prevent pregnancy after unprotected sex or a contraceptive mishap. Many doctors are unaware of the morning-after pill, never having learned about it during medical training. If your doctor is one of them, contact your local Planned Parenthood office. You can also request a prescription for postcoital pills in advance, in case of an emergency. You may experience nausea and vomiting when you take the pills, and your next period may begin later or earlier than usual; if you don't get your period within three weeks, see your doctor.

Contraception in Your 30s

At age 30, half of all U.S. women do not intend to have any more children. For this reason sterilization is the number-one contraceptive choice of women in their thirties. Women who choose sterilization usually have tubal ligations, which, unlike many reversible contraceptive methods, are covered by most health insurance plans. (Vasectomy is just as effective, safer, simpler, less invasive, easier to recover from, and less costly.)

But sterilization is a surgical procedure with attendant risks; in addition there is always the chance that a woman might regret her decision. A divorce, death of a partner, remarriage, or simply advancing age may spark a renewed desire for a child. Medical experts say that the younger a woman is at the time she is sterilized, the more likely she is to regret it later on, whether she's had children or not.

For many women who have delayed marriage and pregnancy, the thirties are an active childbearing time. Still, roughly half of the pregnancies in over-30 women are accidental, reports the Alan Guttmacher Institute. For women in their thirties who wish to prevent unplanned pregnancies—or to space out the birth of children that are planned—the Pill is an excellent choice, because it provides trustworthy contraception with little hassle and offers many health benefits.

Approximately 11 percent of women in their thirties use the condom for contraception, 7 to 8 percent choose the diaphragm, and 3 to 4 percent use spermicides. For women who aren't in long-term, mutually monogamous relationships, condoms offer STD protection; for all women the barrier methods are easy to use, relatively inexpensive, and contain no hormones, which some women can't tolerate physically. (Nausea, headaches, depression, high blood pressure, and breast tenderness are a few of the side effects that may accompany hormone use.)

Along with the Pill, barriers, and the one-year Progestasert IUD are excellent choices if your goal is to space out your children's births. Longer-term methods aren't the most cost-effective way to postpone children; if they're removed early, you won't get the full value of Norplant or the ParaGard Copper T 380A IUD, and if you use Depo-Provera, your fertility may not return for up to one year after the shots are discontinued. Since fertility starts to decline naturally after 30, this Depo-delay could mean the difference between having a child or not.

The long-term methods may be attractive to women who are breastfeeding, particularly if they've just had their last child: The IUD, Norplant, and Depo-Provera are considered safer than the Pill for nursing women and their babies because they don't contain estrogen, which may alter the composition of breast milk. The Pill also decreases milk flow; Depo-Provera may increase it. Norplant, Depo-Provera, and the ParaGard IUD are also attractive to women who are finished with childbearing but don't want to be sterilized. IUD use peaks among women in their thirties and forties, and those who have chosen IUDs are highly satisfied with them, according to a survey of nearly 8,000 women conducted by the Ortho Pharmaceutical Corporation in 1991.

IUDs are considered safe if they are used by appropriate candidates. According to World Health Organization data of 23,000 IUD insertions worldwide, the overall chance of pelvic infection with IUD use is only 0.4 percent. The risk of infection is greatest in the first 20 days after the device is inserted—a risk that can be countered by ensuring that the patient doesn't have an STD at the time of insertion and, to a certain degree, by taking antibiotics.

Contraception in Your 40s

Ironically, unintended pregnancy is as big a problem after age 40 as it is among teenagers: Although the number of pregnancies drops dramatically to nine per 1,000 women, a whopping eight in ten pregnancies in women over age 40 are unplanned. Most of these end in abortion or miscarriage. But doctors say that if the morning-after pill—which is safe for most women over 40—were more widely used, emergency contraception could reduce the number of unintended pregnancies in the United States by 1.7 million and the number of abortions by 800,000.

Another morning-after contraceptive is in the offing: in the mid-1990s the University of California at San Francisco announced it would study RU-486, the so-called abortion pill, as a morning-after contraceptive. The aim of the study is to determine the optimal dose for pregnancy prevention.

Of course, some women in their forties are bearing children. But for most women in this age group, preserving fertility isn't a major concern: They are finished with reproduction and ready to be done with menstruation and pregnancy risks. About 7 percent of women between 40 and 44 opt for sterilization as their method of birth control. Aside from the convenience, this may be because they feel they have few viable alternatives—for example, they may have a medical disorder that makes using some hormonal methods inadvisable, such as elevated cholesterol levels.

Among those who do not choose sterilization, barrier methods rank high: Fifteen percent of women 40 to 44 use condoms, the diaphragm, or spermicides. A woman over 40, who is naturally less fertile and typically less sexually active than a younger woman, is less likely to get pregnant if a condom breaks or she forgets to put spermicide in with her diaphragm than a woman in her twenties.

Condoms are especially handy for women over 40 who are in a solo phase of life—whether as the result of divorce, widowhood, or of never having married—because they offer protection against both pregnancy and STDs. Previously married women need to be particularly careful, as studies show that they tend to have more sexual partners than never-married women, and they also have the highest rate of unintended pregnancies.

Though the *1988 National Survey of Family Growth* indicates that the Pill is used by only 3 percent of women in their forties, it's likely that statistics haven't yet caught up with actual Pill use in the 1990s.

In the past, when estrogen doses of the Pill were higher, women were told to stop taking it at age 35 because oral contraceptives were believed to be potentially dangerous to their health. Today, healthy women who don't smoke can use low-dose oral contraceptives until menopause. And many are: According to the most recent Ortho Pharmaceutical Corporation survey, 9 percent of women between the ages of 40 and 44 who use contraceptives take the Pill. Yet the survey also found that only 35 percent of reproductive-age women in their thirties are aware that birth control pills are an option for them.

Besides its contraceptive value, using the Pill throughout the forties can make the transition to menopause easier for women. Pill use can regulate periods and prevent hot flashes, and appears to protect against bone loss. As a woman nears the age of 50, doctors may perform blood tests to determine if hormone levels are changing—a sign of impending menopause—and switch her to hormone replacement therapy, an even lower-dose regimen than oral contraception.

Because chronic medical conditions tend to develop with age, a woman in her forties who has diabetes, for instance, and any woman who smokes, will be advised not to take the Pill. On a case-by-case basis, however, many doctors may be willing to prescribe a progestin-only method (Norplant, Depo-Provera, the Progestasert IUD, or the mini-pill) for women with medical disorders that would be made worse by the estrogen component of birth control pills. Even women who smoke cigarettes may be able to use these contraceptives.

Like the Pill, the long-term progestin-only methods may prevent hot flashes as menopause nears—Depo-Provera definitely does, Norplant may. But these methods may be more trouble than they're worth. Norplant and Depo-Provera can both cause irregular bleeding. In a 20-year-old, that kind of bleeding is almost certainly due to the contraceptive, but in a 40-year-old, any irregular vaginal bleeding should be evaluated for uterine cancer. In addition, removal of the six Norplant tubes has reportedly caused problems for some women. In the mid-1990s a class action lawsuit was brought by 400 women against the manufacturer, Wyeth-Ayerst Laboratories, claiming that Norplant removal caused severe pain and scarring. On the plus side, Depo-Provera, and sometimes Norplant, can bring a halt to menstrual periods during use, which can be a welcome side effect if a woman knows she isn't pregnant.

As life options have expanded for women in terms of when and if to have children, so too have birth control options. Women can now protect themselves against unplanned pregnancies and prevent STDs.

In the future, more contraceptives and different delivery systems—
hormone-releasing vaginal rings, fewer implantable rods for Norplant,
and others—should enable them to worry less and enjoy their sexuality more.

Nancy Monson is a freelance writer living in Pomona, N.Y. Medical experts consulted for this piece include Jacqueline Darroch Forrest, Ph.D., vice president for research at the Alan Guttmacher Institute; Andrew Kaunitz, M.D., professor of obstetrics and gynecology at the University of Florida Health Science Center in Jacksonville; Herbert Peterson, M.D., chief of the Women's Health and Fertility Branch at the Centers for Disease Control and Prevention; and Felicia Stewart, M.D., coauthor of the birth control manual "Contraceptive Technology."

Chapter 15

Over-the-Counter Birth Control Made Easy

—by Lynne Vickery

Many women choose different birth control methods at different times in their lives. This chapter offers a review of some of the over-the-counter methods of birth control. Since they are relatively inexpensive and easy to obtain, over-the-counter methods offer a unique way to experiment.

There are two varieties of non-prescription methods, barrier and spermicidal. A barrier method blocks sperm from getting into the opening of the cervix (the part of the uterus that extends into the vagina). A spermicide kills sperm which if left on their own, try to get through the uterus and to an egg. When just one sperm penetrates the egg, the egg is fertilized and the pregnancy process begins. The most effective over-the-counter (OTC) birth control does both; it blocks *and* kills sperm.

Some methods of birth control have the added advantage of protecting against sexually transmitted diseases, including HIV/AIDS. The very best way to try to prevent pregnancy and protect against disease is a combination of barrier method and a spermicide.

You can try the various methods and see what works best for you. Birth control works most effectively when the users are comfortable with the method and use it regularly.

One way to make sex more enjoyable is to incorporate birth control and safer sex supplies into your sex play. So, read on, then, grab a friend and go play in the pharmacy!

Spermicides

Spermicides come in lots of different forms: *jellies, creams, film, suppositories, and foam*. Consistent and correct use is the key to using them effectively.

- **Vaginal Contraceptive Film (VCF) and suppositories** are dry but melt when inserted into the vagina at least 20 minutes prior to intercourse. They then become creamy or gel-like and create a chemical barrier over the cervix. Some people have problems with suppositories (shaped like small eggs or capsules) not melting. Film melts easily and doesn't cause the "drippy" feeling of some spermicides, but it may be more difficult to insert properly over the cervix.

- **Creams and jellies** were originally manufactured for use with diaphragms and cervical caps. They can be used in several ways. They can be inserted into the vagina with an applicator similar to a tampon applicator except it's washed and reused. Creams and jellies can also be put on the inside of an unrolled condom or on the outside of a condom once it is rolled onto the penis, or both. Some men have said the wetness inside the condom enhances their pleasure, and the extra lubrication on the outside of the condom can be enjoyable for the woman as well. Some jellies or creams taste bitter or have a strong smell so oral sex may not be as enjoyable after you've applied the spermicide.

- **Foam** has a consistency like shaving cream and is also inserted into the vagina with an applicator. Foam is odorless, but bitter tasting. Complaints of "drippy-ness" after sex with foam are more common than with other methods.

With all of these spermicides, it is important to insert more each time you have intercourse if it's been longer than a half-hour from the time you originally inserted the spermicide until you have intercourse.

Some manufacturers sell single-use applicators of foam, cream, or jelly which can be handy for traveling or dates. If you are buying spermicide for home use, it's probably less expensive to purchase the bigger containers and the applicators that are reusable.

Today Contraceptive Sponge

[*Note: The Today Sponge has been removed from the market and cannot currently be found in stores in the USA. Allendale Pharmaceuticals hopes to have it back on store shelves in 2001.*]

The Today Sponge is a polyurethane sponge containing nonoxynol-9. Inserted to cover the cervix, it acts as both a spermicide, killing sperm continuously over as much as a 24-hour period, and as a kind of barrier; sperm have to pass through the spermicide-soaked sponge to enter the cervix.

Because the Sponge contains such a large amount of spermicide, it is not necessary to apply more each time you have intercourse. Some women have reported that the quantity of spermicide causes vaginal irritation. The Sponge should be left in for 6–8 hours after the last time you have sex—an uncomfortable length of time for women who have experienced severe irritation. Another complaint is difficulty removing the Sponge. It has a cloth loop but sometimes the Sponge turns over inside the vagina and the loop is hard to reach. Some women say the Sponge feels so much like vaginal tissue that it's hard to get a hold of it.

The difficulty with reaching and distinguishing the Sponge probably plays a part in its lower effectiveness among users because it cannot be consistently placed over the cervix. It is not a barrier but only a spermicide if it does not block the entrance to the uterus. Women who use cervical caps or diaphragms, which are prescription female barrier methods, report similar problems with placement. A proper cervical cap or diaphragm fitting includes instruction and practice of placement. Cap and diaphragm users probably will have less difficulty placing a Sponge properly. Some women use the Sponge in combination with a condom, which greatly increases effectiveness.

Condoms for Women

The "female condom" is a relatively new option for women. Unfortunately, they may be hard to find on store shelves. As the consumer demand increases, female condoms will become more accessible.

The female condom is a plastic pouch, longer than a traditional condom, with two polymethane rings, one on each end. The smaller ring fits inside the vagina and rests against the cervix; the other stays outside the vagina and holds the mouth of the condom open. It keeps the condom from being pushed inside the vagina. Like other condoms, it is meant to used once and thrown away.

Lubrication seems to be the key to successful use. They come with a small amount inside, and a small bottle of (non-spermicidal) lubricant to add later if desired. It is necessary that the condom be well lubricated inside so the penis may slip in and out without pulling the condom out of the vagina. During intercourse, make sure the penis goes inside, not beside, the condom. Adding another of the spermicides discussed in this chapter will increase the female condom's effectiveness.

The female condom offers some features otherwise unavailable. Since it is made from polyurethane, it is an alternative for latex-sensitive folks. Polyurethane, unlike latex, conducts heat. It will warm up quickly against human skin and stay warm longer than rubber. It does prevent the transmission of HIV and other sexually transmitted diseases and offers another alternative for safer sex.

Condoms for Men

Male condoms are probably the easiest method of birth control to find. In addition to pharmacies, grocery and convenience stores, they can also be found in vending machines in laundromats, bathrooms (usually in the men's room), gas stations, and sometimes rest stops. Although convenient, it is not wise to buy condoms stored in hot laundromat bathroom vending machines or infrequently used rest stops, since heat breaks down latex rubber and spermicides will expire over time. Also, do not store condoms in hot places, including cars in the sun. The stock in grocery and drug stores turns over fast enough to provide the freshest condoms. Check the expiration date on both the outside package and condom wrapper. Don't rely upon one that has expired.

Condoms range in price, but are generally inexpensive. They usually come in packages of three, six, or twelve. Clinics have them for less than retail stores and can usually sell them individually. Lots of safer-sex programs have them on display in stores, bars, and schools for a small donation. Many education and disease prevention programs give them away for free.

Condoms are made from either animal membranes (called "natural skin" condoms) or latex rubber. Natural skin condoms prevent pregnancy as well as latex condoms but **do not** provide the same protection from sexually transmitted diseases (STDs), including HIV/AIDS. The membrane (usually from the intestines of goats or lambs) is porous and while these pores are too small to let sperm through, viruses, such as herpes and HIV, can pass through these microscopic openings.

Latex condoms come with spermicidal lubrication, non-spermicidal lubrication, or without any lubrication. Most condoms that are spermicidally lubricated use nonoxynol-9, an agent shown to kill HIV in a laboratory setting. Many people use these condoms to prevent STD transmission but an additional spermicide should be used if condoms are your only method of birth control. If a condom breaks, the small amount of spermicide provided by the manufacturer is not enough to prevent pregnancy. Condoms with spermicide can often have a strong smell and usually taste bitter.

Non-spermicidally lubricated condoms usually say "lubricated" or "sensitive" on the package. Read it carefully to tell the difference between spermicidally lubricated and plain lubricated condoms. Now that most people know about HIV/AIDS, manufacturers emphasize their nonoxynol-9 content. Condoms without spermicide may be a good option for women who use a separate spermicide, or are using the Pill or diaphragm.

Non-lubricated condoms have a light dusting of powder in them to keep the rubber from sticking to itself in the package. They don't have much of a smell or taste. To help prevent STD transmission during oral sex, place some spermicide on the inside of a non-lubricated condom. Non-lubed condoms are good for folks who want to add their own or who use them for oral sex.

Condoms come in a variety of shapes, sizes, and colors. While most condoms are one-size-fits-all, there are large and small sizes. Condoms also come in contoured (shaped like a circumcised penis), reservoir, or plain-end. Reservoir-tipped condoms have a small nipple at the end, designed to catch the sperm.

Some people think condoms break easily; but in fact, they are very strong when properly lubricated. Sufficient lubrication is the key to preventing most breakage. To increase lubrication, add K-Y jelly, any water-based lubricant, or spermicide. Do not use Vaseline or other oil-based lubricants as they will cause breakdown of the condom fabric.

Instructions

Spermicides

- Read the package carefully
- Wash and dry your hands well
- Add more spermicide for each act of intercourse (except with the Sponge)

Foam

Shake the can very well. Place the applicator on the top of the can and press down or to the side, depending on the package directions. The plunger will rise as the applicator fills. Insert the applicator about two or three inches into your vagina and press the plunger to deposit the foam over your cervix. As you withdraw the applicator, be sure not to pull back on the plunger as this will suck some foam back into the applicator. Insert the quantity recommended on the package.

Suppositories

Insert a suppository into your vagina and up to your cervix. Wait at least 20 minutes before having intercourse.

Vaginal Contraceptive Film (VCF)

Open the foil wrapper and fold one VCF square in half. Fold it in half again, over your finger. Insert your finger into your vagina and deposit the VCF over your cervix. Your finger must very dry to start with and you must insert it quickly, otherwise the VCF will stick to your finger and come back out when you remove your finger.

Creams and Jellies

Place a small amount inside an unrolled condom or, after the condom is on, rub it over the outside. Or, you can insert cream or jelly into the vagina using an applicator similar to a foam applicator. Creams are opaque and jellies are clear; otherwise, there is little difference between them. Use them the same way.

The Contraceptive Sponge

First, locate your cervix by inserting your finger into your vagina. The cervix feels firmer than your vaginal walls and you may feel the os, the opening to your cervix, as a little dimple. Run warm water over the sponge to wet it. Squeeze it to create suds, but do not rinse these suds out. That is the spermicide. Fold the Sponge in half and insert it into your vagina, dimple up toward your cervix. You may want to squat, sit on a toilet, or raise one leg on a chair. Press the sponge to make sure it is up against your cervix. Leave it in for at least six hours after the last act of intercourse, but no more than 25 hours total. Once removed, throw in the trash. Don't flush; it will clog the pipes.

Barrier Methods

- always read the package insert first
- check the expiration date if it has one
- do not use it if the package has been tampered with

The Female Condom

Carefully peel open the condom package. Stand with one leg on a chair or the toilet. Hold the condom with the open end down and squeeze the inner ring between your thumb and middle finger. Use your index finger to hold the condom steady. While still squeezing the ring, insert the inner ring into your vagina. You may need to add some extra lubrication before you insert it (the manufacturer provides you with some). Push the inner ring high into the vagina and over your cervix. Use your index finger to push the ring past the pubic bone (which you can feel by curving your finger once it is two inches or so inside your vagina). The outer ring stays outside and rests open against your outer vaginal lips. During intercourse, guide the penis into the pouch. You can add lubricant inside or outside the pouch to make it more comfortable.

After sex, do not stand up with the condom in. This may leak sperm into your vagina. While lying down, twist the outer ring to close off the semen inside and pull it out gently. Tie a knot in it and throw in the trash (not the toilet). Use a new condom for each intercourse. For increased pregnancy protection, you can insert extra spermicidal cream, jelly, or foam into the vagina after removing the condom.

The Male Condom

Check the wrapper first; it should have a pocket of air before you open it. After opening the wrapper, do not unroll it until you're ready to place it on the penis. If you want to add spermicidal cream or jelly, place a small amount in the tip of the condom. Twist a half-inch of the tip so that there is a small section of airless space. Hold the twisted part with one hand and roll the condom down the shaft of the penis with the other. With an uncircumcised penis, you must pull back the foreskin before placing the condom on the penis. Once unrolled, check the condom and smooth out any air bubbles.

After ejaculation, hold onto the base of the condom to prevent spilling semen during withdrawal from the vagina. Remove the condom by "milking" it off the penis, tie it in a knot and throw in the garbage. Wash the penis with warm soapy water to remove any semen. Condoms are meant to be used only once.

Over-the-Counter Birth Control Methods Reference Table

Non-prescription birth control methods are listed below. Prices in the following chart were researched by Syrenka in June, 1996.

Method	Price	Effectiveness*
sponge	N/A**	72–82%
foam	$8 per can (about 20 uses)	75–90%
suppository	$7–9 for 10 capsules	75–90%
vaginal contraceptive film	$8 for 12 films	75–90%
jelly/cream	$8–10 per tube	75–90%
female condom	3 for $8	75–87%
male condom—latex	6 for $7–10	90%
male condom with foam	see above	99+%
male condom—natural skin	12 for $25	90%

*Effectiveness rates vary enormously. By combining two or more methods, birth control effectiveness increases greatly. The primary factors affecting effectiveness are correct and consistent usage. Other factors include age, number of previous childbirths, and frequency of sex.

**temporarily removed from market

Prices based on survey of Fred Meyer, Bartell's, and Planned Parenthood in the Seattle area June of 1996.

This information was originally researched and prepared by Lynne Vickery, who was a healthworker and birth control counselor at Cedar River Clinic from 1992 to 1996. Lynne has Bachelor Degrees in Human Sexuality and Counseling and Women's Studies from the University of Massachusetts at Amherst.

Chapter 16

Methods of Contraception for Women 15–44 Years of Age, According to Race and Age: United States, 1982, 1988, and 1995

Centers for Disease Control and Prevention, National Center for Health Statistics, Division of Vital Statistics, 1998. Data from the *National Survey of Family Growth*, 1995.

Methods of contraception for women 15–44 years of age, according to race and age: United States, 1982, 1988, 1995

Method of contraception and age	All Races			White			Black		
	1982	1988	1995	1982	1988	1995	1982	1988	1995
Number of women in thousands									
15–44 years	54,099	57,900	60,201	45,367	47,076	47,981	6,985	7,679	8,460
15–19 years	9,521	9,179	8,961	7,815	7,313	6,838	1,416	1,409	1,454
20–24 years	10,629	9,413	9,041	8,855	7,401	7,015	1,472	1,364	1,386
25–34 years	19,644	21,726	20,758	16,485	17,682	16,609	2,479	2,865	2,861
35–44 years	14,305	17,582	21,440	12,212	14,681	17,516	1,618	2,041	2,758
All methods									
Percent of women using contraception									
15–44 years	55.7	60.3	64.2	56.7	61.8	65.5	52.0	56.7	61.5
15–19 years	24.2	32.1	29.8	23.4	32.2	30.0	30.0	35.1	34.5
20–24 years	55.8	59.0	63.5	56.6	60.2	63.3	52.5	61.1	66.9
25–34 years	66.7	66.3	71.1	67.7	67.7	72.6	64.0	63.8	66.4
35–44 years	61.6	68.3	72.3	63.1	70.2	73.4	52.3	58.9	68.0
Female sterilization									
Percent of women using contraception									
15–44 years	23.2	27.5	27.7	22.1	26.1	25.7	30.0	38.1	39.9
15–19 years	–	*1.5	*0.3	–	*1.6	–	–	*1.6	–
20–24 years	4.5	4.6	4.0	*3.8	3.9	3.5	9.8	9.1	7.2
25–34 years	22.1	25.0	23.8	20.2	23.2	21.3	33.5	39.9	40.3
35–44 years	43.5	47.6	45.0	41.9	44.7	41.7	56.8	70.5	66.3

Method of contraception and age	All Races			White			Black		
	1982	1988	1995	1982	1988	1995	1982	1988	1995
Male sterilization									
15–44 years	10.9	11.7	10.9	12.2	13.6	12.7	*1.4	*0.9	1.7
15–19 years	*0.4	*0.2	—	*0.5	*0.3	—	—	—	—
20–24 years	*3.6	*1.8	*1.1	*4.2	*2.3	*1.3	*0.5	—	0.2
25–34 years	10.1	10.2	7.8	11.3	11.7	8.9	*1.4	*1.1	*1.5
35–44 years	19.9	20.8	19.4	21.6	23.7	22.1	*3.1	*1.5	3.1
Birth control pill									
15–44 years	28.0	30.7	26.9	26.7	29.8	28.0	38.0	38.0	23.8
15–19 years	63.9	58.8	43.8	62.1	55.9	47.5	70.8	74.2	33.2
20–24 years	55.1	68.2	52.1	53.5	67.9	55.4	65.0	70.3	41.5
25–34 years	25.7	32.6	33.3	24.8	32.4	35.0	33.7	35.7	23.6
35–44 years	3.7	4.3	8.7	3.7	4.5	8.9	*5.1	*4.2	9.6
Intrauterine device									
15–44 years	7.1	2.0	0.8	6.9	1.8	0.8	9.1	3.1	*0.8
15–19 years	*1.3	—	—	*0.5	—	—	*4.9	—	—
20–24 years	4.2	*0.3	*0.3	*3.5	*0.3	*0.4	6.2	*0.9	*0.2
25–34 years	9.7	2.1	0.8	9.4	1.7	0.7	13.0	*4.1	*1.5
35–44 years	6.9	3.1	1.1	7.0	3.0	1.2	*6.5	*4.3	*0.6

Method of contraception and age	All Races			White			Black		
	1982	1988	1995	1982	1988	1995	1982	1988	1995
Diaphragm									
15–44 years	8.1	5.7	1.9	8.8	6.2	2.1	3.5	1.9	*0.8
15–19 years	*6.0	*1.0	*0.1	*7.1	*1.3	*0.2	*1.8	–	–
20–24 years	10.2	3.7	*0.6	11.3	4.1	*0.6	*2.8	*1.6	*0.7
25–34 years	10.3	7.3	1.7	11.3	8.0	1.8	*3.0	*1.7	*1.0
35–44 years	4.0	6.0	2.8	3.8	6.2	3.2	*6.0	*3.3	*0.9
Condom									
15–44 years	12.0	14.6	20.4	12.7	14.9	19.7	6.2	10.3	20.5
15–19 years	20.8	32.8	36.7	22.6	34.2	36.8	*12.6	22.7	37.8
20–24 years	10.7	14.5	26.4	11.4	15.8	23.8	*6.4	9.6	33.8
25–34 years	11.4	16.7	21.1	12.0	14.0	20.6	5.3	9.4	17.7
35–44 years	11.3	11.2	14.7	12.0	11.3	14.6	*4.5	7.0	12.2

(Data are based on household interviews of women in the childbearing ages)

– Quantity zero.
*Relative standard error greater than 30 percent

Notes: Method of contraception used in the month of interview. If multiple methods were reported, only the most effective method is shown in the table.

Chapter 17

Facts in Brief: Contraceptive Use

Who Needs Contraception?

- 60 million U.S. women are in their childbearing years (15–44).

- 15% of these women are aged 15–19, 15% are 20–24, 34% are 25–34, and 36% are 35–44.

- 30 million are married (49%), 23 million have never been married (38%), and 8 million (13%) are separated, divorced, or widowed.

- 1 in 6 of these women have a household income below 150% of the federal poverty level. (In 1995, the poverty level was $15,569 for a family of four.)

- 42 million, or 7 in 10 women of reproductive age, are sexually active and do not want to become pregnant, but could do so if they or their partner fail to use a contraceptive method.

- A woman who wants only two children will need to practice contraception for at least 20 years of her life.

- Nevertheless, health insurance coverage for contraceptive services lags far behind coverage for obstetric care, abortion, and sterilization, which are included in most health care plans.

Who Uses Contraceptives?

- Overall, 64% of the more than 60 million women aged 15–44 practice contraception.

- 31% of these 60 million women do not need a method because they are sterile for noncontraceptive reasons; are pregnant, postpartum, or trying to become pregnant; have never had intercourse; or are not sexually active.

- Thus, only 5% of women aged 15–44 in need of contraception are not using a method.

- When only fertile, sexually active women who do not want to become pregnant (39 million) are considered, 9 in 10 are practicing contraception.

Who Has Unintended Pregnancies?

- More than 3 million unintended pregnancies occur every year in the United States.

- The 3 million women who use no contraceptives account for almost half of these pregnancies (47%), while the 39 million method users account for 53%.

- The majority of unintended pregnancies among contraceptive users result from inconsistent or incorrect use.

Who Uses Which Methods?

- 61% of reproductive-age women who practice contraception use reversible methods such as oral contraceptives or condoms. The remaining women rely on female or male sterilization (28% and 11%, respectively).

- Female sterilization, the pill, and the condom are the most widely used methods in the three major racial and ethnic groups. However, black women and Hispanic women are most likely to rely on female sterilization, while white women are most likely to use the pill.

- Female sterilization is most commonly relied on by women who are older than 34, are previously married, have less than a high school education, or have a household income below 150% of the federal poverty level.

- 50% of all women aged 40–44 who practice contraception have been sterilized and another 20% have a partner who has had a vasectomy.

- Of the 2.7 million teenage women who use contraceptives, 44%—more than 1 million women—rely on the pill.

- The pill is the method most widely used by women in their 20s.

- The women most likely to use the pill have never been married and have at least some college education.

- More than one-third (37%) of teenage women using contraceptives choose condoms as their primary method. Condom use declines as women grow older and marry.

- Of the 9.8 million women using barrier contraceptives such as the male condom, the female condom, and the diaphragm, one-third report not using their method every time they have intercourse.

Chart A

Almost half of the 6.3 million pregnancies in the United States each year are unintended.

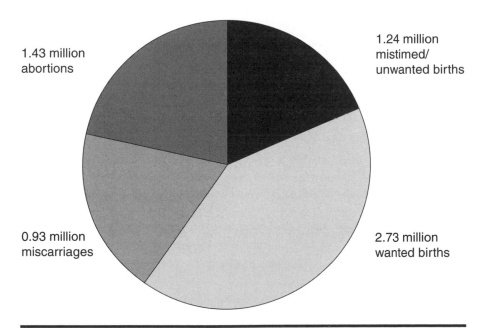

1.43 million abortions

1.24 million mistimed/ unwanted births

0.93 million miscarriages

2.73 million wanted births

- Fewer than 1% of contraceptive users say their primary method is the female condom.

- In 1995, the first year national data were collected on the injectable and the implant, women younger than 24 were the age-group most likely to rely on those methods. Among women aged 15–17, for example, 15% were using the injectable and 4% were relying on the implant.

- Women with a household income below 150% of the federal poverty level are almost twice as likely to use the injectable as those with a higher income, and about three times as likely to use the implant.

Chart B

Unintended pregnancies among women who do not use a method are almost as likely to end in abortion as in birth.

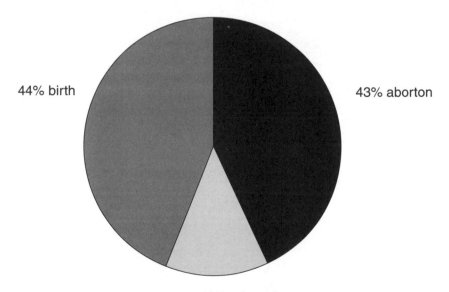

44% birth

43% aborton

13% miscarriage

Has Contraceptive Use Changed?

- The proportion of women aged 15–44 practicing contraception rose from 56% in 1982 to 64% in 1995.

- 76% of women used a contraceptive at first intercourse in the 1990s, compared with 50% before 1980.

- The percentage of women who are sexually active but not using a method declined by 30% between 1982 and 1995.

- The percentage of nonusers among sexually active women declined by 49% among blacks, by 34% among Hispanics, and by 19% among whites during that period.

- In 1988, women aged 22–44 who had a household income below 150% of the federal poverty level were 12% less likely to use a contraceptive method than were those with a higher income (60% vs. 67%); in 1995, 71% of both groups were using a method.

- Contraceptive use among women aged 22–44 who had less than a high school education rose from 60% in 1988 to 73% in 1995, more than equaling prevalence among women with more education (70–72%).

- The proportion of female contraceptive users relying on condoms increased between 1988 and 1995—from 15% to 20% among all women, from 20% to 30% among never-married women, and from 33% to 37% among adolescents.

- During the same period, the proportion of use accounted for by the pill declined slightly, from 31% to 27%.

- 28% of contraceptive users relied on female sterilization in both 1988 and 1995.

- Use of the diaphragm declined (from 6% of all users in 1988 to 2% in 1995).

- The proportion of users relying on the IUD also decreased, from 2% in 1988 to fewer than 1% in 1995.

Method	Perfect use	Average use
No method	85.0	85.0
Spermicide	6.0	30.0
Withdrawal	4.0	24.0
Periodic abstinence	9.0	19.0
Cervical cap	9.0; 26.0*	18.0
Diaphragm	6.0	18.0
Condom	3.0	16.0
Pill	0.1	6.0
IUD	0.8	4.0
Tubal sterilization	0.5	0.5
Injectable	0.3	0.4
Vasectomy	0.1	0.2
Implant	0.05	0.05

*9% for nulliparous women; 26% for parous women.

Sources of Data

The information in this fact sheet is the most current available. All of the data are from research conducted by The Alan Guttmacher Institute and the National Center for Health Statistics and/or were published in *Family Planning Perspectives* or *Contraceptive Technology*. This fact sheet was prepared, in part, with support from the Office of Population Affairs of the U.S. Department of Health and Human Services.

Method (in 000s)	No. of users	% of users
Tubal sterilization	10,727	27.7
Pill	10,410	26.9
Male condom	7,889	20.4
Vasectomy	4,215	10.9
Withdrawal	1,178	3.0
Injectable	1,146	3.0
Periodic abstinence	883	2.3
Diaphragm	720	1.9
Other	670	1.8
Implant	515	1.3
IUD	310	0.8
TOTAL	38,663	100.0

Chapter 18

Facts about Title X, the National Family Planning Program

Overview

The national family planning program, Title X (ten) of the Public Health Service Act, was established in 1970 with broad bipartisan support. The original measure was introduced by then Representatives James Schauer (D-NY) and George Bush (R-TX), and Senators Joseph Tydings (D-MD) and Charles Percy (R-IL). The program provides federal funds for project grants to public and private nonprofit organizations for the provision of family planning information and services which:

- improve maternal and infant health;
- lower the incidence of unintended pregnancy;
- reduce the incidence of abortion; and
- lower rates of sexually transmitted diseases (STDs).

The program's FY 1999 appropriation of $215 million (a $12 million increase over the FY 1998 funding level) will enable approximately 4.5 million Americans to receive services at the over 4,400 Title X-funded clinics nationwide.

What Services Does Title X Provide?

Services supported by Title X include contraceptive information and the provision of all contraceptive services, as well as gynecological examinations, basic lab tests, and other screening services for STDs and HIV, high blood pressure, anemia, and breast and cervical cancer. Also provided are pregnancy testing, sterilization services, natural family planning, and community education and outreach. Title X prohibits the use of federal funds to pay for abortions.

Where Do People Receive Services?

Title X clinic sites include state and local health departments, hospitals, university health centers, Planned Parenthood affiliates, independent clinics, and other public and non-profit agencies. Although we refer to these providers as a network, it is not one uniform system, but represents adaptation to the unique health care delivery systems and needs of different states and localities across the country. Thus, Title X clinics are community-based providers. Title X-funded clinics are located in every state, three-quarters of U.S. counties, and virtually every congressional district in the nation. They serve as the entry point to the health care system and the only source of service for millions of Americans.

Who Receives Services through Title X?

Title X clinics primarily serve low-income Americans. Eighty-three percent of Title X clients had incomes below 150 percent of the federal poverty level in 1997. The vast majority of Title X clients are uninsured and do not qualify for Medicaid. Title X clinics provide services free of charge to clients whose incomes do not exceed 100 percent of the federal poverty level and services are offered on a sliding fee scale for clients with incomes up to 250 percent of the federal poverty level.

Why America Needs a National Family Planning Program

Family Planning Works!

Recent data show that the U.S. teen pregnancy rate has dropped 17 percent since peaking in 1990. About 20 percent of the decrease since the late 1980s is due to a decrease in sexual activity, and 80 percent is due to more effective contraceptive practice among teenagers. Between 1995 and 1996, the teenage pregnancy rate (including births, abortions, and miscarriages) declined by four percent, the teenage birthrate declined by four percent, and the abortion rate declined by three percent. (*Teenage Pregnancy: Overall Trends and State-by-State Information*, Alan Guttmacher Institute [AGI], April 1999)

This is a step in the right direction, but we still have a long way to go. Title X is a critical component of a strategy to ensure that unintended pregnancy rates continue to decline.

- Approximately one million unintended pregnancies were averted among women who received services at Title X-funded clinics in 1994. (*Title X and the U.S. Family Planning Effort*, AGI, 1997)

- As unintended pregnancies have declined and contraceptive use has improved, the number of abortions in our country has dropped. According to data from the Centers for Disease Control, the 1995 abortion rate in the U.S. declined five percent since 1994, and 15 percent since 1990.

- Title X family planning services help reduce the need for abortion. Federal law specifies that "None of the funds appropriated under this title shall be used in programs where abortion is a method of family planning." (P.L. 91-572, Family Planning Services and Population Research Act)

- Family planning is a basic preventive health service which is a key contributor to healthy families and healthy babies. Infant deaths could be reduced by 10 percent, and the incidence of low birthweight babies could be reduced by 12 percent, if all pregnancies were planned. (*Troubling Trends: The Health of America's Next Generation*, National Commission to Prevent Infant Mortality, 1990)

- Publicly funded family planning services provided between 1982 and 1988 prevented 20,000 low-birth weight deliveries, 6,500 infant deaths, and 5,500 neonatal deaths. (*American Journal of Public Health*, Vol. 84, pp. 1468–1472, 1994)

- Title X provides services to women and adolescents *before* they become pregnant unlike Medicaid, which generally provides family planning services only *after* a pregnancy has occurred.

- Title X family planning clinics provide confidential screening and treatment for STDs, which affect 15.3 million Americans annually. (American Social Health Association, 1998) One quarter of new cases occur in teens 15–19 years old, and two-thirds of cases occur in people ages 15–24. (AGI, 1993)

- Visits to Title X clinics involving testing and treatment for STDs rose by 30 percent between 1980 and 1990. (*Title X and the U.S. Family Planning Effort,* AGI, 1997)

- *Americans support federally funded family planning.* In a poll conducted by the firm of Hickman-Brown in October of 1995, 64 percent of the survey participants said they would be more likely to vote for a candidate who would support "continued funding for federal family planning programs."

- Over three-fourths of Americans favor funding for "birth control for unmarried women on welfare." (CBS/New York Times poll, April 1995)

Family Planning Is Cost-Effective

- Each public dollar spent to provide family planning services saves an average of $3 in Medicaid costs for pregnancy-related and newborn care alone. (*Title X and the U.S. Family Planning Effort,* AGI, 1997)

- Because pregnancy is so costly, all available contraceptive methods are extremely cost-effective when compared with no contraception. Each year, out of 100 typical women who engage in sex without using contraception, 85 will get pregnant. (*American Journal of Public Health,* April 1995)

Title X Framework

- The Title X program provides the framework for family planning service delivery throughout the United States through a national network of clinics and its uniform federal regulations and guidelines. These uniform regulations and guidelines guarantee women access to contraceptive counseling, a range of contraceptive options, confidentiality of services, and referral for other health and social services when necessary. The federal regulations and guidelines often serve as the blueprint for state family planning programs.

- Title X funds comprise approximately one-third of the budget for clinics providing federally subsidized family planning services. These funds are critical in maintaining the family planning service delivery infrastructure in the United States.

- Title X allows states and communities flexibility in tailoring family planning services to meet local needs and priorities while promoting quality of care and access. Title X ensures that family planning services are delivered at the local level by a diverse array of providers, including state health departments, hospitals, community-based non-profit organizations, and Planned Parenthood affiliates.

Title X Funding

- Current Title X funding is inadequate to meet the needs of all eligible Americans. The Title X program serves less than half of those currently eligible for services.

- In constant dollars, funding for the Title X program declined by over 65 percent between 1980 and 1994. In 1980, the Title X program was funded at $162 million. Had the program's funding increased at the rate of inflation as determined by the medical care services index, Title X would currently be funded at more than $500 million, more than twice its current funding level of $215 million.

- As funding for Title X declined in the 1980s, health care costs soared, the number of eligible patients increased, and the cost of contraceptive supplies rose dramatically.

- Some clinics have been forced to curtail services. The decline in funding (in constant dollars) and the rise in health care costs and patient loads has forced some family planning clinics to curtail hours of operation and place patients on waiting lists for the most effective and longest lasting family planning methods, such as the IUD, Depo-Provera®, and Norplant®.

Congressional Support for Title X Remains High

- Recent legislative proposals to impose restrictions on access to Title X services have not become law. For the first time, the House, on October 8, 1998, approved a proposal to condition teens' access to confidential family planning services on written parental consent or advance parental notification by a vote of 224–200. This provision was not approved by the Senate and was not included in the final version of the Labor/HHS spending bill for FY 1999.

- In August 1995, the House voted 224–204 to reverse a decision made by the House Appropriations Committee to eliminate Title X funding. Similar shows of support for access to family planning services took place in July 1996 and September 1997, when the House of Representatives voted 232–198 and 220–201, respectively, to support amendments requiring Title X clinics to encourage family participation in a teen's decision to seek family planning services.

Key Reproductive Health Indicators

The need for continued and increased federal funding for family planning services is clear when key reproductive health indicators are examined. Title X provides services that are critical in helping to combat unintended pregnancy, teen pregnancy, and the high rates of STDs in our country.

Unintended Pregnancy

- In the United States, almost half of all pregnancies are unintended. Half of unintended pregnancies end in abortion. (AGI, 1998)

- The 10 percent of American women at risk of unintended pregnancy (those who do not want to be pregnant but are sexually active and fertile) who do not practice contraception account for 53 percent of all unintended pregnancies. (Institute of Medicine, 1995)

- By the age of 45, American women, on average, will have had 1.42 unintended pregnancies. ("Unintended Pregnancy in the United States," *Family Planning Perspectives,* AGI, 1998)

- Women spend more than 75 percent of their reproductive lives trying to avoid pregnancy. (*Hopes and Realities: Closing the Gap Between Women's Aspirations and Their Reproductive Experiences,* AGI, 1995)

Teen Pregnancy

- Each year, 1 in 8 women aged 15 to 19 in the United States becomes pregnant, resulting in over half a million births. Two-thirds of these births are unintended. (*Contraceptive Technology,* Robert Hatcher et al., 1998, p. 701–702)

- The teenage pregnancy rate in the United States is much higher than in many other developed countries—twice as high as in England and Wales, France, and Canada; and nine times as high as in the Netherlands or Japan. (*Teenage Reproductive Health in the United States,* AGI, 1994)

- Without publicly funded family planning services, an additional 386,000 teens would become pregnant each year, resulting in 155,000 more teen births and 183,000 more teen abortions. (*Title X and the U.S. Family Planning Effort,* AGI, 1997)

- Over three-quarters of teen pregnancies are unintended. (AGI, 1998)

Sexually Transmitted Diseases

- Family planning clinics can play a critical role in addressing our national STD epidemic.

- Women bear a disproportionate burden of STD-associated complications, including infertility, ectopic pregnancy, and chronic pelvic pain. Women are particularly vulnerable to STDs because they are biologically more susceptible to certain STD infections than men and are more likely to have asymptomatic infections that commonly result in delayed diagnosis and treatment.

- A conservative estimate of the public and private costs of STD treatment each year in the United States is at least $8.4 billion. (*STDs in America: How Many and At What Cost?,* Kaiser Family Foundation and ASHA, 1998)

- Half of the 10 most frequently reported infections to the Centers for Disease Control and Prevention (CDC) are STDs, including the most common, chlamydia. (CDC, 1998) The prevalence of chlamydia among teenagers often exceeds 10 percent among girls and 5 percent among boys. (Mertz, CDC, 1998)

- STD infections increase susceptibility to HIV by three to five times. (ASHA, 1998) However, a third of Americans (36 percent) are not aware that having an STD increases a person's risk of HIV infection. (Kaiser Family Foundation/*Glamour* magazine survey, 1998)

- At least one in three sexually active people are estimated to have contracted an STD by the age of 24. (*STDs in America: How Many and At What Cost?,* Kaiser Family Foundation and ASHA, 1998)

- Over one in five Americans over the age of 12 has a herpes infection. The number of people living with herpes, one of the most common incurable STDs, has risen 30 percent since the late 1970s. (*New England Journal of Medicine,* October 16, 1997)

Part Four:

Traditional Methods of Contraception

Chapter 19

Abstinence

Chapter Contents

Section 19.1

Abstinence

"Abstinence: Not Having Sexual Intercourse," Emory University School of Medicine, August 5, 1997; available at http://www.emory/edu/WHSC/MED/FAMPLAN/abstinence.html.

—by Robert A. Hatcher, M.D., M.P.H., Emory University School of Medicine

What Is abstinence?

Abstinence means avoiding sex. Sex can have different definitions for different people. Some people define sex as penis-in-vagina intercourse. Others may include oral sex, anal sex, or even kissing and touching. The way you define "sex" determines what activities to avoid if you want to abstain. For the purpose of this section, we will focus on abstaining from penis-in-vagina intercourse because the goal of this material is to help you prevent pregnancy.

Please remember that it's OK to go through periods of your life, or periods of time within a single relationship, in which you want to abstain and periods in which you want to have sex. The decision to have sex is YOUR decision, each and every time.

Advantages:

- Abstinence is free and available to everyone.
- It's extremely effective at preventing both pregnancy and infection.
- It can be started at any time in your life.
- Abstinence may encourage people to build relationships in other ways.
- It may be the course of action which you feel is right for you and makes you feel good about yourself.

Disadvantages:

- If you're counting on abstinence, and you change your mind in the heat of the moment, you might not have birth control handy. *Some people would like to be prepared* and have a condom or spermicide available in case they change their mind. *Others feel that having a contraceptive available might tempt them.*
- Some people find not having sex frustrating.

Where Can I Learn More?

What you do sexually is an important decision. Start by thinking it through carefully by yourself. You may want to discuss your decision with another person whom you respect. You may want to pray, meditate, or talk it over with your partner. Some churches and sex education programs have organized support groups or curricula for young people wanting to wait until marriage before having intercourse.

Section 19.2

Outercourse

"Outercourse!," Emory University School of Medicine, August 5, 1997; available at http://www.emory/edu/WHSC/MED/FAMPLAN/outercourse.html.

—by Robert A. Hatcher, M.D., M.P.H.,
Emory University School of Medicine

What Is Outercourse?

Outercourse usually refers to types of sexual intimacy which do not involve the penis entering the vagina or anus. Some examples of outercourse include:

- holding hands
- hugs
- kisses

- mutual masturbation
- oral-genital contact
- petting above the waist
- petting below the waist
- touching

Outercourse does take some discipline! Both partners must be commited to this method, or these exciting forms of sexual intimacy can lead to traditional intercourse. Many people choose to practice outercourse because of the risk of infection. It works better if there has been communication about using this method in advance. Decide in advance what sexual activities you will say "yes" to and discuss these with your partner. Tell your partner very clearly what activities you will not do. At the same time learn more about the methods of safer sex and birth control so that you will be ready if you change your mind.

Advantages:

- Outercourse is always an option ... no supplies are necessary and it's free!
- It's fun and there is no worry about pregnancy. For some it's more fun than traditional intercourse.
- There is no exchange of fluids [with the exception of oral sex]. This provides some protection against infection.
- There are no medical complications associated with outercourse.
- Outercourse can increase emotional closeness between individuals.

Disadvantages:

- Oral sex can spread some infections.
- One partner may really want to have intercourse. This can cause stress.
- This method may cause either partner to wonder, "Is this going to go farther than I want?" Such concern may decrease enjoyment.

Chapter 20

Withdrawal (Coitus Interruptus)

What Is Withdrawal?

Withdrawal is a method in which the man takes his penis out of the woman's vagina just before his climax.

Is It Effective?

Withdrawal is effective when it is used every time the man has sexual intercourse.

Note: Withdrawal does not provide protection against HIV infection and other sexually transmitted diseases. Aside from abstinence, latex condoms offer the best protection against these infections.

How Does It Work?

Withdrawal works by not allowing the man's sperm to enter the woman's vagina. If the man's sperm do not enter the woman's vagina, she will not get pregnant.

"Withdrawal: Answers to Your Questions" and "Is Withdrawal the Right Method for Me?," © 1998 AVSC International; available at http://www.avsc.org/contraception/cwit2.html and http://www.avsc.org/contraception/cwit1.html; reprinted with permission.

How Do I Use Withdrawal?

When you feel that you are about to ejaculate, remove your penis from inside the vagina. Make sure that ejaculation takes place away from the entrance to the vagina.

What Are the Advantages and Disadvantages of Withdrawal?

Advantages:
- Withdrawal does not require medication or supplies.
- Withdrawal can be used when other methods are not available.
- Withdrawal has no side effects.
- Withdrawal is permitted by some religions and cultures that do not permit other methods.
- Withdrawal can be discontinued by the man on his own.
- A woman who has just delivered a baby or had an abortion may start using withdrawal with her partner as soon as they start having sexual intercourse again.

Disadvantages:
- Withdrawal does not provide protection against HIV infection and other sexually transmitted diseases.
- Withdrawal requires the man's self-control.
- Withdrawal may reduce the pleasure of sexual intercourse.
- When withdrawing, even though the man takes his penis out, some sperm may have already gotten into the woman's vagina.

Is Withdrawal the Right Method for Me?

There are a number of factors you should consider to determine whether withdrawal is the right contraceptive method for you. As with any contraception, you should first talk to your doctor or a counselor at your local clinic or hospital before using withdrawal as a contraceptive method.

Withdrawal May Be an Appropriate Method for You

If any of the following is true:

- You find other contraceptive methods unacceptable for religious or other reasons.
- You prefer a method you can discontinue yourself.
- You are concerned about the side effects of other methods.
- You have sexual intercourse only occasionally and do not need or want ongoing contraception.
- You feel that the man should share responsibility for family planning.
- You or your partner have medical precautions for the use of other contraceptive methods.
- You and your partner have just had a baby. You may start using withdrawal as soon as you resume sexual intercourse after delivery.
- Your partner has just had an abortion. You and your partner may start using withdrawal as soon as you resume sexual intercourse after the abortion.

Withdrawal May Not Be an Appropriate Method for You

If any of the following is true:

- You are at risk of exposure to, or transmission of, sexually transmitted diseases, including HIV infection. Withdrawal does not provide protection against these infections. Aside from abstinence, latex condoms offer the best protection against these infections.
- Either you or your partner are not willing to cooperate in using this method.

Withdrawal Is Not an Appropriate Method for You

If the following is true:

- You desire very effective contraception.

Chapter 21

Fertility Awareness Methods: Ways to Chart Your Fertility Pattern

There are days when a healthy woman is fertile, days when she is infertile, and some days when fertility is unlikely, but possible. A woman's fertile period depends on the life span of sperm as much as it does on the life span of her egg. The egg lives for about a day. A man's sperm can live inside a woman's body for about five days—possibly seven. Fertilization of a woman's egg is more likely from intercourse before or during ovulation than from intercourse following ovulation. It usually occurs during a six-day period that ends in ovulation.

In total, a woman has a good chance of becoming pregnant from unprotected vaginal intercourse over the course of about nine days of her menstrual cycle—as long as seven days before the release of an egg (ovulation), the day of ovulation, and, possibly, the day after ovulation. She is less likely to become pregnant from unprotected intercourse in the day or two following ovulation, but it is possible.

Understanding her monthly fertility pattern can help a woman avoid an unintended pregnancy. It can also help her plan a pregnancy. The key is for her to know when fertilization may occur by estimating the time of ovulation as nearly as possible. This must be done care-

"Ways to Chart Your Fertility Pattern," text adapted from *Ways to Chart Your Fertility Pattern*, © revised version July 1996 Planned Parenthood® Federation of America, Inc., original copyright 1997 PPFA, PPFA Web Site © 1998, Planned Parenthood® Federation of America, Inc.; available at http://www.plannedparenthood.org/BIRTH-CONTROL/WaysToChart.HTM; reprinted with permission.

fully because the timing of ovulation varies greatly from one woman to another and, for some women, from one month to the next.

Women who monitor their fertility to prevent pregnancy may choose to abstain from vaginal intercourse for at least one-third of each menstrual cycle or to use barrier methods or withdrawal during that time. **Periodic abstinence** and **fertility awareness methods** are the two methods of contraception that depend on charting your fertility pattern.

Couples who want to prevent pregnancy using **periodic abstinence** do not have vaginal intercourse during their "unsafe days"— the days during which the fertile phase may occur. Although they abstain from vaginal intercourse during the fertile days, they may enjoy other forms of sex play.

Couples who use **fertility awareness methods (FAMs)** use withdrawal or barrier contraceptives—condoms, vaginal pouches, diaphragms, or cervical caps—during their fertile or "unsafe days."

Understanding Your Menstrual Cycle

Understanding your menstrual cycle is essential for your good health. It is especially important if you want to chart your fertility pattern as a method of contraception.

The monthly pattern that occurs regularly in most women, from puberty to menopause, is called the menstrual cycle. Every cycle is divided into two parts—*before* ovulation and *after* ovulation. In a 28-day cycle, the pattern usually follows this timing:

- The beginning of the cycle, called Day 1, is the day bleeding begins. The flow usually lasts about three to five days. Usually by Day 7, certain hormones cause some of the eggs in the ovaries to start ripening. Between Days 7 and 11, the lining of the uterus begins to thicken. The influence of additional hormones after Day 11 causes the egg that is most ripe to be released on about Day 14 in women who have a 28-day cycle. The other ripening eggs stop growing and dry up. That's part one.

- In the second part, the egg travels down the fallopian tube toward the uterus. If a single male sperm unites with the egg while it is in the tube, the fertilized egg may attach to the spongy lining of the uterus. Pregnancy begins if this "implantation" occurs. If fertilization doesn't take place, the egg cell will break apart in a day or two. About Day 25, hormone levels drop.

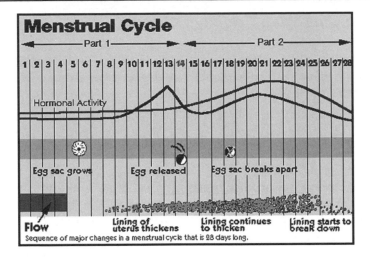

This causes the lining of the uterus to break down and in a few days it is shed in a menstrual period. Another cycle has begun.

For some women, cycles recur fairly regularly every 28 days. But the number of days in each cycle can vary from woman to woman, from every 21 to every 35 days. In fact, a few women have only three or four cycles a year.

The first part of the cycle, from menstruation to ovulation, may vary from 13 to 20 days in length. The length of the first part is not only different from one woman to another, but also differs in some women from month to month. It is during this critical first part of the cycle that fertilization can occur. Such common circumstances as sickness, worry, physical exertion, and even sudden changes in climate may occasionally upset a regular pattern by shortening it or extending it.

The second part of the cycle, from ovulation to menstruation, is about the same length in all women. The egg is released consistently 14 to 16 days before the onset of menstruation, regardless of the length of a woman's menstrual cycle.

There are a few women who believe they can tell when the egg has been released from the ovary. Some report having a slight pain in the back, or on the right or left side of the lower abdomen. A few may also have some increased vaginal discharge—a little blood-tinged or clear discharge from the vagina. But it is generally accepted that none of these is a sure signal that an egg has been released—the same symptoms can be caused by other factors.

Ways to Chart Your Fertility Pattern

Here are brief descriptions of the changes you can chart to predict when you ovulate in order to plan or prevent pregnancy. More complete descriptions follow.

- For the ***temperature method:*** Take your temperature every morning before getting out of bed. Your temperature rises between 0.4°F and 0.8°F on the day of ovulation. It remains at that level until your next period.

- For the ***cervical mucus method:*** Observe the changes in your cervical mucus. You must do so all through the first part of your menstrual cycle, until you are sure you have ovulated. Normally cloudy, tacky mucus will become clear and slippery in the few days before ovulation. It also will stretch between the fingers. When this happens you are in your most fertile phase. You must abstain from vaginal intercourse or use a barrier contraceptive during this time.

- For the ***calendar method:*** Chart your menstrual cycles on a calendar. You may be able to predict ovulation if your periods are the same every month. You must abstain or use a barrier method during your "unsafe days." It will be more difficult to predict the day of ovulation if the length of your cycle varies from month to month. In that case, you will have more "unsafe days." **It is best not to rely on this method alone.**

It is best to combine the **temperature method**, the **cervical mucus method**, and the **calendar method**. The combination of these methods is called the **symptothermal** method.

Temperature Method

One of the changes that ordinarily take place in a woman's body as part of her menstrual pattern is that her body temperature is lower during the first part of the cycle. In most women it usually rises slightly with ovulation and remains up during the second part until just before her next period. Recording each day's temperature helps to indicate when ovulation has occurred.

The temperature method requires charting your basal body temperature (BBT), the temperature your body registers when you're completely at rest. BBT varies slightly from person to person. For most

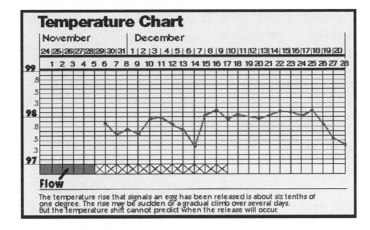

Temperature Chart

The temperature rise that signals an egg has been released is about six tenths of one degree. The rise may be sudden or a gradual climb over several days. But the temperature shift cannot predict when the release will occur.

women, 96 to 98 degrees taken orally is considered normal before ovulation and 97 to 99 after. The changes are small fractions—from 1/10 to 1/2 degree. So it's best to get a special, large-scale, easy-to-read thermometer that registers only from 96 to 100 degrees. A rectal or oral basal temperature thermometer can be bought in most drug stores for about $10. Generally, rectal readings are more reliable. But whichever you choose, take your temperature the same way every day.

Taking Your Temperature

Each morning take your temperature, as soon as you wake up—before getting out of bed, talking, eating, drinking, having sex, or smoking. Either insert the thermometer in your rectum or place it in your mouth for a full five minutes. Read the temperature to within 1/10 of a degree and record the reading.

Charting Your Temperature Pattern

Each reading must be recorded. Charts for this purpose may be obtained from your clinician or women's health center. As each day's temperature is plotted on the graph, you will learn to recognize your own pattern. Your temperature rise may be sudden, gradual, or in steps. The pattern may vary from cycle to cycle.

You must also realize that your BBT can be influenced by physical or emotional upsets or even lack of sleep. In addition, illness, emotional distress, jet lag, disturbed sleep, smoking, drinking an unaccustomed amount of alcohol the night before, and using an electric blanket may

211

affect your body temperature. Noting such events on the chart helps to interpret the readings.

In the beginning, you should get help in reading your BBT chart from a physician, nurse, or family planning specialist. In time, under supervision, you'll gain the knowledge and confidence to use the chart by yourself. Be sure to chart your temperature for at least three months before relying on this method.

The Safe Times

After the temperature rise has lasted for at least three days, you can assume that your safe days have begun. They will last until the temperature drop that usually comes just before the onset of your next menstrual period. For complete protection, consider unsafe all the days between the start of your period and the start of the fourth day of the next temperature rise. That is because the temperature method is quite accurate in detecting when ovulation has occurred, but can't predict when it's about to happen. And there's another important reason why the whole first part of the cycle must be considered unsafe— the lifetime of a man's sperm.

Sperm generally remain capable of fertilizing an egg for two to three days after ejaculation. There are even instances of sperm remaining active five or more days after intercourse. So if you have sexual intercourse several days before ovulation, there's a good chance that live sperm could still fertilize a newly released egg. Combining BBT with another method may help in trying to calculate ovulation in advance.

When you become confident about using your BBT to determine your safe days, you may not need to take your temperature between the start of the infertile time and the beginning of your next menstrual period.

Cervical Mucus Method

The cervical mucus method is based on another change that occurs during the menstrual cycle. The hormones that control menstrual cycle phases also act on the glands of the cervix that produce mucus secretions. The mucus secreted by the cervix collects in the cervix and vagina. It changes in quality and quantity just before and during ovulation. With proper personal instruction, many women can learn to recognize the changing characteristics. Instruction in the cervical

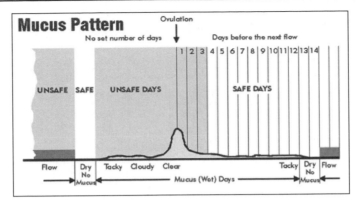

mucus method is usually given on a one-to-one basis. The cervical mucus method is also known as the **ovulation method** or the **Billings method.**

The Mucus Pattern

- The cycle begins with menstruation. During vaginal bleeding, the flow disguises the mucus signs.

- The menstrual period is usually followed by a few days when no mucus is present—these are "dry days."

- As an egg starts to ripen, mucus increases in the vagina and appears at the vaginal opening. It is generally yellow or white, and it is cloudy and sticky.

- The greatest amount of cervical mucus usually occurs immediately before ovulation during the "wet days." The mucus takes on a clear and slippery quality that resembles raw egg whites. When the mucus can be stretched between the fingers, it is called *spinnbarkeit*—German for stretchable. This is the peak period of fertility.

- About four days after the wet days begin, mucus may abruptly become cloudy and sticky, reduce sharply in volume, and a few dry days may return before your period starts.

Charting Your Mucus Pattern

As with the other methods, records need to be kept. It's suggested that a woman chart her observation daily on a calendar. Mark the days of your menstrual period, the dry days, sticky days, and wet days. It's best for a woman to avoid intercourse for at least one whole cycle when

Charting Your Mucus Pattern

August

Sunday	Monday	Tuesday	Wednesday	Thursday	Friday	Saturday
		Sticky 1	Dry 2	Wet 3	Wet 4	Flow 5
Flow 6	Flow 7	Flow 8	Dry 9	Dry 10	Tacky 11 white	Sticky 12
Creamy 13	Milky 14 more	Clear 15 spinn	Wet 16	Sticky 17 less	Sticky 18 yellow	Sticky 19 scant
Dry 20	Tacky 21	Dry 22	Dry 23	Dry 24	Dry 25	Tacky 26
Dry 27	Sticky 28	Wet 29	Wet 30 milky	Flow 31		

you start to use the mucus method for birth control. Get someone with experience to help you become familiar with your own pattern until you are able to interpret the changes yourself.

A woman can check her mucus in several ways, depending on which is most comfortable for her. She can:

- Wipe the vaginal opening with toilet tissue before urination
- observe the discharge on underpants
- obtain some of the mucus by placing her fingers (making sure they are clean) in the vagina.

She should check several times a day when there is any sign of mucus.

This method is less reliable for women who produce little mucus or if the natural mucus pattern is altered by:

- using douches, "feminine hygiene" products, or contraceptive foams, creams, jellies, or suppositories
- surgery that is performed on the cervix—especially if cryotherapy or a loop electrosurgical excision procedure is used
- vaginitis
- sexually transmitted infections
- breastfeeding
- perimenopause
- recent use of hormonal contraceptives.

Women who ovulate on Day 7 or 8 may produce too little mucus to use this method.

The Safe Times

- It is considered unsafe to have vaginal intercourse during menstruation, especially during shorter cycles. Vaginal bleeding can disguise the mucus signs. Non-menstrual vaginal bleeding around the time of ovulation may be mistaken for a menstrual period.

- Intercourse may take place during the brief period of safe dry days that may follow menstruation in a long cycle.

- The fertile phase begins at the first sign of wetness after menstruation, but it may also begin a day or two before wetness begins. Intercourse must be avoided on any wet day, unless you are trying for a pregnancy—fertilization is most likely to occur during this phase. Otherwise, you must refrain from sex for at least three days after ovulation or until the wet days end, whichever is the longer number of days.

- It is considered safe to have sex after ovulation when mucus sharply decreases in volume and becomes cloudy and sticky again. It is considered even safer to have intercourse during the dry days that may follow before your period begins.

Fewer pregnancies occur when intercourse takes place only on the dry days following ovulation.

The Calendar Method

The calendar method attempts to predict ovulation using a woman's menstrual history. A written record is kept—an ordinary calendar can be used to note each cycle, counting from the first day of one menstrual period up to, but not including, the first day of the next. The day bleeding starts is Day 1, and you mark this by circling that date on the calendar. Continue to circle Day 1 for at least 8 months (12 is better). Then you count the days in each cycle.

Of course, you have no assurance that your cycle variations will remain the same. So you must continue to circle each Day 1 and list the length of your last cycle.

Cycle Record

First Day of Period	Number of Days in Preceding Cycle	First Day of Period	Number of Days in Preceding Cycle
Jan. 20	29	May 12	26
Feb. 18	29	June 9	28
Mar. 18	28	July 9	30
Apr. 16	29	Aug. 5	27

The Role of the Calendar Method

These rules can only help you to find out a couple of days in advance when you *probably* will ovulate. Calendar records should always be used with other methods explained in this chapter. Always be guided by any sign that says you may be fertile. The calendar method is especially chancy if your cycles are not always the same length.

Charting Your Pattern

Keep a record of the number of days in each cycle. When bleeding starts, circle the date on your calendar.

To find the first day you are likely to be infertile, check your record of previous months, find the shortest cycle, and subtract 18 from the total number of days. For example, if the shortest cycle is 26 days long, subtract 18 from 26, which leaves 8. Starting with the date you circled (the first day of your current cycle) count ahead eight days and draw an X through that second date. That's the first day you're likely to be fertile and, therefore, the first day of abstinence or contraceptive use. But if your temperature chart shows even a slight shift before that, don't have unprotected intercourse until three full days after your temperature rise.

To find the last day you must abstain or use contraception with the calendar method, subtract 11 days from your longest cycle. Draw an X through that date also. Remember, you need to chart your cycles for at least eight months before you can calculate your safe times. Be sure to confirm this with other methods.

The Safe Times

Safer times are likely from the first day of menstruation, Day 1, which you have circled, to the first X. They are also likely from the second X to the next circle. Unsafe days appear between the two X's.

Remember: if all your cycles are shorter than 27 days, don't try to use calendar estimates at all. The first part of any cycle may be irregular. Trying to add a few days of intercourse in the early part of your cycle can be risky when attempting to prevent an unplanned pregnancy. Learning the meaning of changes in your normal vaginal discharge may reduce miscalculations. But always be guided by any sign that says you may be fertile.

Using These Methods Together

Using all three methods—temperature, cervical mucus, and calendar—is called the **symptothermal method.** The symptothermal method allows a woman to be more accurate in predicting her safe days than if she uses any one of the methods alone. When using these methods together, the signs of one can serve to confirm those of the other. For example, a record of the mucus pattern can be useful because temperature rises resulting from illness or emotional stress may be confusing. Combining methods also permits sexual relations during the early dry days, and shortens the period of abstinence necessary for complete protection when using the temperature method alone.

In the **post-ovulation method,** couples abstain from vaginal intercourse or use withdrawal or a barrier method from the beginning of the woman's period until the morning of the fourth day after her predicted ovulation. A woman is much less likely to be fertile after ovulation has occurred (post-ovulation). However, couples who practice the post-ovulation method must abstain from vaginal intercourse or use withdrawal or a barrier method for more than half of the woman's menstrual cycle.

How Well These Methods Work

Of 100 couples who use any of these methods for one year, 20 women will become pregnant with *typical* use. The failure rate is higher for single women. Combining the various methods with careful and consistent use and having no unprotected vaginal intercourse during the fertile phase can give better results.

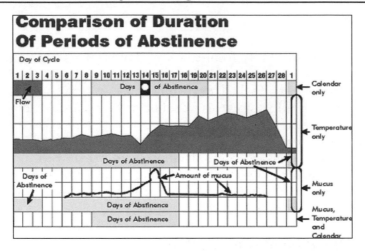

Comparison of Duration Of Periods of Abstinence

Of 100 couples who use the **temperature method** for one year with *perfect* use, two women will become pregnant.

Of 100 couples who use the **cervical mucus method** for one year with *perfect* use, three women will become pregnant.

Of 100 couples who use the **calendar method** for one year with *perfect* use, nine women will become pregnant.

Few couples, however, are able to use these methods perfectly. These methods require keeping consistent and accurate records. Some skill is required in figuring, and the margin for error depends on how accurately signs and records are interpreted and followed. It is most important that original explanations, early coaching, and frequent follow-up be done by a professional instructor or successful users. These methods work better for women whose cycles are always the same length.

Some couples chart the woman's fertility pattern to prevent pregnancy because it is economical, safe, and can be discontinued easily when pregnancy is desired. Little equipment is needed, and calendars, thermometers, and charts are widely available. No medication is involved, which is especially appealing to women who have physical or health conditions that might make other forms of birth control less desirable or unsuitable. Medical checkups are not required, although professional instruction is important. Periodic abstinence is acceptable to most religious groups. However, if a couple decides to have vaginal intercourse during the fertile period, pregnancy is likely to occur unless they use barrier methods such as a combination of condom and foam.

Charting fertility patterns requires dedication, education, and practice. It is most effective when both partners are mature, responsible, and committed to making them work. That's why it is very important for both partners to learn the fundamentals and support each other in observing the abstinence or contraceptive use that is required.

Women who are breastfeeding or approaching menopause may find it more difficult to chart their fertility. Their fertile signs may vary in unpredictable ways due to irregular hormonal fluctuations. Likewise, multiorgasmic women are also likely to ovulate unpredictably.

If you are taking the Pill or any other hormonal method, you'll have to stop taking it and use another method of contraception that has no hormones, such as a barrier method (condoms, diaphragm, cervical cap), while learning fertility awareness methods. Hormones in the Pill alter the natural menstruation and fertility cycle.

Do Not Depend on Charting Your Fertility Pattern If:

- you have irregular periods
- your partner is unwilling to observe periods of abstinence from vaginal intercourse, practice withdrawal, or use barrier methods at unsafe times
- you have a sexually transmitted infection or frequent abnormal discharges
- you cannot keep careful records.

Products for Use with These Methods

At this time no device exists that can simplify or ensure greater success with any of these methods. From time to time announcements are made of patented items to help in calendar calculation or to test mucus change by chemically treated paper, or of other products under development for this purpose. None has proven any more reliable for *contraceptive* purposes. Success in the use of any of these methods for predicting fertility is the result of good initial instruction, persistence, accuracy in keeping records, and cooperation by both partners in the discipline involved.

Test kits that attempt to predict ovulation are available for home use. They may be useful for planning pregnancies but are not reliable for purposes of birth control. Sperm can live in the fallopian tubes for about up to seven days. So, pregnancy often results from unprotected vaginal intercourse during the six days *before* ovulation.

Charting Your Fertility Pattern Can Work for You If:

- You have received careful instruction in the methods.
- You have only one sex partner and he is equally committed to the methods you want to use.
- You have the self-discipline required to check and chart your fertility signs and observe the rules.
- You don't mind abstaining or using withdrawal or barrier methods for the first part of the cycle.

Charting Your Fertility Pattern May Not Be Appropriate for You If:

- You have more than one sex partner.
- Your sex partner isn't equally committed to the methods you want to use.
- You are temperamentally unsuited for keeping close track of your fertile days.
- You have doubts about being able to abstain from vaginal intercourse for at least 10 days each month or to use a barrier method on "unsafe" days.
- You wouldn't consider having an abortion although you have a medical condition that poses a grave danger for you if you become pregnant.
- You take medication that may affect your cervical mucus, body temperature, or menstrual regularity.

Cost

Charts for graphing fertility signs cost little or nothing. They are available at family planning clinics and from private instructors and organizations. Basal body temperature thermometers cost about $10 to $12. You may have to pay a fee for classes to learn fertility awareness techniques. In some states, Medicaid will cover the cost of classes taken at a clinic or when authorized by a private physician.

Finding a Teacher

Couples can learn how the woman's body signs serve as the basis of their contraceptive method by taking a course or being counseled by a health professional trained to teach methods to monitor fertility. Both partners should attend the sessions so each will be aware of precisely how these methods work. Not only will learning the methods together increase their effectiveness, but many couples report that cooperating on contraception helps them become more intimate.

Classes on charting fertility patterns for contraception are offered by many family planning health centers, church-affiliated instructors, and at Catholic hospitals, often at little or no cost.

Instruction in a religious setting may reflect the tenets of that religion in regard to other methods of contraception. For nonsectarian instruction, ask for a referral from a Planned Parenthood health center, a women's clinic that is not affiliated with a religious group, or your state or county health department.

An information packet that includes a basic overview, a book list, addresses of resource organizations, and information on how to find a teacher is available for $4 and a self-addressed, stamped business envelope from the Fertility Awareness Center, P.O. Box 2606, New York, NY 10009.

Chapter 22

Lactational Amenorrhea Method (Breastfeeding)

Chapter Contents

Section 22.1

Lactational Amenorrhea Method (LAM)

What Is the Lactational Amenorrhea Method (Lam) of Family Planning?

LAM is a contraceptive method that is based on the natural postpartum infertility that occurs when a woman is amenorrheic and fully breastfeeding.

How Does LAM Work? (Mechanism of Action)

The infant's suckling suppresses the production of the hormones that are necessary for ovulation. Without ovulation, pregnancy cannot take place.

Who Can Use LAM?

Women who have all three of the following criteria present:
- Exclusively or almost exclusively breastfeeding
- Have not had menses since giving birth
- Are less than six months postpartum

To use LAM, a woman should breastfeed:
- Soon after delivery
- Frequently, upon request, not on schedule
- Without bottles or pacifiers
- Without long intervals between feeds, both day and night
- Without supplementation
- Even when mother and/or baby are ill

Advantages

- Highly effective (at least 98%)
- Easy to use
- Begins immediately postpartum
- No supplies required
- Does not interfere with intercourse
- No side effects
- Has health benefits for mother and infant
- Builds on established cultural and religious practices

Disadvantages

- Not an option for women who do not breastfeed
- Breastfeeding pattern may be difficult to maintain
- Duration of method limited
- No protection against STDs/HIV

Follow-up and Counseling

- Initial counseling involves detailed instructions on how to establish optimal breastfeeding practices and how to ensure effectiveness of LAM
- Help women choose another method of contraception and provide it to them before LAM expires

Section 22.2

Is Breastfeeding an Effective Contraceptive?

Is breastfeeding an effective contraceptive? Research has shown that breastfeeding suppresses fertility. Yet many women know someone who became pregnant when breastfeeding—or became pregnant themselves during breastfeeding. Service providers are sometimes reluctant to allow women to rely on breastfeeding for pregnancy protection, and have in certain settings discouraged breastfeeding in favor of initiating a modern method of contraception.

In 1988, a group of scientists met in Bellagio, Italy, to define a set of guidelines that a woman could use to predict her return to fertility during breastfeeding. The scientists reviewed data from studies regarding return to fertility and determined that breastfeeding can provide up to 98% effective contraception if three criteria are met:

- The mother has not experienced the return of her menstrual periods (bleeding up to the 56th postpartum day is considered part of the postpartum recovery process and is not counted as menstrual bleeding);

- The mother is fully or nearly fully breastfeeding; and

- The baby is less than six months old.

These guidelines later defined a new method of family planning called the Lactational Amenorrhea Method or LAM. Recent clinical trials and a new 1995 Consensus Statement have shown that LAM is

Efficacy of LAM Reported from Several Clinical Trials

Country	Number of Women Studied	Number of Pregnancies	LAM Failure Rate
Chile	422	1	0.45%
Pakistan	391	1	0.58%
Philippines	485	2	0.96%

at least as effective as the Bellagio scientists predicted it would be. Fewer than 1% of LAM users in three clinical trials became pregnant when all the three LAM criteria were met.

Of the three LAM criteria, the return of menses is the most important indicator of fertility. The studies conducted by Family Health International in Pakistan and the Philippines have shown that pregnancy is rare even beyond six months and the end of full breastfeeding among women who do not experience vaginal bleeding. Only 1.1% of the women in Pakistan and 2.6% of the women in the Philippines conceived during 12 months of lactational amenorrhea.

The pattern of breastfeeding exerts a strong effect on the resumption of menstruation and fertility. However, defining what is meant by "full" breastfeeding can be difficult. The following definitions are currently being used by family planning counselors who are teaching LAM:

- Full breastfeeding can be *exclusive* (no other liquid or solid is given to the infant) or *almost exclusive* (vitamins, water, juice, or ritualistic feeds are given infrequently to the infant).

- Nearly full breastfeeding means that the vast majority of feeds (at least 85%) are breastfeeds. There can be some supplementation with another liquid or food, but supplementation never replaces or delays a breastfeed.

A mother can maximize the contraceptive effect she receives from breastfeeding by following the guidelines for optimal breastfeeding behaviors.

The Lactational Amenorrhea Method is, however, a temporary method of family planning. To continue effective pregnancy protection, a woman who uses LAM must be ready to switch to another family planning method when any one of the LAM criteria changes. She should be made aware that:

- Once her periods return, breastfeeding will no longer protect her from a new pregnancy. She should consider any vaginal bleeding (after the 56th postpartum day) to be a warning that her fertility is returning, even if that bleeding does not resemble her regular menses.

- If she starts to give the infant any food or drink on a regular basis or experiences disruptions in her breastfeeding routine, such as returning to work or ceasing to breastfeed at night, she is no longer protected from pregnancy.

- Once the infant is older than six months, the chance of becoming pregnant, even before her periods return, is increased.

If any of these changes occur, a woman should choose another contraceptive method if she wants to be protected from pregnancy. There is no need to discontinue breastfeeding, however. Family planning methods that are recommended for breastfeeding women include barrier methods, IUDs, male or female sterilization, and hormonal methods that contain only progestin, such as progestin-only pills ("minipills"), injectables, and Norplant®. Contraceptive pills containing both estrogen and progestin (the most common kind of birth control pill) have been associated with reduced breastmilk production and should be considered a last-choice method.

Optimal Breastfeeding Behaviors for Child Health and Child Spacing

- Begin breastfeeding as soon as possible after the child is born.
- Breastfeed exclusively for the first six months.
- After the first six months, when supplemental foods are introduced, breastfeeding should precede supplemental feedings.
- Breastfeed frequently, whenever the infant is hungry, day and night.
- Continue breastfeeding even if the mother or the baby become ill.
- Avoid using a bottle, pacifiers or other artificial nipples.
- Continue to breastfeed up to two years and beyond.
- Eat and drink sufficient quantities to satisfy the mother's hunger.

Conclusions

Breastfeeding is best for both mothers and babies and should be encouraged. Breastfeeding can also provide natural, safe, effective contraceptive protection, if certain conditions are met, for up to six months postpartum. Women who are interested in using the natural protection of breastfeeding should have access to information about LAM and about other available family planning methods suitable for breastfeeding women.

Part Five:

Barrier Methods of Contraception

Chapter 23

Male Condoms

Chapter Contents

Section 23.1

The Condom

The sex drive is one of the most powerful in human nature. It is normal to want to enhance intimacy and love by having sex. And it is normal to want to have sex without causing pregnancy—and without getting a sexually transmitted infection.

The only foolproof way to avoid pregnancy is not to do anything that could bring semen in contact with the vagina or vulva.

The only foolproof way to avoid sexually transmitted infections (STIs) is not to be sexually intimate with anyone.

The condom helps women and men express themselves sexually and responsibly by greatly lowering the risk of unintended pregnancy and sexually transmitted infection.

What It Is

A condom is a sheath that fits over the penis. It is made of latex, plastic, or animal tissue. It is also called a rubber, safe, or jimmy. It catches semen before, during, and after a man ejaculates ("comes"). Some condoms have a nipple-shaped tip to hold the semen—others do not.

What It Is for and How Well It Works

The condom makes sex safer. It protects both partners during vaginal, anal, and oral intercourse.

The Condom Prevents Pregnancy

It prevents sperm from entering the vagina. Of 100 women whose partners use condoms, about 12 will become pregnant during the first year of typical use. ("Typical use" refers to failure rates for women and men whose condom use is not consistent or always correct.) Only two will become pregnant with perfect use. ("Perfect use" refers to failure rates for women and men whose condom use is consistent and always correct.)

More protection is possible if contraceptive foams, creams, jellies, films, or suppositories are also used. They can immobilize sperm if the condom breaks. Some condoms are coated with spermicide like nonoxynol-9, which is used in many vaginal contraceptives to increase effectiveness in preventing pregnancy.

The Latex Condom Protects Against Many Sexually Transmitted Infections (STIs), Including HIV—the Human Immunodeficiency Virus That Can Cause AIDs

The latex condom offers better protection against STIs than any other birth control method. It blocks exchange of body fluids that may be infected.

Condoms Work!

In a 1987–91 study of couples in which one partner had HIV, all 123 couples who used condoms every time for four years prevented transmission of HIV. In 122 couples who did not use condoms every time, 12 partners became infected.

A similar 1993 study showed that using condoms every time prevented HIV transmission for all but two of 171 women who had male partners with HIV. However, eight out of ten women whose partners didn't use condoms every time became infected.

Latex condoms offer good protection against:

- vaginitis caused by infections like trichomoniasis and bacterial vaginosis
- pelvic inflammatory disease (PID)
- gonorrhea
- chlamydia
- syphilis
- chancroid
- human immunodeficiency virus.

Latex condoms also offer some protection against:

- human papilloma virus (HPV) that can cause genital warts
- herpes simplex virus (HSV) that can cause genital herpes
- hepatitis-B virus.

Latex condoms may even reduce a woman's chance of getting cervical cancer. They offer some protection against the kinds of HPV infections associated with cervical cancer.

Plastic and animal tissue condoms are not recommended for protection against STIs. There have not been sufficient tests of plastic condoms. Some viruses, such as hepatitis-B and HIV, may be small enough to pass through the pores of animal tissue.

The Pill, IUD, Norplant®, Depo-Provera®, vasectomy, and tubal sterilization offer greater protection against pregnancy than condoms, but no protection against STIs. Many people use latex condoms along with these and other methods for the best protection against both pregnancy and STIs.

How to Use Condoms

Handle condoms gently. Store them in a cool, dry place. Long exposure to air, heat, and light makes them more breakable. Do not stash them continually in a back pocket, wallet, or glove compartment.

Use lubricant inside and outside the condom. (Many condoms are pre-lubricated.) Lubrication helps prevent rips and tears, and it increases sensitivity. Use only water-based lubricants, such as K-Y® jelly, with latex condoms. Oil-based lubricants like petroleum jelly, cold cream, butter, or mineral and vegetable oils damage latex.

Putting On a Condom

For pleasure, ease, and effectiveness, both partners should know how to put on and use a condom. To learn without feeling pressured or embarrassed, practice on your penis or a penis-shaped object like a ketchup bottle, banana, cucumber, or squash.

Remember: Practice Makes Perfect

Put the condom on before the penis touches the vulva. Men leak fluids from their penises before and after ejaculation. Pre-ejaculate ("pre-cum") can carry enough sperm to cause pregnancy. It can also carry enough germs to cause STIs.

Use a condom only once. Use a fresh one for each erection ("hard-on"). Have a good supply on hand.

Condoms usually come rolled into a ring shape. They are individually sealed in aluminum foil or plastic. Be careful—don't tear the condom while unwrapping it. If it is brittle, stiff, or sticky, throw it away and use another.

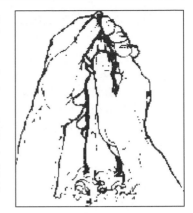

- Put a drop or two of lubricant inside the condom.
- Place the rolled condom over the tip of the hard penis.
- Leave a half-inch space at the tip to collect semen.
- If not circumcised, pull back the foreskin before rolling on the condom.
- Pinch the air out of the tip with one hand. (Friction against air bubbles causes most condom breaks.)

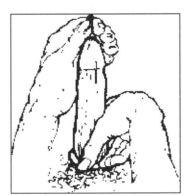

- Unroll the condom over the penis with the other hand.
- Roll it all the way down to the base of the penis.
- Smooth out any air bubbles.
- Lubricate the outside of the condom.

Taking Off a Condom

- Pull out before the penis softens.
- Don't spill the semen—hold the condom against the base of the penis while you pull out.
- Throw the condom away.
- Wash the penis with soap and water before embracing again.

If a Condom Breaks...

- ...during intercourse, pull out quickly and replace it. Men should be able to tell if a condom breaks during intercourse. To learn what it feels like, men can break condoms on purpose while masturbating.
- ...and semen leaks out, wash the semen away with soap and water.
- ...and semen leaks into the vagina during a woman's fertile period, ask a reproductive health clinician for information about emergency contraception.

Don't Let Embarrassment Become a Health Risk

Nearly as many women as men buy and carry condoms. And many people use them—every time they have sexual intercourse. If you are embarrassed to talk with your partner about using condoms, practice before you are in a sexual situation. Then, choose the right time to talk—don't wait until the heat of passion takes over. It may overwhelm your good intentions.

Don't be shy—be direct. Be honest about your feelings and needs. Talking with your partner about using condoms makes it easier for you both. It can help create a relaxed mood to make sex more enjoyable.

It may be difficult to talk about using condoms. It will be easier if you are in a loving relationship that makes you feel happy and good about yourself and your partner. In any case, don't let embarrassment become a health risk.

Don't Be Afraid of Being Rejected.

Remember, when people are given the choice of intercourse with a condom or no intercourse at all, most people will choose to use a condom. Besides, the partner who doesn't care about protecting your health and well-being is not worth your sexual involvement.

Benefits of Condom Use

- Condoms let men help prevent pregnancy.
- Condoms let men help prevent sexually transmitted infections.
- Condoms are easy to get.
- Condoms are inexpensive.
- Condoms are lightweight and disposable.
- Condom use does not need medical supervision.
- Condoms may help a man stay erect longer.

Disadvantages of the Condom

- Condom use requires high motivation and a strong sense of responsibility.
- Condom use may interrupt sex play.
- Condoms may dull sensation for either partner.

Side Effects of Condoms

Condoms have no side effects except for people who are allergic to rubber. Five to 7 percent of women and men have such allergies. They may use animal tissue or plastic condoms instead. Although animal tissue and plastic may not protect as well as latex against viruses like HSV, HPV, HIV, and hepatitis-B, they do offer some protection.

Sex Play, Pleasure, and the Condom

Many women and men say they have better sex when they use condoms. They are able to focus on their sexual pleasure without distractions about unintended pregnancy and STIs. Some couples put the condom on as part of their foreplay. Many men stay hard longer when they use condoms.

However, other men and women feel that the condom dulls sensation. Others become frustrated and lose some of their sexual excitement when they stop to put on a condom.

Some men are self-conscious about using condoms. They feel pressured about having to maintain an erection to keep the condom on.

Others feel pressured to ejaculate. Many overcome these pressures and learn to enjoy using condoms by using them during sex play before intercourse.

The Condom and Vaginal Contraceptives

Vaginal contraceptives are chemical and barrier methods of birth control. They include contraceptive foams, creams, jellies, films, suppositories, diaphragms, and cervical caps.

If you use the condom with any of these methods, you will greatly increase your protection against pregnancy. Read the directions in packages of over-the-counter methods. Diaphragms and cervical caps are fitted and prescribed by a clinician.

Contraceptive foam is often used with condoms. It increases protection against pregnancy. Apply before intercourse and immediately again if a condom breaks.

The Vaginal Pouch

The vaginal pouch, or "female condom," is the newest barrier method for women. The pouch fits inside the vagina like the diaphragm and also covers the vulva. It has the advantage of not requiring a man to maintain an erection during use. Although it is not as effective as the condom, the vaginal pouch is a valuable option for women who want to prevent sexually transmitted infection or unintended pregnancy.

Choosing and Buying a Condom

All condoms are tested for defects. But, like rubber bands, condoms deteriorate with age. If properly stored, condoms can be used five years after the date of manufacture or until the expiration date that is printed on the wrapper of each condom.

Condoms may be transparent or opaque, tinted, nipple-ended, rippled, studded, contoured, dry, powdered, or lubricated, with spermicide or without. Read labels on "novelty" condoms to be sure they protect against pregnancy and sexually transmitted infections.

Usually, size is not marked on the package. But condoms come in different lengths, widths, and thickness. Try different brands and styles to find out which fits best.

Condoms are usually available in packages of three or a dozen. Plain, nonlubricated condoms can cost as little as 20 to 30 cents each. Other styles and brands can cost from 60 cents to $2.50 each. For lubricated condoms, the average price per dozen is about $6. Animal tissue and plastic condoms cost about $25 per dozen.

You can get condoms in drugstores and drug departments of other stores. They also are available in Planned Parenthood health centers and other family planning clinics where they may be less expensive or free. Many drugstores display condoms and vaginal contraceptives. If they are not in sight, ask for them.

Don't be embarrassed by the thought of going into a store and asking for condoms. Be proud. Buying condoms says that you are responsible and that you accept your sexuality as a normal part of living.

HIV Risk Comparisons

HIV is the most deadly STI. Sex partners who want to avoid HIV must practice "safer sex."

"Safer-sex" activities lower our risk of exchanging blood or semen—the body fluids most likely to spread HIV.

Each of us must decide what risks we will take for sexual pleasure. Here are some common sex behaviors grouped according to relative risk.

Very Low Risk
No reported cases due to these behaviors:
- Masturbation—mutual masturbation
- Touching—massage
- Erotic massage—body rubbing
- Kissing—deep kissing
- Oral sex on a man with a condom
- Oral sex on a woman with a dental dam, plastic wrap, or cut-open condom (Don't worry about getting vaginal secretions, menstrual flow, urine, or semen on unbroken skin away from the vulva.)

Low Risk
Rare reported cases due to these behaviors:
- Oral sex
- Vaginal intercourse with a condom or vaginal pouch

- Anal intercourse with a condom or vaginal pouch
- (Try not to get semen or blood into the mouth or on broken skin.)

High Risk
Millions of reported cases due to these behaviors:
- Vaginal intercourse without a condom
- Anal intercourse without a condom

Some of the Drugs That Encourage Taking Risks with Sex
- Alcohol
- Speed
- Poppers
- Marijuana
- Cocaine
- Crack
- Ecstasy

Some of the Feelings That Encourage Taking Risks with Sex
- Desire to be swept away
- Fear of losing a partner
- Insecurity
- Shame
- Embarrassment
- Low self-esteem
- Need to be loved
- Anger

Section 23.2

Breakage and Slippage of Male Condoms: What Do We Know?

How frequent is condom breakage/slippage? Recent international research indicates that male condom breakage ranges from 0 to 12 percent, with many of the U.S.-based studies falling in the 2 to 5 percent range. The percent of condoms that slip off the penis during or after intercourse is in a similar range.

A Family Health International (FHI) study has shown that most condom users rarely experience condom breakage and/or slippage. A small group of users is often responsible for a majority of the breaks and slips. In the study, 177 couples used 1,947 condoms and reported a combined breakage/slippage rate of 8.7 percent. If every couple were equally likely to experience condom breakage/slippage, then each couple would have been expected to have about 1 out of 11 condoms either break or slip off. However, in this study, 16 couples (less than 10 percent of participants) were responsible for 50 percent of all the breakage/slippage. Well over half the couples did not experience any condom breakage/slippage among the 11 condoms each couple used.

Observed vs. Expected Number of Condom Breakage/Slippage 177 Couples

Number per Couples	Observed # of Couples	Expected # of Couples
0	110	65
1	26	68
2	17	33
3	8	9
4+	16	2

In this study, four factors for men were significantly associated with increased condom breakage and slippage:

- no condom experience in the past year;
- condom breakage in the past year;
- not living with partner;
- 12 or fewer years of schooling.

Several other reasons for condom failure have been mentioned in the literature:

- opening the package with sharp objects or teeth;
- incorrect methods of putting on the condom, such as pulling it on like a sock;
- use of oil-based lubricant;
- lengthy and vigorous intercourse;
- using condoms for non-vaginal intercourse;
- not holding rim of condom during withdrawal;
- re-use of condoms.

In addition to presenting overall percentages of breakage and slippage, it also may be informative to present their distribution among study participants (i.e., the percentage of users with no breaks, the percentage with one break, etc.). This illustrates that for a majority of condom users, condom breakage and slippage are rare events.

It is equally important to understand that not all breakage/slippage exposes the condom user to the same risks. Researchers have begun to distinguish between clinical and nonclinical breakage. Clinical breakage occurs when condoms break during intercourse or withdrawal and are the only type of break that directly put the couple at risk of pregnancy and/or sexually transmitted diseases (STD). Nonclinical breaks occur when opening the package and putting on the condom and do not expose the couple to pregnancy or STD. In a recent review of ten FHI condom studies, about one-third of the breaks were classified as nonclinical.

Although the condom literature mentions relatively high breakage and slippage rates, it is important to remember that:

- these rates may be caused by certain behaviors and certain characteristics of a very small proportion of users;

- about one-third of the breaks do not put the users at risk of pregnancy and disease transmission because they occur prior to intercourse.

Condoms are an effective method of preventing pregnancy and sexually transmitted diseases if they are used correctly and consistently during each act of intercourse. The dissemination of condom use instructions must be a high priority in service delivery programs to assure that maximum protection is provided by the use of condoms.

Condom Instructions

A multitude of condom instructions have been developed over the years by various organizations. The following instructions are based on recent FHI research findings.

Follow These Guidelines for Proper Use
- Carefully open package so condom does not tear.
- Do not unroll condom before putting it on.
- Put the condom on end of hard penis.
- Unroll condom until it covers all of penis.
- Always put condom on before entering partner.
- After ejaculation (coming), hold rim of condom and pull penis out before penis gets soft.
- Slide condom off without spilling liquid (semen or come) inside.
- Throw away or bury condom.

Other Considerations
- Do not use grease, oils, lotions or petroleum jelly to make condoms slippery, only use a jelly or cream that does not have oil in it.
- Use a condom each time you have sex.
- Use a condom only once.
- Store condoms in a cool, dry place.

- Do not use condoms that may be old or damaged; do not use a condom if:
  — the package is broken
  — the condom is brittle or dried out
  — the color is uneven or changed
  — it is unusually sticky

Chapter 24

Female Condoms

—*by Robert A. Hatcher, M.D., M.P.H.,*
Emory University School of Medicine

What Is the Female Condom?

Reality female condoms are made of a thin plastic called polyurethane. This is NOT latex or rubber. The condom is placed in the woman's vagina. It is open at one end and closed at the other. Both ends have a flexible ring used to keep the condom in place. Among typical couples who initiate the use of Reality condoms, about 21% will experience an accidental pregnancy in the first year. If these condoms are used consistently and correctly, about 5% will become pregnant.

Advantages

- Female condoms give women more control and a sense of freedom.
- Women don't need to see a clinician to get it. No prescription or fitting is necessary.
- It can be inserted several hours in advance.

"The Reality Female Condom: A Condom for Women," Emory University School of Medicine, updated August 5, 1997; undated graphic from Family Health International (FHI). Available at http://www.emory.edu/WHSC/MED/FAMPLAN/reality.html; reprinted with permission.

- The female condom is safe and fairly effective at preventing both pregnancy and infection.
- Your partner can insert it and make it part of love-making.
- Any lubricant can be used with the female condom (including oil-based lubricants) since it is made of plastic rather than latex. Lubricant is provided in the package.
- Polyurethane transmits heat well. This may make sex more fun.
- The female condom can be used if either partner is allergic to latex.

Disadvantages

- The female condom is large and some feel it is unattractive or odd-looking. Although it looks different and may appear unusual at first, its size and shape allow it to protect a greater area. Many of the couples who have used it like the way it feels.
- Some women may not want to touch their own vagina.
- It will not work if the man's penis is placed outside the female condom (between the condom and the woman's vagina).
- It may make rustling noises prior to or during intercourse. Using a lubricant may decrease noises.
- It takes practice to use it correctly. Some people complain that it is hard to use.
- Female condoms are not sold in as many stores as male condoms. They may be hard to find, so call the store in advance.
- Female condoms are about three times more expensive than male condoms.

Where Can I Get Reality Female Condoms?

- Reality female condoms are sold at most drugstores and some supermarkets. Call in advance to be sure.
- Female condoms are sold in packs of three or six. Each condom costs $2 to $3.
- The package comes with a leaflet that explains how to use female condoms.

- To learn more about the Reality condom, speak with your clinician or call 1-800-274-6601.

- The Female Health Company, which manufactures the Reality female condom, has its own website which you can access for more information: http://www.femalehealth.com.

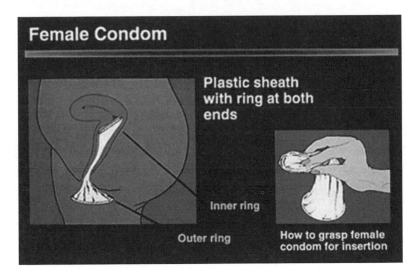

Female Condom

Plastic sheath with ring at both ends

Inner ring

Outer ring

How to grasp female condom for insertion

Chapter 25

Spermicides

What Is a Spermicide?

A spermicide is a chemical agent (Nonoxynol-9 or Octoxynol-9) which kills the sperm inside the vagina before it can get through the uterus to fertilize an egg. Spermicides are 79% effective. Their effectiveness increases to 97% when used along with a barrier method such as a condom, diaphragm, or cervical cap. Spermicides come in lots of different forms: jellies and creams, foams, suppositories, and film. Spermicides can be inserted up to 1 hour before intercourse and must be reapplied before each encounter. Do not douche after sex when using a spermicide. It takes 6–8 hours for the spermicide to kill the sperm, so it must be left inside the body.

How to Use Spermicide

Foam: Shake the can well. Place the applicator on top of the can and press down. The plunger will rise as the applicator fills. Insert the applicator two or three inches into your vagina and depress plunger. With plunger still depressed, remove applicator. Wash the applicator with soap and water.

Cream/jelly: Insert cream or jelly into the vagina using an applicator similar to a foam applicator. Some manufacturers sell single-use applicators which can be handy for travel and dates. Creams are opaque and jellies are clear; otherwise there is little difference.

Film: Remove film square from wrapper and fold in half. Fold it in half again over your finger. Insert your finger into your vagina and deposit the film over your cervix. Your finger must be dry to start with and you must insert it quickly, otherwise it will stick to your finger and come back out when you remove your finger.

Suppository: Remove suppository from wrapper. Using your index finger, insert deep into the vagina near the cervix. Wait at least 10 minutes before having intercourse.

What Are the Advantages?

- Easy to use
- No hormonal side effects
- Inexpensive
- Available without prescription at your local retail store
- Acts as a lubricant
- May protect against some sexually transmitted diseases

What Are the Disadvantages?

- Possible allergic reaction (burning or rash)
- Interrupts sex play
- Can be messy
- May taste bitter or have a strong smell, making oral sex less enjoyable after application

Chapter 26

Diaphragms and Cervical Caps

Diaphragms and cervical caps are soft rubber barriers that cover the cervix. Both must be used with a spermicide cream or jelly. The diaphragm is a shallow, dome-shaped cup with a flexible rim. It fits in the vagina and over the cervix. The cervical cap is thimble-shaped and smaller than the diaphragm. It fits snugly onto the cervix.

How They Work

Diaphragms and caps keep sperm from joining the egg.

- They block the opening to the uterus and prevent sperm from entering.
- The contraceptive cream or jelly applied to the diaphragm or cap immobilizes sperm.

How Well They Work

Of 100 women using diaphragms or cervical caps, about 18 will become pregnant during the first year of use. Of 100 women who use them correctly and consistently, about six will become pregnant in the first year of use.

PPFA Web Site © 1998, Planned Parenthood® Federation of America, Inc.; available at http://www.plannedparenthood.org/BIRTH-CONTROL/ DIAPHRAGMS.HTM; reprinted with permission.

Protection may be increased by:

- checking that the diaphragm or cap covers the cervix before vaginal intercourse every time
- using a fresh application of contraceptive cream or jelly if intercourse is repeated
- using a condom.

How to Get Them

A pelvic examination by a clinician is needed to determine the correct size. The clinician will also provide instruction for use, insertion, and removal. Most women can be fitted with diaphragms or cervical caps.

Diaphragms are available in a wide variety of sizes. A different size diaphragm may be needed after:

- a full-term pregnancy
- abdominal or pelvic surgery
- miscarriage or abortion after 14 weeks of pregnancy
- weight gain or loss of 10 pounds or more.

Cervical caps are available in only four sizes. They also need to be refitted in some of the circumstances listed above.

Women should have pelvic examinations once a year. During these examinations the diaphragm or cervical cap can be checked for wear and size.

Some Conditions That May Rule Out the Use of Diaphragms

- poor vaginal muscle tone
- tipped or sagging uterus
- vaginal obstructions
- history of toxic shock syndrome
- recurrent urinary tract infections.

Some Conditions That May Rule Out Use of Cervical Caps

- correct size unavailable
- insertion too difficult for some women
- abnormal Pap test
- history of toxic shock syndrome
- presence of sexually transmitted or reproductive tract infection
- inflammation of the cervix.

Advantages

Diaphragms and cervical caps offer some protection against certain sexually transmitted infections, including gonorrhea and chlamydia.

- They offer some protection against pelvic inflammatory disease (PID).
- The diaphragm may reduce the risk of developing cervical cancer.
- They do not interrupt sex play if inserted ahead of time.
- They generally cannot be felt by either partner.
- They can be carried conveniently in pocket or purse.

Disadvantages

- It may be difficult for some women to insert diaphragms or cervical caps.
- A woman must be willing to insert the diaphragm or cap every time she has vaginal intercourse.
- Diaphragms require refitting every year or two to see if a different size is needed.
- Diaphragms may become dislodged if the woman is on top during intercourse.

Possible Side Effects

Some women who use diaphragms develop frequent bladder infections. Those who do may: have their clinician check the fit of the diaphragm; urinate before inserting the diaphragm; urinate after intercourse.

Rare cases of toxic shock syndrome (TSS) have been reported with diaphragm use. The symptoms of TSS include: sudden high fever; diarrhea, vomiting; sore throat, aching muscles and joints; dizziness, faintness, weakness; a sunburn-type rash.

If such symptoms occur, remove the diaphragm or cap and contact your clinician.

Rarely, abnormal cell growth may occur in the cervix during the first few months of cap use. This condition usually corrects itself, but sometimes requires medical treatment. Women who are allergic to rubber may not be able to use the diaphragm or cervical cap. Those who experience mild allergic reactions to the contraceptive jelly or cream may switch brands to try to clear up the problem.

Check with your clinician if any of the following symptoms occur:

- discomfort when the diaphragm or cap is in place
- burning sensations while urinating
- irritation or itching in the genital area
- unusual discharge from the vagina
- irregular spotting or bleeding.

How to Use the Diaphragm

- Insert up to six hours before intercourse.
- Put about a teaspoonful of contraceptive cream or jelly in the cup and spread some around the rim. (Never use Vaseline or cold cream. They damage rubber and do not kill sperm.)
- Find a comfortable position—stand with one foot on a chair, sit on the edge of a chair, lie down, or squat.
- Separate the labia with one hand and, with the other, pinch the rim of the diaphragm to fold it in half. Place index finger in center of fold for a firmer grip. The contraceptive cream or jelly must be inside the fold.

- Push as far up and back in the vagina as possible, tuck behind the pubic bone, and make sure the cervix is covered.

It may be inserted several hours in advance of vaginal intercourse and must stay in place six to eight hours after the last intercourse.

- If intercourse is repeated or occurs more than six hours after insertion, leave the diaphragm in place and insert another application of contraceptive cream, jelly, or foam into the vagina.
- To remove, hook a finger over the top of the rim to break the suction; then pull the diaphragm down and out.
- Do not leave the diaphragm in place for more than 24 hours.
- Women who have difficulty inserting the diaphragm may need to use a special inserter to help with correct placement and removal.
- Do not use during vaginal bleeding.

How to Use the Cervical Cap

- Fill the dome of the cap 1/3 full of spermicide.
- Find a comfortable position—stand with one foot on a chair, sit on the edge of a chair, lie down, or squat.
- Locate your cervix.
- Separate the labia with one hand and squeeze the cap rim together with the other.
- Hold the cap dome side down, slide it into the vagina, and push it up and onto the cervix.
- Press the rim into place on the cervix, pinch the rounded end to create suction, then twist the cap like the lid of a jar.
- Sweep a finger around the cap to make sure the cervix is completely covered and there are no gaps.
- The cap must stay in place eight hours after the last intercourse.
- To remove, push the rim away from the cervix to break the suction and pull the cap out.
- Do not leave the cap in place for longer than 48 hours.
- Do not use during vaginal bleeding.

Practice Makes Perfect

The better a diaphragm or cervical cap fits and is inserted, the better it will stay in place, and the better it will protect against pregnancy. After your fitting, the clinician will watch you insert and remove your diaphragm or cap to be sure you are doing it correctly. Practice inserting and removing it at home, too.

Care of Diaphragms and Cervical Caps

With proper care, diaphragms and caps can last about two years. The FDA suggests that diaphragms and caps be replaced every year.

- After removal, wash with mild soap (no detergents, no perfumed soap) and warm water.
- Let dry in the open air.
- Do not use powders—they can cause infections. Scented powders and oil seed lubricants, like Vaseline, can damage rubber.
- Examine regularly against a light for small holes or weak spots.

Diaphragms and caps can still be used if the rubber becomes discolored. However, if the rubber puckers, especially near the rim, it has become dangerously thin. Pin holes can be spotted by holding the diaphragm up to the light and stretching the rubber gently between the fingers.

Where to Get Them and What They Cost

Visit a private doctor or a family planning clinic for an examination and prescription. Diaphragms and caps may be purchased at a drugstore or clinic. An examination costs from $50 to $120. Diaphragms and caps average from $13 to $25. A kit of spermicide cream or jelly costs from $8 to $17.

Part Six:

Hormonal Methods of Contraception

Chapter 27

Birth Control Pills
(Oral Contraceptives)

Chapter Contents

Section 27.1

You and the Pill

The Basics

"The Pill" is the common name for oral contraception. There are two basic types—combination pills and progestin-only pills. Both are made of hormones like those made by a woman's ovaries—estrogen and progestin. Combination pills contain both hormones. Progestin-only pills contain only progestin. Both kinds of pills require a medical evaluation and prescription.

Both kinds of pills are intended to prevent pregnancy. But they work differently. Combination pills usually work by preventing a woman's ovaries from releasing eggs (ovulation). Progestin-only pills also can prevent ovulation. But they usually work by thickening the cervical mucus. This keeps sperm from joining with an egg. Combination pills also thicken cervical mucus. Both types of pill may also prevent fertilized eggs from implanting in the uterus (womb).

Effectiveness

The Pill is one of the most effective reversible methods of birth control. Of 100 women who use the Pill, only five will become pregnant during the first year of typical use. ("Typical use" refers to failure rates for women whose use is not consistent or always correct.)

Combination pills are somewhat more effective than progestin-only pills. Fewer than one out of 100 women who use combination pills will become pregnant with perfect use. ("Perfect use" refers to failure rates for women whose use is consistent and always correct.) Five out of 100 who use progestin-only pills will become pregnant with perfect use.

Certain medicines, including the antibiotic rifampin and certain drugs used to control seizures, may make the Pill less effective. Vomiting and diarrhea may also keep the Pill from working. Ask your clinician for advice. Until you are sure, use an additional method of birth control.

It is very important to remember that the Pill does not protect against sexually transmitted infections. Use a latex or female condom along with the Pill for protection against STIs.

Getting the Right Pill

You must see a clinician to tell whether you can take the Pill and what dosage is right for you. The clinician will discuss your medical history with you, check your blood pressure, and give you any other medical exam that may be needed.

If the Pill is right for you, you likely will be given the lowest amount of hormone needed to protect you against pregnancy. Your clinician will adjust the prescription if you continue to experience side effects after a few months. Be sure to have checkups at least once a year. Your prescription may need to be changed as your health needs change. See your clinician right away if any problem develops.

Remember to tell any other clinician you may see that you take the Pill.

The Cost

The cost of an examination by a private doctor may range from $50 to $125. Family planning clinics usually charge according to your income. Pills vary in price depending on the type and brand. A prescription filled at a drugstore costs about $20–$35 a month. Pills usually cost less in a clinic.

Conditions That Affect Who Can Use the Pill

Some women cannot take the Pill. These include women who:
- smoke more than 15 cigarettes a day and are 35 or older
- have high blood pressure
- have had blood clots or inflammation of the veins
- have unexplained bleeding from the vagina
- have had an abnormal growth or cancer of the breast or uterus
- have very high cholesterol levels
- have a severe liver disease or have had growths of the liver

- certain conditions associated with diabetes mellitus
- think they might be pregnant

Some women may be advised to take the Pill under close medical supervision because they are very overweight or have:

- a high risk for heart disease
- slightly high cholesterol or slightly increased blood pressure
- migraine headaches
- a seizure disorder that requires taking anticonvulsant medication
- had diabetes—including diabetes associated with pregnancy
- a skin cancer called malignant melanoma
- a certain cancer of the nervous system called meningioma

For most women with these conditions, the risk of pregnancy is far greater than the risks associated with taking the Pill.

Women with a history of depression may not be able to continue to take the Pill if it worsens the problem.

Some Benefits

Taking the Pill is simple and convenient. Many women who take the Pill have more regular, lighter, and shorter periods.

The Pill does not interfere with having sex. Many women say the Pill has improved their sex lives. They say they are free to be more spontaneous and do not have to worry about becoming pregnant.

The Pill offers many health benefits, including some protection against:

- infection of the fallopian tubes (pelvic inflammatory disease), which commonly leads to infertility
- ectopic pregnancy
- non-cancerous breast growths
- ovarian cysts
- cancer of the ovaries
- cancer of the lining of the uterus
- troublesome menstrual cramps
- iron deficiency anemia that results from heavy menses

- rheumatoid arthritis
- acne

In fact, protection against developing cancer of the ovary or the lining of the uterus can last up to 15 years after stopping the Pill. Protection against endometrial cancer increases with each year of use—women who use the Pill for eight years reduce their risk of getting endometrial cancer by up to 80 percent.

Some Risks

As with all drugs, there may be some undesirable side effects for some women taking the Pill. However, the Pill is much safer than pregnancy and childbirth for healthy women—except among smokers age 35 and older.

Some side effects that usually clear up after two or three months of use include:

- bleeding between periods
- weight gain or loss
- breast tenderness
- nausea—rarely, vomiting
- depression.

These reactions often clear up in three months. Nausea and vomiting often can be reduced or eliminated by taking the Pill with the evening meal or at bedtime. (Do not stop taking the Pill if you feel sick to your stomach.) Irregular spotting and bleeding happens more frequently with progestin-only pills than with combination pills.

Once in a while, menstruation is irregular or absent for as long as six months after stopping the Pill. This generally occurs if periods were irregular before starting the Pill.

Serious problems do not occur very often. Pill users have a slightly greater chance of certain major disorders than non-users. The most serious is the possibility of blood clots in the legs, lungs, heart, or brain.

Women on the Pill who undergo major surgery seem to have a greater chance of having blood clots. Blood clots in the legs occur with increased frequency for women and men who:

- have one or both legs immobilized
- are confined to their beds.

It is important to stop taking the Pill about four weeks before a scheduled major operation. Do not start again while recuperating or while a leg or arm is in a cast.

Rarely, high blood pressure may develop in women who take the Pill. The rise usually is slight. But it may worsen over time. Stopping the Pill almost always brings blood pressure back to normal. Be sure to have your blood pressure checked after your first three months on the Pill. Have it checked at least once a year after that.

Very rarely, liver tumors, gallstones, and jaundice (yellowing of the skin or eyes) occur in women who take the Pill. Though very rare, liver tumors occur most often in women who have used the Pill five years or more. They usually subside when the Pill is stopped. Occasionally, surgery is required. Most pill-related cases of jaundice and gallstones occur within the first year of use.

In *extremely rare* cases, heart attack or stroke associated with Pill use can threaten life. The chances increase with age among women who have had blood vessel disorders or who have other health problems. These problems include diabetes, high cholesterol, high blood pressure, and, most of all, smoking. Pill-related risks of heart attack or stroke go away once the Pill is stopped.

Heavy smoking (more than 15 cigarettes a day) is the greatest risk factor related to taking the Pill. Women over 35 must not smoke and take the Pill.

If the Pill is stopped to solve these or other such problems, another method of birth control must be used to prevent pregnancy.

More detailed information about the use and risks of the Pill is provided in an insert included with each pill pack.

Most experts agree that taking the Pill does not increase the overall risk of developing breast cancer—no matter how long a woman takes the Pill or even if she has a close relative with breast cancer.

Early Warning Signs

Serious problems usually have warning signs. Watch for them. If one occurs, report it to your clinician as soon as possible. These warning signs include:

- sudden or constant pain or redness and swelling in the leg
- pain in the abdomen, chest, or arm
- sudden shortness of breath or spitting up blood
- severe headaches
- eye problems such as blurred or double vision
- worsening depression
- yellowing of the skin or eyes (jaundice)

Staying on Schedule Is Very Important

Correct and consistent use of the Pill increases your protection against pregnancy.

It is very important not to skip pills, even if you:
- have spotting or bleeding between periods
- do not have vaginal intercourse very often

Pills come in monthly packs. Combination pills come in 28-day packs that are taken without interruption. The first 21 pills in the pack of combination pills are called "active"—they contain hormones that prevent pregnancy. The last seven pills in the pack of combination pills are called "reminder" pills. They do not contain hormones. They are taken during the fourth week, including during menstruation.

Combination pills also come in 21-day packs. All 21 of the pills are "active." The pills are taken for three weeks. No reminder pills are taken during the fourth week, when menstruation usually occurs. A new pack of pills is started seven days after the last pack is completed.

Progestin-only pills come only in 28-day packs. All progestin-only pills are "active."

Menstruation usually occurs during the fourth week, no matter which series is used.

Be sure to follow the instructions on the package. Your clinician will explain how to use your pill pack—either the 28-day or 21-day pack.

You will also be advised whether you should start on a Sunday or on the first day of your period.

Taking the Pill at the same time each day makes it more effective. It also helps you remember to stay on schedule. Pick a time of day that will be easy to remember.

If You Are a "Sunday Starter":

- Take the first active pill of the first pack on the Sunday after your period starts—even if you are still bleeding. If your period begins on Sunday, start the pack that same day.

- Continue taking pills daily according to the schedule provided in the pack. If you are using a 28-day pack, take one every day until the pack runs out, then start a new pack on the next day. If you are using a 21-day pack, take one every day until the pack runs out, then take seven days off before starting the next pack.

- Use another method of birth control if you have vaginal inter-course during the first week of pill use—anytime from the Sunday you start your first pack until the next Sunday. Good back-up methods include the latex or female condom, diaphragm or cervical cap, and contraceptive foam, cream, jelly, or film. Protection will begin after seven days and continues as long as the Pill is taken on schedule.

- Twenty-eight-day pack users should start the next pack the day after finishing the previous pack—regardless of when menstruation takes place. Twenty-one-day pack users should start the next pack seven days after finishing the previous pack.

If You Are a "First-Day Starter":

- Take the first active pill of the first pack during the first 24 hours of your period.

- You will not need to use a back-up method of birth control. You are protected against pregnancy immediately. Protection continues as long as the Pill is taken on schedule.

What to Do If You Forget...

If you forget ONE active combination pill: Take it as soon as you remember. Take the next pill at the usual time. (This means you may take two pills in one day.) Finish that series and start the next pack on time.

If you forget TWO active combination pills in a row in the first two weeks: Take two pills on the day you remember. Then take two pills on the next day. Take one pill every day until the pack is finished. Use a back-up method for seven days after the pills are skipped. Call your clinician if you do not get your period.

If you forget TWO active combination pills in a row in the third week—or you forget THREE or more active combination pills in a row during the first three weeks:

"Sunday Starters"

Take one active pill every day until the next Sunday. Throw away the rest of the pack and start a new pack the same day (Sunday). Use a back-up method for seven days after the pills are skipped. You may not have your period this month, but this is expected. Call your clinician if you do not get your period two months in a row.

"First-Day Starters"

Throw away the rest of the pack. Start a new pack the same day. Use a back-up method for seven days after the pills are skipped. You may not have your period this month, but this is expected.

Call your clinician if you do not get your period two months in a row.

If you forget ANY of the seven reminder pills in the fourth week: Throw away the pills you missed. Take one of the remaining reminder pills each day until the pack is empty. Start the next pack on time.

If you forget EVEN ONE progestin-only pill: Take it as soon as you remember. Take the next pill at the usual time. (This means you may take two pills in one day.) Continue to take the rest of the pack on schedule. Use a back-up method of birth control for the rest of the month. Start the next pack on time.

If you are still not sure what to do about the pills you have missed: Use a back-up method anytime you have vaginal intercourse. Take one active pill each day until you can talk with your clinician.

Missing pills can cause spotting or light bleeding—even if you make up the missed pills. You also may feel a little sick to your stomach when you take two pills to make up for missed pills.

Pregnancy and the Pill

There is a very slight chance that you will become pregnant even if you take the Pill regularly, especially if you vomit, have diarrhea, or take medicines that make the Pill less effective. Talk with your clinician about this.

A missed period does not always mean you are pregnant, especially if you have not skipped any pills. But it is important to see your clinician if you miss a second period. It is unlikely that taking the Pill during early pregnancy will increase the risk of defects in the fetus. However, the likelihood of tubal pregnancy is greater if you become pregnant while taking the progestin-only pill.

If you want to become pregnant, stop taking the Pill. If you want to plan the timing of your pregnancy, use another form of birth control until your period becomes regular. It usually takes about one to three months for periods to become regular.

After childbirth, your clinician can help you decide when to take the Pill again.

Progestin-only pills will not affect your milk during nursing. Combination pills may reduce the amount and quality of milk in the first six weeks of breastfeeding. Also, the milk will contain traces of the Pill's hormones. It is unlikely that these hormones will have any effect on your child.

Emergency Hormonal Contraception

The Pill can also be used for emergency hormonal contraception. Emergency hormonal contraception is designed to prevent pregnancy after unprotected vaginal intercourse. You may decide to use emergency contraception if:

- His condom broke or slipped off, and he ejaculated inside your vagina.

- You forgot to take your birth control pills.
- Your diaphragm or cervical cap slipped out of place, and he ejaculated inside your vagina.
- You miscalculated your "safe" days.
- He didn't pull out in time.
- You weren't using any birth control.
- He forced you to have unprotected vaginal intercourse.

Two increased doses of certain oral contraceptives taken 12 hours apart and within 72 hours of unprotected intercourse are *75% effective*. The closer to ovulation a woman is during unprotected intercourse, the less likely the method will succeed. Severe nausea, vomiting, and cramping are likely side effects. Consult your clinician for more information.

Don't use emergency hormonal contraception if you:
- are pregnant from previous intercourse
- have missed your period or it is late
- are allergic to the medication

Consult your clinician about whether you can take emergency hormonal contraception if you are:
- having migraine headaches
- at high risk of having blood clots

Contact your clinician immediately if you have unprotected intercourse when you think you might become pregnant.

Call toll-free, 1-800-230-PLAN for the nearest Planned Parenthood center and ask about emergency contraception.

Section 27.2

What Is the Correct Way to Use Progestin-only Pills (Mini-Pills)?

Family Health International (FHI), revised August 12, 1998; available at http://resevoir.fhi.org/en/fp/fpfaq/fpfaqs/fpfaq53.html; reprinted with permission.

Progestin-only oral contraceptive pills (POPs) have specific advantages over combined oral contraceptives. Because they do not contain estrogen, they are a good contraceptive choice for breastfeeding women and for women with health conditions that preclude use of combined oral contraceptives (containing both estrogen and progestin). Yet POPs are not as well known or as frequently used as the combined estrogen-progestin oral contraceptives. Only 1 to 10 percent of the oral contraceptives sold are POPs. They can be an increasingly valuable part of any family planning program, if providers are well informed about POP characteristics and make sure that their clients know how to take pills correctly.

How Progestin-only Pills Work

Progestin-only oral contraceptives have very low doses of progestin, lower than combined pills. POPs prevent pregnancy in two main ways:

- They prevent ovulation in about half the cycles.

- They cause a thickening of the cervical mucus, which prevents sperm from reaching the egg.

POPs also produce changes in the endometrium so that it becomes less receptive to implantation in the unlikely case that ovulation occurs, and POPs slow the movement of the egg through the fallopian tube.

These multiple mechanisms of action, along with the low doses of progestin required, create most of the advantages, and the few disadvantages, of POPs.

Advantages of Progestin-only Pills

POPs are indicated most strongly for women who prefer oral contraceptives but should not be taking estrogens.

They are especially recommended for:

- breastfeeding mothers;
- women over age 35, including smokers;
- women with hypertension (high blood pressure).

POPs may also be recommended for women with:

- migraine (vascular) headaches;
- thromboembolism;
- cardiovascular disease;
- diabetes;
- sickle cell disease.

Like all progestin-only methods, POPs do not have most of the estrogen-related side effects of oral contraception. For example, the nausea, headaches and other symptoms associated with starting the combined pill are minimal. Side effects of POPs are few. Menstrual irregularities, especially more frequent bleeding, are the most commonly reported side effects. Informing women of this possibility will help allay concerns if such problems develop.

Once POPs are discontinued, fertility returns rapidly. Unlike other progestin-only methods (especially injectables and implants), POPs are inexpensive and user controlled at all times. They can be bought over-the-counter in many countries.

Cautions with POPs

Only three categories of women should not use POPs. These include women with:

- known or suspected pregnancy (as for any drug);
- known or suspected breast cancer;
- undiagnosed abnormal genital bleeding, which could indicate a reproductive tract cancer (or other conditions requiring medical care).

271

POPs must be taken every day, without interruption for bleeding. When a woman takes POPs, her progestin levels build up rapidly after taking a pill, then return to baseline levels in 24 hours. Therefore, POPs should be taken at the same time every day. If a POP is taken three or more hours late, a back-up method of contraception, such as the condom, is needed until 48 hours after pill-taking resumes. Although this means a back-up method may be needed more often for POPs than for combined pills, it is only needed for two days, not seven days as for combined pills.

Ectopic pregnancies, while rare, are more likely to occur among POP users than among women using other contraceptive methods. Symptoms include abdominal pain and amenorrhea.

Specific drugs that may interfere with POPs' effectiveness include most anticonvulsants and rifampicin, used primarily to treat tuberculosis. POPs offer no protection against AIDS and STDs. Therefore, women at risk for AIDS and STDs should consider the use of latex condoms.

Special Advantages of POPs for Breastfeeding Mothers

POPs can be a good contraceptive choice for breastfeeding mothers who wish to use hormonal contraception. Progestins administered alone do not interfere with breastmilk production. Also, because such small amounts enter the infant's system (resulting in infant plasma levels of 1 to 6% of the levels in maternal plasma), no adverse effects on the health, growth, or development of the infant have been found.

In addition, breastfeeding mothers have less need for back-up contraceptive methods. Women who are fully breastfeeding already have the back-up protection of their breastfeeding and, therefore, do not need to use a second back-up method when a single pill is taken late.

Conclusion

POPs are a safe, effective method of contraception. When discussing contraception, providers should inform clients of the special advantages of POPs, including safety for breastfeeding mothers and women who want hormonal contraception but cannot take combined pills. Because these pills must be taken at the same time each day to be effective, counseling clients about correct use is especially important.

Section 27.3

The Pill: When Do I Need a Backup Method?

"The Pill (Oral Contraceptives): When Do I Need a Backup Method?" Virginia Tech University Student Health Service Pharmacy, revised September 1997; available at http://healthed2.shs.vt.edu/pillbackup.html.

What Is a Drug Interaction?

A drug interaction results when someone takes two or more drugs together or within a short time span of one another and an undesired reaction occurs. In fact, a drug's intended effects may be drastically altered when it is combined with other drugs. **Alert!** Alcohol Blood Level/Effect may be increased by "the pill."

Are There Any Drug Interactions with Oral Contraceptives?

Yes, various interactions may occur. You should check with your doctor and pharmacist if you are taking any other prescription or non-prescription medicines.

Are There Any Drugs That May Reduce the Effectiveness of the Pill?

Yes, these include (this list may not be complete, check with your practitioner):

- Laxatives
- Tranquilizers:
  - A.C. w/ Butalbital (Florinal)
  - Belladonna PB (Donnatal)
  - Phenobarbital
  - Phenytoin (Dilantin)
  - Secobarbital (Seconal)
- Antiepileptics:
  - Carbamazepine (Tegretol)
  - Ethosuximide (Zarontin)

273

— Primidone (Mysoline)

- Antibiotics: Reduced effectiveness of "the pill" caused by antibiotics is a rare occurrence. However, several case reports exist where women who were taking their birth control pills regularly become pregnant after taking an antibiotic.

  — Ampicillin (Principen)

  — Griseofulvin (Gris-Peg)

  — Amoxicillin (Amoxil)

  — Isomazid (INH)

  — Cefaclor (Ceclor)

  — Metronidazole (Flagyl)

  — Cephalexin (Keflex)

  — Nitrofurantoin (Macrodantin)

  — Chloramphenicol

  — Oxacillin (Prostaphlin)

  — Clindamycin (Cleocin)

  — Penicillins (Pen Vee K)

  — Co-Trimoxazole (Septra, Bactrim)

  — Rifampin (Rifadin)

  — Dicloxacillin (Dynapen)

  — Sulfisoxazole (Gantrisin)

  — Doxycycline (Vibramycin)

  — Tetracycline (Sumycin)

  — Erythromycin (E-Mycin)

Diarrhea or vomiting also may decrease the effect of "the pill."

What Happens If I Take a Medication or Have Diarrhea/ Vomiting That Reduces the Effectiveness of Oral Contraceptives?

1. Breakthrough bleeding may occur during the particular cycle of pills which may indicate a reduction in the pill's effectiveness.

2. "Pill Failure" or pregnancy has occurred in some women while taking these medications with oral contraceptives.

What Should I Do?

1. Proceed as usual taking "the pill" daily as directed.

2. Use an additional method of birth control such as abstention, or condoms and spermicide, from that point on and through the first 7 days of the next package of oral contraceptives.

3. If you need to take an interfering medication on a long-term basis, be sure to discuss this potential interference with your health care professional.

4. Consider yourself at risk of pregnancy and use the above back-up method procedure. Remember today's lower dosage "pill" (as effective as it might be) leaves no room for mistakes.

Remember: This same procedure applies anytime you miss a pill or take it 4 hours late.

I Am Taking Antibiotics Daily for Acne, Should I Be Careful?

After long-term use of antibiotics (4–6 weeks), it appears that no interaction occurs; however, as with short-term use, one should remember to use an alternate method of birth control for the first month of antibiotic use.

Have Drug Interactions with Oral Contraceptives Always Been a Major Concern?

No, until recently this has not been recognized as a significant problem. In the past, "the pill" contained higher levels of estrogen and progesterone. These active components of "the pill" in high doses intensified the side effect of oral contraceptives. Today, "the pill" contains lower levels of these components to reduce the side effects. Because of this, the effectiveness of birth control pills may be altered more easily.

Are There Drugs Whose Effects May Be Changed by Taking the Pill?

Yes, these include drugs used for the following:
- Seizure Disorders

- Anxiety
- High Blood Pressure
- Asthma
- Diabetes Mellitus
- Depression
- Blood Clotting Disorders

What Should I Do If I Am Taking One of These Drugs and Begin Taking Oral Contraceptives?

If you are taking any of these prescribed medications and begin taking "the pill," you should talk to your health care provider to decide what, if anything, should be done.

Remember

- Be sure to inform anyone prescribing your drugs of any and all other medications that you are also taking (make sure that you tell your dentist if she/he asks). This is especially important if you depend on oral contraceptives for birth control.
- Read your package insert at least once.
- For Prevention of STDs always use **condoms** as back-up method.

Section 27.4

7 Myths about the Pill

Myth #1

I've heard the birth control pill doesn't work very well.

The Truth

Women who take the Pill consistently and correctly—without fail—have less than a one-in-one-hundred chance of becoming pregnant.

Nevertheless, many women hear claims that the Pill is not very effective. They may not know that many women who say they are taking the Pill don't always take it consistently or correctly. Here are the facts:

- Only 28 percent of women always take the Pill correctly.
- Only 42 percent take the Pill every day.
- At least 16 percent have pills left at the end of the month.
- About 25 percent stop using the Pill before a year has passed and do not use another method.
- About 33 percent of teen women missed a pill in a three-month period.
- About 17 percent do not take the pills in the right order.

These are the typical reasons that women become pregnant while "using the Pill."

Myth #2

I've heard that women should "take a rest" from taking the Pill after every nine months.

The Truth

There is no medical reason to take a "rest" from the Pill.

Taking a rest from the Pill is unnecessary because:
- There are no medical benefits.
- Taking a rest from the Pill can lead to unintended pregnancy.
- Discontinuing and restarting the Pill may cause another round of the unpleasant side effects that may be associated with the first few months of Pill use.
- Women who discontinue the Pill sacrifice the non-contraceptive benefits of the Pill.

Myth #3

I've heard that women gain weight when they take the Pill.

The Truth

Some women gain weight while using the Pill. Some women lose weight while using the Pill.
- Hormones in the Pill may cause changes in appetite. These changes occur over several years and may cause some weight loss or gain.
- Some women have temporary fluid retention during the first month or so after starting the Pill.
- Some women gain weight as a side effect of estrogen use. This weight gain develops in the hips, thighs, and breasts. It is usually noticed after several months on the Pill.
- The Pill may aggravate depression for some women. This may lead to increased eating.

Changes in workplace, exercise habits, lifestyle, and diet may also lead to weight gain or loss. It may not be possible to isolate one single cause.

Myth #4

I've heard that the Pill isn't safe.

The Truth

Having a child has twice the risk of death as using the Pill.

Nevertheless, more than 60 percent of women mistakenly believe that oral contraception is more risky or as risky as childbirth.

Myth #5

I've heard that the Pill causes cancer.

The Truth

The Pill protects against cancer of the ovaries and cancer of the lining of the uterus.

Most experts also agree that taking the Pill does not increase the overall risk of developing breast cancer—no matter how long a woman takes the Pill—even if she has a close relative with breast cancer.

Claims that the Pill causes cancer of the liver or cervical cancer have not been proven.

Myth #6

I've heard that the Pill causes heart attack, stroke, and blood clots.

The Truth

There is no increase in the risk of heart attack or stroke among healthy women who use the Pill and who do not smoke.

There is a small increase in the risk of blood clots in the legs and arms. The risk increases from 5–20 per 100,000 women for a year to 15–20 per 100,000 women for a year.

Myth # 7

I've heard that the Pill causes birth defects.

The Truth

The Pill does not cause birth defects or affect the health of future children—even if a woman becomes pregnant while taking the Pill.

Where Do All These Myths Come From?

Some myths come from misunderstandings about side effects and the fact that only some women experience them.

Some myths are rumors started by people and organizations that don't want women to plan their families by using birth control.

Other myths are based on the experience of women who used "old-fashioned" pills that had very high doses of estrogen and progestin.

The first pill was called Enovid®. Its makers wanted to be very certain that it worked. They used what we now know were unnecessarily high levels of hormones. Enovid contained 10 milligrams (10,000 micrograms) of progestin and 150 micrograms of estrogen.

The pills that most women use today have much lower doses. They have only a fraction of those used in the first pill. Today's pill contains from 50–150 micrograms of progestin and 20–35 micrograms of estrogen.

Section 27.5

The Pill Revisited: Benefits Beyond Birth Control

Mayo Clinic Health Oasis, August 13, 1998; originally published in *Mayo Clinic Women's Health Source*, August 1998; © 2000 Mayo Foundation for Medical Education and Research; available at http://www.mayohealth.org/mayo/9808/htm/thepill.htm; reprinted with permission.

What if there were a pill that could stop the hot flashes, night sweats, insomnia, and vaginal dryness which occur in the years leading up to menopause? What if that pill could also cut a woman's risk of several cancers and osteoporosis and eliminate heavy and irregular periods?

That pill—yes, the Pill—not only exists, it's nearing its 40th birthday. Yet, its benefits as a reliever of early menopausal symptoms and a preventive of long-term disease are still virtually unknown to most women. Surveys show that more than half of all women are unaware of the pill's noncontraceptive health benefits, and nearly as many still believe—incorrectly—that taking birth control pills is risky, especially after age 35. It's time to put those misconceptions to rest and gain a broader understanding of the pill's benefits.

The Shrinking Birth Control Pill

Birth control pills have come a long way since they were introduced. The original pill contained about five times more estrogen and ten times more progesterone than today's versions. If you took the pill back then, you probably remember morning sickness-like nausea and feeling as bloated as a Thanksgiving Day parade balloon. You may also remember distressing stories about how the pill caused a dramatic increase in the risk of heart disease if used past the age of 35—a concern that proved to be overblown unless you also happened to be a smoker. It's still true that smoking and the pill don't mix because the combination significantly increases your risk of stroke and heart attack.

Today, because of much lower dosages, most women find the pill far easier to tolerate. Women also have a number of preparations to choose from. Regimens may offer a constant dose of the hormones estrogen and progesterone, increasing doses of estrogen with a constant dose of progesterone, or increasing doses of progesterone with a constant dose of estrogen. If one produces unpleasant side effects, you can try another. But they all offer benefits beyond preventing pregnancy.

Surprising Health Benefits

Your doctor may recommend the pill during what's called perimenopause—when you experience menopausal symptoms that commonly occur in the years before your period stops completely. Or your doctor might prescribe it to help eliminate premenstrual syndrome, painful periods, or acne. What you may not realize, however, is that the pill can also provide other important—even life-saving—health benefits. It can reduce your risk of:

- **Ovarian cancer**—The longer you're on the pill, the greater your protection. After more than ten years on the pill, your risk may be reduced by 60 percent to 80 percent. This protective effect appears to last at least 15 years after you stop using the pill. Researchers theorize that the pill may work in part by inhibiting ovulation.

- **Endometrial (uterine) cancer**—The risk may be reduced by as much as 50 percent. This protection also lasts at least 15 years after you stop taking the pill.

- **Colorectal cancer**—The risk may be reduced by about 35 percent. Researchers believe the protective effect may be due to a reduction in the concentration of bile acids (which help digest fats) in the colon.

- **Pelvic inflammatory disease (PID)**—Although rarely fatal, this infection can lead to infertility from scarring of the fallopian tubes. The pill cuts the risk of PID by half. Doctors believe the pill works by making cervical mucus an unfriendly environment for disease-causing bacteria.

- **Osteoporosis**—The estrogen in the pill protects bones the same way that estrogen in hormone replacement therapy does. So when you take the pill, you strengthen your bones. Then when you enter menopause—a time of accelerated bone loss—you're ahead of the game.

- **Benign ovarian cysts**—Taking the pill for several cycles may be all that's needed to shrink a benign ovarian cyst. The pill also decreases the development of cysts.

The Pill and Breast Cancer—Easing Fears

An analysis of 54 studies conducted in 25 countries found no increased risk of breast cancer ten or more years after women had stopped taking the pill, compared with women who never took it. This was true even for women with a family history of breast cancer.

The analysis did find that women who had never used the pill had a slightly lower incidence of breast cancer than women who were current users and women who had stopped taking the pill within the last ten years. But researchers don't believe the pill caused the cancer. It's more likely that the pill enhances the growth of an existing tumor, rather than initiating a new one.

The Other Side of the Pill

No medication is without risks, but the pill has a far better track record than its reputation indicates, especially since the introduction of low-dose varieties. These risks, though small, are still associated with the pill:

- **Blood clots**—Unless a woman has a history of developing blood clots in her veins, her risk with the pill is very small. At most, it may increase from 1 in 10,000 to 2 in 10,000.
- **Stroke**—The risk while taking the pill is negligible—barely more than not taking the pill at all.
- **Higher blood pressure**—A study in the April 1998 issue of the *Journal of Women's Health* found that postmenopausal women who had taken the pill for five years or less in their lifetimes had slightly increased blood pressures. Their diastolic blood pressures (the second number) were 3.9 millimeters of mercury higher than women who had never taken birth control pills.

Who Shouldn't Take the Pill?

Although the pill is remarkably safe for most women, you shouldn't take it if you:

- Smoke cigarettes, particularly if you're older than 35.
- Have a history of strokes or blood clots.
- Have liver disease.

Talk with your doctor about taking the pill if you have any of these conditions, since there are pros and cons depending on your personal health risks, You may still be able to take the pill if you:

- Have diabetes.

- Have high blood pressure.

- Have risk factors for cardiovascular disease, such as a family history and high cholesterol.

Pill Pluses

The birth control pill isn't just for birth control anymore. After almost four decades of use, doctors now know that this tiny pill is not only safe but packs a powerhouse of good—from treating the annoying symptoms that occur in perimenopausal years to protecting against cancer.

Section 27.6

Oral Contraceptives and Cancer Risk

CancerNet, National Cancer Institute, February 2000; available at http://
cancernet.nci.nih.gov/clinpdq/risk/
Oral_Contraceptives_and_Cancer_Risk.html.

Oral contraceptives (OCs) first became available to American women in the early 1960s. The convenience, effectiveness, and reversibility of action of birth control pills (which are popularly known as "the pill") has made them the most popular form of birth control in the United States. However, a correlation between estrogen and increased risk of breast cancer has led to continuing controversy about a possible link between OCs and cancer.

This section addresses only what is known about OC use and the risk of developing cancer. It does not deal with the most serious side effect of OC use—the increased risk of cardiovascular disease for certain groups of women.

Oral Contraceptives

Currently, two types of OCs are available in the United States. The most commonly prescribed OC contains two synthetic versions of natural female hormones (estrogen and progesterone) that are similar to the hormones the ovaries normally produce. Estrogen stimulates the growth and development of the uterus at puberty, thickens the endometrium (the inner lining of the uterus) during the first half of the menstrual cycle, and stimulates changes in breast tissue at puberty and childbirth. Two types of synthetic estrogens are used in OCs, ethinyl estrachol and mestranol.

Progesterone, which is produced during the last half of the menstrual cycle, prepares the endometrium to receive the egg. If the egg is fertilized, progesterone secretion continues, preventing release of additional eggs from the ovaries. For this reason, progesterone is called the "pregnancy-supporting" hormone, and scientists believe it to have valuable contraceptive effects. The synthetic progesterone used in OCs is called progestogen or progestin. Norethindrone and levonorgestrel are examples of synthetic progesterones used in OCs.

The second type of OC available in the United States is called the minipill and contains only a progestogen. The minipill is less effective in preventing pregnancy than the combination pill, so it is prescribed less often.

Because medical research suggests that cancers of the female reproductive organs sometimes depend on naturally occurring sex hormones for their development and growth, scientists have been investigating a possible link between OC use and cancer risk. Medical researchers have focused a great deal of attention on OC users over the past 30 years. This scrutiny has produced a wealth of data on OC use and the development of certain cancers, although results of these studies have not always been consistent.

Breast Cancer

A woman's risk of developing breast cancer depends on several factors, some of which are related to her natural hormones. Hormonal factors that increase the risk of breast cancer include conditions that allow high levels of estrogen to persist for long periods of time, such as early age at first menstruation (before age 12), late age at menopause (after age 55), having children after age 30, and not having children at all. A woman's risk of breast cancer increases with the amount of time she is exposed to estrogen.

Because many of the risk factors for breast cancer are related to natural hormones, and because OCs work by manipulating these hormones, there has been some concern about the possible effects of medicines such as OCs on breast cancer risk, especially if women take them for many years. Sufficient time has elapsed since the introduction of OCs to allow investigators to study large numbers of women who took birth control pills for many years beginning at a young age and to follow them as they became older.

However, studies examining the use of OCs as a risk factor for breast cancer have produced inconsistent results. Most studies have not found an overall increased risk for breast cancer associated with OC use. In June 1995, however, investigators at the National Cancer Institute (NCI) reported an increased risk of developing breast cancer among women under age 35 who had used birth control pills for at least six months, compared with those who had never used OCs. They also saw a slightly lower, but still elevated, risk among women ages 35 to 44. In addition, their research showed a higher risk among long-term OC users, especially those who had started to take the pill before age 18.

A 1996 analysis of worldwide epidemiologic data, which included information from the 1995 study, found that women who were current or recent users of birth control pills had a slightly elevated risk of developing breast cancer. However, ten years or more after they stopped using OCs, their risk of developing breast cancer returned to the same level as if they had never used birth control pills.

To conduct this analysis, the researchers examined the results of 54 studies conducted in 25 countries that involved 53,297 women with breast cancer and 100,239 women without breast cancer. More than 200 researchers participated in this combined exhaustive analysis of their original studies, which represented about 90 percent of the epidemiological studies throughout the world that had investigated the possible relationship between OCs and breast cancer.

The return of risk to normal levels after ten years or more of not taking OCs was consistent regardless of family history of breast cancer, reproductive history, geographic area of residence, ethnic background, differences in study designs, dose and type of hormone, and duration of use. The change in risk also generally held true for age at first use; however, for reasons that were not fully understood, there was a continued elevated risk among women who had started to use OCs before age 20.

One encouraging aspect of the study is that the slightly elevated risk seen in both current OC users and those who had stopped use less than ten years previously may not be due to the contraceptive itself. The slightly elevated risk may result from the potential of estrogen to promote the growth of breast cancer cells that are already present, rather than its potential to initiate changes in normal cells leading to the development of cancer.

Furthermore, the observation that the slightly elevated risk of developing breast cancer that was seen in this study peaked during use, declined gradually after OC use had stopped, then returned to normal risk levels ten years or more after stopping, is not consistent with the usual process of carcinogenesis. It is more typical for cancer risk to peak decades after exposure, not immediately afterward. Cancer usually is more likely to occur with increased duration and/or degree of exposure to a carcinogen. In this analytical study, neither the dose and type of hormone nor the duration of use affected the risk of developing breast cancer.

Ovarian and Endometrial Cancers

Many studies have found that using OCs reduces a woman's risk of ovarian cancer by 40 to 50 percent compared with women who have not used OCs. The Centers for Disease Control and Prevention's (CDC) Cancer and Steroid Hormone Study (CASH), along with other research conducted over the past 20 years, shows that the longer a woman uses OCs, the lower her risk of ovarian cancer. Moreover, this lowered risk persists long after OC use ceases. The CASH study found that the reduced risk of ovarian cancer is seen in women who have used OCs for as little as three to six months, and that it continues for 15 years after use ends. Other studies have confirmed that the reduced risk of ovarian cancer continues for at least ten to 15 years after a woman has stopped taking OCs. Several hypotheses have been offered to explain how oral contraceptives might protect against ovarian cancer, such as a reduction in the number of ovulations a woman has during her lifetime, but the exact mechanism is still not known.

Researchers have also found that OC use may reduce the risk of endometrial cancer. Findings from the CASH study and other reports show that combination OC use can protect against the development of endometrial cancer. The CASH study found that using combination

OCs for at least one year reduced the risk of developing endometrial cancer to women who never took birth control pills. In addition, the beneficial effect of OC use persisted for at least 15 years after OC users stopped taking birth control pills. Some researchers have found that the protective effect of OCs against endometrial cancer increases with the length of time combination OCs are used, but results have not been consistent.

The reduction in risk of ovarian and endometrial cancers from OC use does not apply to the sequential type of pill, in which each monthly cycle contains 16 estrogen pills followed by five estrogen-plus-progesterone pills. (Sequential OCs were taken off the market in 1976, so few women have been exposed to them.) Researchers believe OCs reduce cancer risk only when the estrogen content of birth control pills is balanced by progestogen in the same pill.

Cancer of the Cervix

There is some evidence that long-term use of OCs may increase the risk of cancer of the cervix (the narrow, lower portion of the uterus). The results of studies conducted by NCI scientists and other researchers support a relationship between extended use of the pill (five or more years) and a slightly increased risk of cervical cancer. However, the exact nature of the association between OC use and risk of cervical cancer remains unclear.

One reason that the association is unclear is that two of the major risk factors for cervical cancer (early age at first intercourse and a history of multiple sex partners) are related to sexual behavior. Because these risk factors may be different between women who use OCs and those who have never used them, it is difficult for researchers to determine the exact role that OCs may play in the development of cervical cancer.

Also, many studies on OCs and cervical cancer have not accounted for the influence of human papillomaviruses (HPVs) on cervical cancer risk. HPVs are a group of more than 70 types of viruses, some of which are known to increase the risk of cervical cancer. Compared to non-OC users, women who use OCs may be less likely to use barrier methods of contraception (such as condoms). Since condoms can prevent the transmission of HPVs, OC users who do not use them may be at increased risk of becoming infected with HPVs. Therefore, the increased risk of cervical cancer that some studies found to be caused by prolonged OC use may actually be the result of HPV infection.

There is evidence that pill users who never use a barrier method of contraception or who have a history of genital infections are at a higher risk for developing cervical cancer. This association supports the theory that OCs may act together with sexually transmitted agents (such as HPVs) in the development of cervical cancer. Researchers continue to investigate the exact nature of the relationship between OC use and cancer of the cervix.

OC product labels have been revised to inform women of the possible risk of cervical cancer. The product labels also warn that birth control pills do not protect against human immunodeficiency virus (HIV) and other sexually transmitted diseases such as HPV, chlamydia, and genital herpes.

Liver Tumors

There is some evidence that OCs may increase the risk of certain malignant (cancerous) liver tumors. However, the risk is difficult to evaluate because of different patterns of OC use and because these tumors are rare in American women (the incidence is approximately 2 cases per 100,000 women). A benign (noncancerous) tumor of the liver called hepatic adenoma has also been found to occur, although rarely, among OC users. These tumors do not spread, but they may rupture and cause internal bleeding.

Reducing Risks

After many years on the U.S. market, the overall health effects of OCs are still mixed. The most serious side effect of the pill continues to be an increased risk of cardiovascular disease in certain groups, such as women who smoke; women over age 35; obese women; and those with a history of high blood pressure, diabetes, or elevated serum cholesterol levels. Information about the increased risk of cardiovascular disease is available from the National Heart, Lung, and Blood Institute (NHLBI). The NHLBI Information Center can be reached at:

P.O. Box 30105
Bethesda, MD 20824-0105
Telephone: 301-592-8573
Fax: 301-592-8563
E-mail: NHLBIinfo@rover.nhlbi.nih.gov
Internet Web site: http://www.nhlbi.nih.gov

The NCI recommends that women in their forties or older get screening mammograms on a regular basis, every one to two years. Women who are at increased risk for breast cancer should seek medical advice about when to begin having mammograms and how often to be screened. A high-quality mammogram, with a clinical breast exam (an exam done by a professional health care provider), is the most effective way to detect breast cancer early.

Women who are or have been sexually active or are in their late teens or older can reduce their risk for cervical cancer by having regular Pap tests. Research has shown that women who have never had a Pap test or who have not had one for several years have a higher-than-average risk of developing cervical cancer.

Women who are concerned about their risk for cancer are encouraged to talk with their doctor. More information is also available from the Cancer Information Service at 1-800-4-CANCER (1-800-422-6237).

Section 27.7

Low Dose Oral Contraceptives Do Not Pose Major Increase in Stroke Risk

National Institute of Child Health and Human Development, *NICHD News Notes*, July 3, 1996.

According to a study funded by the National Institute of Child Health and Human Development (NICHD), the modern, low-dose oral contraceptive formulations now in use do not increase the risk of stroke.

The study, which appeared in the July 4 *New England Journal of Medicine*, was conducted by researchers at the Kaiser Permanente Medical Program in both Pasadena and Oakland, California.

"We conclude that, as used by the women in this study, currently available low-estrogen oral contraceptives are generally safe with respect to the risk of stroke," the study authors wrote.

The study was undertaken because of concern that oral contraceptives could increase the risk of stroke in the women who took them.

This concern originated when studies conducted in the 1970s confirmed a link between stroke and oral contraceptive use. However, the results of studies conducted since that time have been inconclusive.

The researchers noted that the stroke risk found in the 1970s studies could have been due to the much higher doses of estrogen contained in oral contraceptives commonly prescribed at the time. Studies at that time were based on the use of oral contraceptive preparations that contained from 80 to 100 micrograms of estrogen. Current oral contraceptive preparations in use in the United States contain from 30 to 35 micrograms of estrogen. The researchers added that the absence of risk observed in the present study could also reflect the practices of physicians in prescribing for the study population. Generally, women with hypertension and diabetes were not given oral contraceptives.

The researchers identified the women in Kaiser's Northern and Southern California programs who had suffered strokes between 1991 and 1994. In all, 295 stroke cases were analyzed in the study. These cases were compared to 774 women who were similar to the stroke cases, but did not themselves suffer stroke.

The researchers calculated the risk for all types of stroke among current oral contraceptive users as 1.16, meaning that oral contraceptive users had a 16 percent increase in the risk of having a stroke. However, the results of the study are compatible with the interpretation that the use of low-dose oral contraceptives is not associated with any increased risk of stroke in women adequately screened for safe use of the pill.

> "This study establishes the low incidence of stroke among women of childbearing age," the authors wrote. "Even if the small increase we observed was due directly to the use of oral contraceptives, the number of excess cases of stroke in healthy women would be small."

The researchers added that there was no increased risk of stroke among women who had used oral contraceptives in the past but had since discontinued their use.

The authors of the study were Diana B. Petitti, M.D., Sheldon Wolfe, M.D., and Harry K. Ziel, M.D., of the Kaiser Permanente Medical Care Program, Southern California, in Pasadena, and Stephen Sidney, M.D., Allan Bernstein, M.D., and Charles Quesenberry, Ph.D., Kaiser Permanente Medical Care Program, Northern California, in Oakland.

Chapter 28

Answers to Your Questions about Norplant® Implants

*[**Note:** In the fall of 2000, routine testing revealed lower-than-expected release rates of levonorgestrel in certain lots of recently manufactured Norplant implants, which could reduce the effectiveness of contraceptive protection. Women using suspect lots of Norplant were advised to use a contraceptive backup method. Until the manufacturer, Wyeth-Ayerst, concludes the investigation, no additional Norplant kits will be made available for reinsertion.]*

General Information

1. What Are Norplant® Implants?

Norplant is an effective, long-acting, reversible contraceptive for women that protects for up to five years. Six thin, flexible capsules made of a soft, rubberlike material, filled with a synthetic progestin, are inserted just under the skin of a woman's upper arm in a minor surgical procedure. The implants do not contain estrogen. Protection is generally provided within 24 hours after the insertion and the woman rapidly returns to her normal fertility when the implants are removed. The most common side effect is change in menstrual bleeding patterns.

Population Council, July 1995; available at http://www.popcouncil.org/rhpdev/norplantfaq.html; reprinted with permission.

2. How Do Norplant Implants Work?

Pregnancy is prevented in Norplant users by a combination of mechanisms. The most important of these are the inhibition of ovulation and the thickening of the cervical mucus, which makes it impermeable to sperm. Other mechanisms may add to these contraceptive effects.

3. What Are the Capsule's Components?

Norplant implants are made with silicone rubber tubing filled with a synthetic hormone. This contraceptive is not made of new ingredients; the tubing has been used in surgical applications since the 1950s and the hormone released by the implants, levonorgestrel, has been used in combined oral contraceptives and in the minipill for more than 20 years. What is new about the Norplant implants method is the way it delivers the contraceptive drug to the body.

Each of the six Norplant capsules is 34mm long and 2.4mm in diameter (about the size of a pocket match) and contains 36 mg of levonorgestrel, released at a low, steady rate.

4. How Effective Are Norplant Implants?

The Norplant implant method is one of the most effective reversible contraceptives available. For every 100 women who use Norplant implants for a year, less than one will become pregnant. During the first two years of use, Norplant implants have a lower failure rate than the pill or most IUDs and its efficacy can be compared to surgical sterilization. The cumulative pregnancy rate for the entire five years is 3.9 per 100 users.

The Population Council data are based on capsules made from two different kinds of tubing, one denser than the other.

The softer tubing, which is now used everywhere, is more effective over a five-year span, because of a higher release rate of levonorgestrel into the bloodstream. Recently published data show that the softer tubing has a cumulative failure rate of less than 2.0 percent.

5. How Long Are Norplant Implants Effective?

Norplant implants provide contraceptive protection for five years. All six capsules have to be inserted during the same procedure, even if the method is to be used for fewer than five years. At the end of the fifth year, when the implants should be removed, a new set may be inserted for continued protection.

6. Who Can Use Norplant Implants?

Norplant implants may be used by almost any woman in her fertile years who wants to avoid getting pregnant. It is suitable for women who are seeking continuous, yet reversible, contraception; who want to space their children; who cannot use methods that contain estrogen; who do not want to be sterilized; and/or who desire a method that is convenient and not related to sexual intercourse. There have been no differences in reactions to Norplant implants based on a woman's race, age, or ethnic group.

7. Who Should Not Use Norplant Implants?

Norplant implants should not be used by women who have: active thromboembolic disorders, such as blood clots in the legs, lungs or eyes; undiagnosed genital bleeding; acute liver disease; or known or suspected carcinoma of the breast. Also, women who are pregnant should not use Norplant implants. Women who have had previous blood clots or other thromboembolic disorders should consult with their healthcare provider whether to use the method.

8. Can Heavier Women Use It?

Yes. Even among heavier women (over 154 lbs.) annual pregnancy rates are below those of oral contraceptives.

9. What Do Women Like Most about Norplant Implants?

Discussions with women using Norplant implants in different countries show they liked the method's convenience, effectiveness, and reversibility best. Other advantages mentioned were the method's long-term duration, limited side effects compared to other methods, and the fact that it was placed in the arm. In some societies, women are reluctant to undergo internal examinations or to touch their bodies.

10. What Do Women Like Least about Norplant Implants?

Menstrual irregularities, a side effect of Norplant that can be troublesome for many women, were cited as the least liked aspects of the method. Prior to insertions and removals, many women were anxious that the procedures might be painful. Some women also were concerned because they could not insert or remove the method themselves. With a provider-dependent method such as Norplant implants, it is most important that women be able to request and receive removal on demand from properly-trained providers.

11. How Many Users Continue Past the First Year?

Continuation rates have been high in clinical studies and field trials of Norplant use. Recently published data for the United States show a continuation rate of 85 percent after the first year. Cumulative continuation rates in seven preintroduction studies averaged 80 percent in the first year. In another study, the rate approached 49 percent at four years.

12. Why Do Women Discontinue Using This Method?

The principal reasons women discontinue using Norplant include: medical reasons and side effects; in order to become pregnant; or for other personal reasons. Studies conducted by the Population Council indicate that the most common side effects causing women to terminate implant use in a five-year period are as follows: menstrual irregularities (17.4 percent); headache (1.9 percent), weight changes (1.7 percent); mood changes (1.1 percent); and depression (0.9 percent).

13. Why Is Counseling Important?

It is important for a woman to know all about Norplant implants and how the method compares with other available contraceptives. Studies have shown that users who receive good counseling are more satisfied with the method they adopt and are more likely to continue using it. Before deciding to use Norplant implants, a woman should understand how the method works, what side effects to expect, and when to have the implants removed. She should know that insertions and removals are simple procedures when performed by trained healthcare providers, and are not painful to most women.

14. Does the Age of the User Matter?

If there are no contraindications, Norplant implants may be used by women throughout their reproductive years. A young woman can start using the method once her period becomes regular, which is usually about two years after the onset of her menses. Older women can use Norplant implants as they approach menopause.

Insertion and Removal

1. Should a Woman Get a Physical Exam before Receiving Norplant?

It is recommended that a woman considering Norplant implants undergo a medical examination. This may include giving a medical history and having a pelvic exam to ensure that she has no diseases or conditions that would make it unsafe for her to use Norplant implants.

2. Can Norplant Implants Be Inserted at Any Time?

To make sure the woman is not pregnant, Norplant implants should be inserted within seven days after the onset of menstrual bleeding, or immediately postabortion. However, Norplant implants may be inserted at any time during the menstrual cycle provided the woman is not pregnant and has effectively used another method for the remainder of the cycle.

3. How Are the Capsules Inserted?

The implants are inserted under the skin of the inner side of the upper arm in a minor surgical procedure. A local anesthetic is injected and the clinician makes a small incision—2mm long. The capsules are placed one at a time in a fan shape using a special hollow needle called a trocar. The procedure should take no longer than 10 to 15 minutes. Because a local anesthetic is used, there should be little or no pain. Usually the incision is covered with a small adhesive bandage and protective gauze.

4. Who Performs the Insertions?

Generally, any specially trained physician, nurse, nurse-midwife, or other healthcare professional can do the insertion. The prevailing laws will determine who is allowed to perform the procedures. Women should confirm that their healthcare provider is properly trained before he or she inserts or removes the Norplant implants.

5. Will the Insertion Site Hurt?

The needle providing the anesthetic may sting briefly. When the anesthetic wears off, there may be some tenderness for a day or two, as well as some discoloration, bruising, and/or swelling in the area for a few days after placement. There have also been reports of tingling and numbness in the arm after the procedure.

6. How Should the Insertion Site Be Cared for?

The insertion site should not be bumped for a few days and the area should be kept dry. The protective gauze bandage should be left in place for three days and the small adhesive bandage should be left on for a day or two longer.

7. Are Norplant Implants Visible?

Since the incision is tiny, Norplant implants do not leave a noticeable scar on most women. The implants are comfortable and barely visible. When they are visible, you can see the outline of the implants under the skin and they resemble colorless veins.

8. Will the Implants Move Around?

The implants do not move around and will remain under the skin where they are placed. They are flexible and cannot break inside the woman's arm. The woman does not have to be concerned if the implants are bumped or if pressure is put on the area during normal activities. After the incision has healed, the skin over the implants can be touched at any time.

9. Can a Woman Work after the Insertion?

Yes. She can resume her normal work and domestic activities, as long as she does not bump the site or get the incision site wet for at least three days.

10. How Soon after Insertion Can the Couple Have Sexual Relations?

Because Norplant becomes effective within 24 hours of insertion, the couple may have sexual relations without a back-up method 24 hours after the implants are inserted. If a woman has the implants inserted during her period, she may resume sexual relations without a back-up method as soon as she wishes.

11. When Should the Woman Return to the Clinic after She Receives Norplant Implants?

The follow-up schedule depends on the practice of the particular clinic or physician's office in which a woman receives the implants. She may be asked to return for periodic health checkups or to report on her experience with the implants. She should be encouraged to return to the same provider or clinic if she has any health problems that worry her; if she wants a child; or if she is moving away and needs the address of a clinic in her new area that provides Norplant implant services.

Annual checkups, besides being good medical practice, offer an occasion to remind women to have their implants removed at five years.

12. How Is Norplant Implant Protection Reversed?

One of the most important characteristics of Norplant implants is their reversibility. The contraceptive action stops within two to three days after the implants are removed during a clinical procedure, under a local anesthetic, similar to the insertion process.

13. When Should Norplant Implants Be Removed?

Norplant implants must be removed at the end of five years when they become less effective. Before that time, however, the woman should be able to request and obtain removal of the implants at any time, for either a personal or medical reason.

14. What Happens if the Implants Are Not Removed after Five Years Have Passed?

More than two-thirds of the hormone remains in the capsules after five years of use. After that time, the implants will gradually become less effective. While the implants should be removed at five years, there is no cause for panic if removal is delayed for a few months.

When pregnancy rates begin to rise, so will the incidence of ectopic pregnancy.

A study in China using the "hard" tubing implants in women with a mean weight of 54 kg showed a cumulative pregnancy rate of 2.3 per 100 women at the end of seven years of Norplant use.

15. Who Should Remove the Implants?

The implants can be removed at the same clinic or office where they were inserted or at another health facility that offers Norplant implants. As with insertion, a woman should confirm that her clinician has been trained in the removal procedure, prior to removing the implants. A woman should also be sure she will have access to a trained provider for removal. Providers should post a schedule of days when removals are performed.

16. Is Removal Painful?

Just as when the capsules were inserted, the health professional will apply a local anesthetic so the woman should not feel pain. It is not necessary to use general anesthesia for this procedure. Clinicians should feel the site to be sure they can locate all six capsules prior to removing them. If they cannot be felt, the implants can be located through x-ray or ultrasound, which are painless procedures.

A small incision—not longer than 4mm—will be made, through which all the implants are removed. When the anesthetic wears off, there may be some tenderness, discoloration, bruising, and swelling in the area for a few days.

This is the procedure used by the Population Council in the Norplant clinical trials. Since then, other techniques have been developed by other organizations and individuals.

17. Are Removals More Difficult than Insertions? How Long Does Removal Take?

Although most removals are not difficult, the removal procedure usually takes longer than insertion. Some implants may be harder than others to locate and remove if they were inserted too deeply or if temporary swelling of the arm occurs during removal. If the clinician is unable to remove all the capsules at one time, the woman should return at another time after her arm heals. Women should be informed of the possibility of needing a subsequent visit for removal and should not be alarmed if this is necessary.

18. How Should Women Care for the Site after Removal?

As with insertion, it is important to avoid rough contact with the removal site for a few days. The area should be kept clean, dry, and bandaged until healed (three to five days) so that the site does not become infected.

19. How Soon Afterwards Can a Woman Become Pregnant?

The reversibility of Norplant implants is one of the important advantages of the method. Once the implants are removed, the contraceptive effect wears off quickly (within two to three days). The woman can become pregnant as rapidly as she would have if she had used another method or if she had used no method during the time Norplant was inserted in her arm.

20. Can Another Set of Implants Be Inserted when the Old Set Is Removed?

Yes. If a woman wants to continue using Norplant, a new set of implants can be inserted when the old set is removed. The second set can be placed through the incision from which the earlier set was removed, in the same or opposite direction, or in the other arm. If a woman does not want to continue with Norplant implants and does not want to become pregnant, she should be offered another contraceptive method before she leaves the clinic.

Side Effects and Health Considerations

1. What Are the Side Effects of Norplant?

The most common side effect of Norplant use is irregular menstrual bleeding. Irregularities vary from woman to woman and may include: prolonged menstrual bleeding during the first months of use (rarely heavy bleeding); untimely bleeding or spotting between periods; no bleeding at all for several months and in some cases, for a year or longer; or a combination of these patterns.

Other side effects experienced with Norplant are frequently associated with use of hormonal methods. Side effects reported by users that are probably related to Norplant implants include: headache (the most frequent complaint after menstrual irregularities); dizziness; adnexal enlargement; itching/rashes; acne; change of appetite; weight gain; breast tenderness; excessive hair growth; hair loss; and discoloration of the skin at the insertion site.

Preexisting conditions of acne or excessive growth of body or facial hair could worsen. Occasionally, an infection may occur at the implant site (which can be treated with an antibiotic), or there may be a brief incidence of pain, itching, numbness, or tingling in the arm of insertion.

2. How Frequently Do Norplant Side Effects Occur in Users?

Bleeding irregularities (including spotting, longer or heavier periods, or no bleeding) are reported by 70 to 80 percent of Norplant users. Both increased and reduced bleeding tend to diminish with time.

Percentages of users reporting the other more common side effects during the first year of use are as follows: headache (18 percent); skin problems including dermatitis and acne (15 percent); nausea (8 percent); and appetite changes, weight changes, and nervousness are each reported by 6 percent of users.

3. Are the Bleeding Irregularities Associated with Norplant Implants Serious?

Most bleeding irregularities associated with Norplant use are not serious, although they may be troublesome for some users. Change in the menstrual bleeding pattern—the most frequently reported side effect—is to be expected with hormonal methods that do not contain estrogen. If a woman experiences heavy bleeding, she should make a follow-up visit to her physician or healthcare provider.

4. What Kind of Bleeding Pattern Can Be Expected?

It is not possible to predict in advance the kind of bleeding pattern a woman will have while using Norplant implants. There is some evidence of a correlation between a woman's weight and the kind of bleeding irregularities she will have, but accurate predictions of how she will react to the method cannot be made. Some studies indicate that very thin women are more likely to be amenorrheic, while heavier women have more bleeding and spotting days. Both increased and reduced bleeding tend to diminish with time. Many women can expect an altered menstrual bleeding pattern to become more regular after six to nine months.

5. Is the Lack of Bleeding Harmful?

Sometimes a woman is concerned about amenorrhea—no monthly bleeding at all. A woman's health or future fertility will not be harmed if she does not have her period while using Norplant; there is no blood "buildup." If a woman wants to make sure she is not pregnant, she can return to the clinic for a pregnancy test. She is probably not pregnant, but the test might reassure her.

6. Does the Use of Norplant Implants Make Women Anemic?

Despite the increased frequency of menstrual bleeding in some women using Norplant, the amount of total blood loss is usually less than normal menses. In some studies, in fact, hemoglobin values of Norplant implant users have been shown to increase. There have been a few rare exceptions of severe blood loss.

7. Should Women Be Given Estrogen to Control Bleeding and Spotting?

Norplant implants are estrogen-free and many women and their healthcare providers choose the method for exactly this reason. Research is being conducted to test the effectiveness of a few treatments for bleeding irregularities, but it is still too early to tell if any will be successful. As of now, the best way to handle irregular bleeding is through sensitive and thorough counseling of women who want the method. Research has shown that women who have been well counseled about what to expect with implants are more likely to find the method acceptable and to continue with it.

8. How Do Norplant Implants Affect the Body's Chemistry?

Extensive clinical pharmacology research has shown no adverse effects of progestin implant use on endocrine patterns, the endometrium, lipoproteins, adrenal function, thyroid function, and a variety of other physiological indicators in healthy women. These studies also have given no indication of cardiovascular, respiratory, central nervous system, or other serious problems, nor is there any evidence of carcinogenicity or teratogenicity associated with Norplant implant use in healthy women.

Certain conditions present before implant use, such as diabetes, may be affected by Norplant use; these women should be carefully monitored. (See additional questions in this section for specific conditions.)

9. What Are Warning Signs of Possible Problems?

A woman using Norplant implants should return to her healthcare provider or clinic right away if she has: severe lower abdominal pain (possible ectopic pregnancy); heavy vaginal bleeding; arm pain; pus or bleeding at the insertion site (an indication of infection); expulsion of an implant (this rarely occurs with proper placement); episodes of migraine, repeated bad headaches; bluffed vision; or delayed menstrual cycles after a long interval of regular cycles.

Failure to have periods after regular cycles may be a sign of pregnancy. If the woman is not bleeding at her expected time and has lower abdominal pain, or symptoms of pregnancy, she should visit the clinic without delay.

10. Are There Other Health Considerations with Norplant Use?

Women with certain health conditions can use Norplant implants, provided they have regular checkups. If a woman has any of the following conditions, she should discuss them with her healthcare provider before using Norplant: breast nodules, fibro-cystic disease of the breast, an abnormal breast x-ray or mammogram; diabetes; elevated cholesterol or triglycerides; high blood pressure; migraine or other headaches; epilepsy; mental depression; gallbladder, heart, or kidney disease; or a history of blood clots, heart attack, or stroke.

11. Does Norplant Cause Heart or Vascular Problems?

Although there have been post-marketing reports of stroke, myo-cardial infarction, and certain vascular problems such as thromboem-bolic disorders (all of which occur among the general population) among Norplant users, no cause and effect relationship between Norplant use and these conditions has been shown.

Thrombophlebitis and superficial phlebitis have also been reported among Norplant users, most commonly occurring in the arm of inser-tion. (See below for more information on stroke and heart attacks among smokers.)

12. Does Norplant Cause Autoimmune Diseases?

Autoimmune diseases such as scleroderma, systemic lupus, and rheumatoid arthritis occur in the general population and more fre-quently among women of childbearing age. There have been rare re-ports of various autoimmune diseases, including the above, in Norplant users; however, the rate is significantly less than the rate among the general population of women of reproductive age. While it is believed that the occurrence of autoimmune diseases among Norplant users is coincidental, health care providers should be alert to the earliest manifestations.

13. Does Norplant Cause Birth Defects?

Although there have been rare reports of birth defects in offspring of women who were using Norplant inadvertently during early preg-nancy, these conditions are not believed to be caused by Norplant use. However, if a woman becomes pregnant while using the implants, they must be removed immediately.

14. Can a Smoker Use Norplant Implants?

Cigarette smoking increases the risk of heart attacks and strokes in users of combined (estrogen-progestin) oral contraceptives. This risk increases with age and with heavy smoking (15 or more cigarettes a day) and is quite marked in women over 35 years old While this is believed to be an estrogen-related effect, it is not known whether a similar risk exists with progestin-only methods such as Norplant implants. Therefore, a woman who chooses to use Norplant implants is advised not to smoke.

15. Do Norplant Implants Protect against Sexually Transmitted Diseases?

No. This form of contraception does not protect against sexually transmitted diseases. If a woman thinks she might be at risk for STDs, she and her partner should use a condom in addition to the implants.

16. Can a Woman Use Norplant Implants if She Is Breastfeeding?

Hormones are not considered the most appropriate contraceptives for breastfeeding women. However, studies have shown no significant effects on the growth or health of infants whose mothers used levonorgestrel implants beginning six weeks after childbirth. There is no experience to support the use of Norplant implants earlier than six weeks after childbirth.

17. Is Sickle Cell Anemia a Contraindication?

Sickle cell anemia is not considered a contraindication for the use of Norplant implants. However, the Council does not have data from clinical trials since women who were anemic were not included in the Council's studies with Norplant implants.

18. Do Other Drugs Interact with Norplant Implants?

Certain drugs may interact with the hormone delivered by Norplant implants to make them less effective in preventing pregnancy. These include drugs used for epilepsy such as phenytoin (like Dilantin), and phenyl-butazone (Butazolidin is one brand). A woman using Norplant implants should tell her healthcare provider if she is taking any of these medications.

19. Is There a Risk of Ectopic Pregnancy?

The risk of ectopic pregnancy (a fetus developing outside the uterus) is very low, because of the high effectiveness of the method. Ectopic pregnancies have occurred among women using Norplant implants at an average rate of 1.3 per 1,000 woman-years, less than the overall ectopic rate of women in the United States during the 1980s. The risk may increase with the duration of Norplant implant use or with increased weight of the user. It is important, therefore, that the implants be removed at the end of five years when they become less effective.

20. Are Ovarian Cysts a Problem for the Users of Norplant Implants?

Functional ovarian cysts or enlarged follicles sometimes occur in Norplant implant users as they do in women who do not use Norplant implants. These enlarged follicles may produce some discomfort in some women, although most users would not be aware of them unless they were found during a physical exam. In the majority of women, enlarged follicles will disappear on their own and should not require surgery. Rarely, they may twist or rupture so that surgery is required.

21. Are Long-term Side Effects Known?

Long-term side effects of Norplant use are not yet known. However, the drug contained in Norplant, levonorgestrel, has been used in oral contraceptives for over 20 years.

To learn more about any possible rare, medium-term health effects related to the method, the World Health Organization, the Population Council, and Family Health International are conducting an international postmarketing surveillance of Norplant implant use. Some 8,000 method users and discontinuers, and an equal number of controls, in eight developing countries are being followed for five years.

Research and Development

1. Why Were Norplant Implants Developed?

The Population Council developed Norplant implants to expand contraceptive options for women, by offering a method that was convenient, long-acting, and reversible. In addition, the implants deliver a very low dose of progestin and contain no estrogen.

2. Where Were Norplant Implants Tested?

Norplant implants were tested in four developing and four developed countries, including the United States. In addition, many countries have conducted preintroduction studies to obtain data on local experience with the method and to train providers in insertion, removal, and counseling techniques. By 1991, when the method became available in the United States, Norplant implants had been studied in clinical trials and preintroduction studies involving over 55,000 volunteers in more than 40 countries.

3. Where Have Norplant Implants Been Approved?

By July 1995, the method was approved in 44 countries, including Sweden, France, the United Kingdom, and the United States. The U.S. Food and Drug Administration approved Norplant for marketing in December 1990.

Chapter 29

Depo-Provera®: The Shot

What Is Depo-Provera®?

Depo-Provera is a synthetic female hormone, a progestin, that is used as a long-acting form of birth control. It is given by injection every 12 weeks (three months) by your clinician. It was originally developed in the late 1950s in Brazil for the purpose of stopping premature labor and miscarriages in women. While it did not work for its original purpose, it was found to make women temporarily infertile. Depo-Provera has been used for years in many countries; it was approved by the Food and Drug Administration (FDA) for use in the United States in October 1992.

How Does Depo-Provera Work?

Each time an injection is given, a high level of progestin is released into the body. This unnaturally high level stops the natural production of both progesterone and estrogen. As a result, the ovary does not prepare an egg and the lining of the uterus is not prepared to support a fertilized egg. In addition, the cervix (opening to the uterus) secretes mucus that blocks sperm from entering the uterus.

"Depo-Provera (The Shot)," copyright 1996 Feminist Women's Health Center; available at http://www.fwhc.org/bcdepo.htm; reprinted with permission.

Depo-Provera is one of the most private methods of contraception a woman can use. There are no supplies to be stored and it cannot be detected by anyone.

How Fast Is Depo-Provera Effective?

Women are usually asked to come get their first shot during their period, which indicates they are not pregnant and probably not ovulating. The clinician will recommend a back-up method of birth control for one to two weeks (condom, cervical cap, diaphragm, foam).

However, if you don't get the shot during your period, using a backup method for two to four weeks is usually recommended.

If you get subsequent shots on time, there should be no need for further backup to prevent pregnancy. (As always, condoms are the best way to prevent sexually transmitted diseases and HIV.)

Is Depo-Provera Safe?

There have been many studies and discussions over the past 20 years about the possible risks and long-term effects on women who use Depo-Provera. Some clinical studies in the 1960s and 1970s on dogs and monkeys linked this drug to cancer of the breast and uterus. In 1987, the FDA changed its regulations and began to require cancer testing in rats and mice instead of dogs and monkeys. Depo-Provera has not been found to cause cancer in these animals.

Studies of the risk of cancer in women using Depo-Provera have been conducted in other countries. The most disturbing results have been in the breast cancer studies. Three studies on Depo-Provera found an increase in the risk of breast cancer in women less than 35 years old. A 1989 New Zealand study showed increased risk of breast cancer for women whose use began under the age of 25 and lasted for two years or more, and for all women who used the drug between the ages of 25 and 34. The highest risk of breast cancer was found in women who used Depo-Provera for more than six years, between the ages of 25 and 34. These studies are not yet conclusive. Many scientists discount the increased risk for young women because they did not find an overall increased risk of breast cancer for all women exposed to Depo-Provera.

The FDA has required the manufacturer of Depo-Provera to conduct studies on the possible loss of bone density during the use of Depo-Provera. One small study found that women appear to lose bone density while on this drug, but may regain some of the bone loss when they stop using Depo-Provera. Bone loss during the reproductive years may make some women more likely to suffer osteoporosis and possible fractures as they age.

What Are the Advantages of Depo-Provera?

- Depo-Provera is 99% effective and it lasts for 12 weeks.
- You do not have to remember to take a pill every day or interrupt sex to use a method of birth control.
- Depo-Provera has been shown to decrease the incidence of cancer in the ovaries and uterus.
- It is highly confidential and no one knows you are using it.

What Are the Disadvantages?

- This method **does not** protect against sexually transmitted diseases (STDs) such as syphilis, gonorrhea, chlamydia, herpes, genital warts, hepatitis B, or AIDS. Only a barrier method of birth control, like condoms, a diaphragm, a cervical cap, or sperm-killing cream or jelly can provide protection from STDs.
- **Every** woman can expect to experience changes in her periods when using Depo-Provera, such as longer periods than usual, spotting between periods, or no periods at all.
- There is no antidote that reverses the effects of Depo-Provera, but the effects eventually wear off as the levels of the drug slowly decline. The side effects may last for several months after the last injection.

What Are the Most Common Side Effects

- Irregular bleeding or no bleeding
- Weight gain of approximately 2–6 pounds during the first year of use
- Fertility may be delayed by as much as 9–24 months after receiving the last injection.
- Less common side effects:

— Headache

— Nausea

— Dizziness

— Depression

— Skin Rash

— Allergic Reaction

— Nervousness

— Change of appetite

— Sore breasts

— Change in sex drive

— Abdominal discomfort

— Hair loss or increased body hair　　·

There is never a time in a woman's reproductive life when her body produces progesterone without estrogen to balance it. Thus, when synthetic progesterone is given alone as a birth control method, women almost always experience changes. The manufacturer of Depo-Provera reports that 70 percent of women who took Depo-Provera in research studies gained weight. After one year on Depo-Provera, 46 percent of the women on Depo-Provera had gained more than five pounds, and 28 percent had gained more than ten pounds.

Menstrual cycles are also disrupted by progestin-only contraceptives. In another study sponsored by the manufacturer, one-third of all women who had one shot of Depo-Provera bled for more than ten days a month. In the manufacturer's study, women who continued receiving Depo-Provera shots eventually bled less. After one year on Depo-Provera, only 12 percent of the women bled for more than ten days, and half of the women had no bleeding at all. (One-third of the women had dropped out of the study by one year, however.)

The manufacturer also reports other side effects which are similar to any hormonal method of birth control such as headaches, nervousness, weakness, and fatigue. It is also possible to have an allergic reaction to Depo-Provera injections.

The National Women's Health Network, working in cooperation with the National Black Women's Health Project, maintained a Depo-Provera Registry, which was most active between 1979 and 1985. Over 600 women reported their experiences with Depo-Provera. In addition to weight gain and irregular periods, women also reported loss of libido, depression (in some cases serious) and bleeding so heavy that physicians removed the uterus.

What Are the Possible Long-term Risks of Depo-Provera?

The possible risk of cancer as a result of Depo-Provera use has been hotly debated for 20 years. Tests on dogs and monkeys conducted in the 1960s and 1970s linked Depo-Provera to cancer of the breast and uterus. In 1987, the FDA changed its regulations and began to require cancer testing in rats and mice instead of dogs and monkeys. Depo-Provera has not been found to cause cancer in these animals.

Studies of the risk of cancer in women using Depo-Provera have been conducted in other countries. The most disturbing results have been in the breast cancer studies. Each of the three studies reported so far has found an increase in the risk of breast cancer in women less than 35 years old. These studies are not yet conclusive, and many scientists discount the increased risk for young women, because they did not find an overall increased risk of breast cancer for all women exposed to Depo-Provera. The Network remains extremely concerned about this possible risk. Long-term use of Depo-Provera may be the most likely to increase the risk of cancer, but very few long-term users were included in the studies.

What Happens when I Stop Using Depo-Provera?

The effects gradually wear off as the levels of the drug slowly decline. The contraceptive effects of the drug cannot be relied upon after three months; however, most women will not resume regular menstrual cycles right away. On the average, it takes ten months after the last shot before women are fertile again. Sometimes the side effects last for several months after the last shot, as well.

What about Depo-Provera and Breast Feeding?

No synthetic progesterones are recommended for use during pregnancy, because they have been associated with serious birth defects. Some women have accidentally been given Depo-Provera before they realized they were pregnant and a few women became pregnant when the drug failed. Studies of children exposed to Depo-Provera during pregnancy have found that low birth weight is more common and fetal growth may be retarded.

Depo-Provera does not reduce the amount of milk a breast feeding women produces. However, the drug is constantly present in the mother's milk, with levels being the highest in the first weeks after each injection. Only one study has followed children who consumed Depo-Provera into adolescence. No problems were found, but the number of children was too few to make definite conclusions.

Do Some Medical Conditions Make Depo-Provera More Risky?

FDA and Upsilon agree that women should not use Depo-Provera if they have experienced any of the following:

- acute liver disease
- breast cancer
- blood clots in the legs, lungs, or eyes
- unexplained vaginal bleeding (currently)

Depo-Provera and Coercion

Because Depo-Provera is a shot that does not have an antidote, it is extremely important that women who are given Depo-Provera are well informed about the drug, as well as other options for contraception. There have been instances, both in the United States and in other countries, of women being pressured into using Depo-Provera, or being given the shot without understanding what it was.

What if I Still Have Questions?

If you still have questions about Depo-Provera, talk to your health care provider. You have a right to have all of your questions answered. There have been instances in the United States and other countries where women have been pressured into using Depo-Provera or have been given the shot without understanding what it was. Only you can decide what the best method of birth control is for you. If you would like information about other methods of birth control that are available, please ask.

Chapter 30

Understanding IUDs

The IUD is the world's most widely used method of reversible birth control for women. The letters "IUD" stand for "intrauterine device." When placed inside a woman's uterus, an IUD helps prevent pregnancy. Not all IUDs are alike. There are several types, and they come in different sizes. The IUD is the most inexpensive long-term reversible method of contraception available in the world.

Unfortunately, years of negative publicity and speculation following lawsuits brought on by the sale and use of a faulty IUD—the Dalkon Shield®—raised many questions about the safety of all IUDs. Some manufacturers even withdrew safe IUDs from the American market. But the IUD is still recognized by the World Health Organization, the American Medical Association, and the American College of Obstetricians and Gynecologists as one of the safest and most effective reversible methods of birth control for women.

What Are IUDs?

IUDs are small devices made of flexible plastic that provide reversible birth control. Those available in the United States contain cop-

Text adapted from *Understanding IUDs*, © revised version July 1996 Planned Parenthood® Federation of America, Inc., copyright PPFA 1978, PPFA Web Site © 1998, Planned Parenthood® Federation of America, Inc.; available at http://www.plannedparenthood.org/BIRTH-CONTROL/IUD.HTM; reprinted with permission.

per or a hormone. IUDs are available by prescription only. A clinician decides which is the right type for each woman and inserts it in her uterus. Two types are now available in the United States. One type, the ParaGard® Copper T 380A, contains copper and can be left in place for ten years. The other, the Progestasert®, continuously releases a small amount of progestin and must be replaced every year. Once inserted, the IUD is immediately effective. When removed, its contraceptive effect is immediately reversed.

How IUDs Work

IUDs usually prevent fertilization of the egg. Scientists are not entirely sure why. IUDs seem to affect the way the sperm or egg moves. It may be that substances released by the IUD immobilize sperm. Another possibility is that the IUD prompts the egg to move through the fallopian tube too fast to be fertilized.

The copper in the ParaGard adds to the effectiveness of the IUD in two other ways. It affects the behavior of enzymes in the lining of the uterus to prevent implantation. It also causes the production of increased amounts of prostaglandins which affect the hormones that support pregnancy.

The progestin in the Progestasert also thickens cervical mucus, providing a barrier that prevents sperm from entering the uterus. It also affects the lining of the uterus in ways that would prevent implantation if an egg were fertilized, which is very unlikely.

Both IUDs have a filament—"string"—that is threaded through a hole in the bottom of the "T" and tied in place with a knot. The string is a monofilament—a single strand of strong plastic. It cannot absorb or "wick" fluid or bacteria into the uterus the way a cotton string could. The string has two purposes. It allows for easier removal by a clinician when the time comes. The string also allows a woman or her clinician to know if the IUD is still in the correct position. If the string seems to shorten or lengthen, the IUD may have moved out of place. If the string can't be located, it may mean that contractions of the uterus have expelled the IUD.

Who Can Use IUDs

An IUD may be right for you if:

- you want a very effective, long-term, reversible method of birth control
- you have not had pelvic inflammatory disease, gonorrhea, or chlamydia within the past 12 months
- you are not at risk for contracting a sexually transmitted infection
- you are breastfeeding
- you cannot use hormonal methods like the Pill because of cigarette smoking or certain conditions like hypertension.

You should not use the IUD if you might be pregnant or if you have:

- a sexually transmitted bacterial infection like gonorrhea or chlamydia
- had postpartum endometriosis or an infected abortion in the past three months
- untreated acute cervicitis or vaginitis, including bacterial vaginosis, until infection is controlled
- abnormal vaginal bleeding
- cancer of the cervix or uterus
- conditions associated with increased susceptibility to infections with micro-organisms, including leukemia, AIDS, and I.V. drug use
- certain anatomical abnormalities of the cervix, uterus, or ovaries that would make insertion difficult or dangerous
- abnormal Pap test results or cancer of the uterus or cervix
- a bacterial infection—such as actinomycosis—of the reproductive tract
- a previously inserted IUD that has not been removed
- a uterus that is shorter or smaller than the IUD
- no access to medical care if problems develop.

Copper IUDs should not be used if you are allergic to copper, if you are having diathermy (heat) treatments, or if you have Wilson's disease. Physical therapy techniques involving the use of heat (diathermy) to transmit energy into deep tissues have been used for many years. Di-

317

athermy has been considered inappropriate for anyone with a pacemaker or another implanted device containing metal, including the copper IUD. The concern is that the copper in an IUD could become hot enough to burn tissue in the uterus and lead to scarring.

Wilson's disease is a rare hereditary disorder associated with the accumulation of potentially dangerous amounts of copper in body tissues.

Special evaluations must be made for women who have a history of heart disease or certain other conditions. These conditions include valvular heart disease, an artificial heart valve, a ventricular septal defect, and an atrial septal defect that hasn't been repaired. There is a possibility that an infection associated with an IUD in a woman with one of these conditions could lead to bacterial endocarditis, a very dangerous infection of the heart and blood.

IUDs are prescribed by licensed health care professionals. Because some women have physical or medical conditions that may rule out IUD use, it is important to have a pelvic examination and a complete medical history taken. The physical examination will let the clinician know if your cervix, vagina, and internal organs are normal. It is also important to make sure you have no pelvic infection. Simple tests will show if you have a sexually transmitted bacterial infection like gonorrhea or chlamydia, a vaginal infection, early cancer, or any other condition that needs to be treated. A blood sample may also be taken to make sure you are not anemic.

Before insertion, discuss any question you have with your clinician. Learn how to watch for possible side effects or other problems. Be sure to read the package insert that comes with the IUD before you decide to have one inserted.

Your clinician will also provide you with a consent form containing detailed information about the risks and benefits of the IUD you are considering. You need to read, understand, and sign this form before your clinician inserts the IUD.

How Well IUDs Work

The chances of avoiding pregnancy when using an IUD are excellent. Only Norplant®, sterilization, and Depo-Provera® are more effective than the IUD in protecting against unplanned pregnancy. Only eight out of 1,000 women using copper IUDs will become pregnant during the first year of use. Only six out of 1,000 become pregnant with perfect use. Fewer than three women in 100 using an IUD with progestin will become pregnant during the first year of use. Fewer than two will become pregnant with perfect use. Fewer pregnancies happen with continued use.

A woman can increase her protection in two ways:

- if she checks for the IUD string regularly and talks with her clinician if it is missing or is longer than before
- if the couple also uses condoms and/or foam for the first two or three months during when she is most likely to be fertile.

IUDs offer no protection against sexually transmitted infections, and they should not be worn by women who are at risk.

How IUDs Are Used

IUDs are inserted into the uterus by trained clinicians. Insertion is often done during menstruation, when the opening of a woman's cervix is softer and she is not likely to be pregnant.

Preparing for Insertion

Your Medical History

If you are considering having an IUD inserted, your clinician will ask you a number of questions about your medical history, including your lifestyle. Being open and honest about your sex life is extremely important because the IUD isn't suitable for all women.

Your clinician will want your assurance, for example, that you have only one sex partner who has no other sex partners, because the IUD provides no protection from sexually transmitted infections.

The Pelvic Exam

An instrument called a speculum is placed in the vagina. It separates the vaginal walls enough so that the vagina and cervix can be seen to make sure both are normal.

The Bimanual Exam

After removing the speculum, the clinician puts one or two fingers of one hand into the vagina. The other hand is placed on the abdomen.

Then both hands are gently pressed together to check the size, shape, and position of the uterus and ovaries.

Scheduling the Insertion

An IUD can be inserted at any time. The most comfortable time may be during a menstrual period, when the cervix is softest. The menstrual fluid also provides lubrication during the insertion. Another good time to have an IUD inserted is midcycle, because the cervix is naturally dilated during ovulation. It is more likely, however, that insertion after menstruation may interrupt or injure a developing pregnancy. This may result in increased bleeding or expulsion.

Insertion

Some clinicians instruct women to take an over-the-counter pain-killer an hour or so before insertion to lessen the cramps that insertion may cause. Because possible infection with IUD use is most often associated with insertion, some clinicians give women an antibiotic to protect against infection during insertion.

To insert the IUD, the clinician holds the vagina open with a speculum—as in a pelvic exam. An instrument called a tenaculum is attached to the cervix to steady the uterus. Then another instrument, called a "sound," may be inserted to measure the length of the cervical canal and uterus.

After the sound is withdrawn, a tube containing the IUD is inserted. The "arms" (T bars) of the IUD bend back as they enter the uterus through the cervix. The IUD is pushed into place by a plunger in the tube. The arms spring open into the T shape when the IUD is in the uterus.

The tube, plunger, tenaculum, and speculum are withdrawn, and the IUD is left in place with the filament hanging down through the cervix into the vagina. The clinician snips the string ends, leaving about an inch to hang out of the cervix. They can't be seen outside the vagina but are long enough to be felt by a finger inserted in the vagina.

During insertion, uterine cramps may be uncomfortable. Some women feel a bit dizzy, and rarely a woman may faint. Deep, relaxed breathing may prevent these events. The cramping eases with a little rest or pain medication. Many women breeze through the insertion feeling nothing more than mild discomfort. Women with sensitive cervical tissue may need to have a local anesthetic injected around the cervix to reduce or prevent the pain.

If you have an IUD inserted, you may want to have someone with you to escort or drive you home. You should plan to rest at home until you are comfortable.

After Insertion

Many women adjust to their IUDs very quickly. Others may take several months to become entirely comfortable. Heavy bleeding and cramping in the first few months may lead women to change their minds and ask their health care providers to remove the IUD. Many clinicians prescribe medication during the first few months to lessen bleeding and cramps during menstruation. Overall, women's level of satisfaction with the IUD is quite strong. More than 60 percent of women who have IUDs inserted continue to use them for more than two years. More than 95 percent of IUD users are pleased with them.

There may be some spotting between periods during the first few months, and the first few periods may last longer, and the flow may be heavier. It is not unusual for a woman to have heavier and longer periods while using an IUD.

Cramping or backache may occur for several days or weeks after insertion. Simple pain medication usually clears up cramping and discomfort. If bleeding or pain is severe and does not seem to lessen, tell your clinician.

You should have a checkup after your first period. Don't wait longer than three months after insertion to make sure your IUD is still in place. Women using an IUD should have checkups at least once a year to make sure everything is all right. This is usually done at the time of your annual physical and Pap test. Your clinician will tell you the type of IUD that is inserted and when it should be replaced. You should write this information down and keep it in a safe place. Otherwise, clinicians you see in the future will not be able to tell which IUD you have or when it needs to be replaced.

Checking Your IUD

Sometimes the uterus pushes out an IUD. "Expulsion" is more common in women who have never been pregnant. The stretching of the uterus during pregnancy may make it less likely to reject the IUD. Expulsion is most likely to happen during the first few months of use, but may occur later. If it does, you must check with your clinician. Until then, use another form of birth control—barrier methods like condoms or vaginal pouches that you can buy over the counter at a drugstore.

Although uncommon, an IUD can be expelled without your knowing it. This is most likely to happen during your period. It is a good idea to check your pads or tampons daily while you are menstruating to see if the IUD has fallen out. The string attached to the IUD hangs from the uterus into the vagina. This makes it easy for you to check if the IUD is still in place. Feel for the string regularly between periods. It is especially important to check every few days during the first few months after insertion.

To Feel for the String:

- Wash your hands. Then either sit or squat down.

- Put your index or middle finger up into your vagina until you touch the cervix. The cervix will feel firm and somewhat rubbery, much like the tip of your nose.

- Feel for the string that should be coming through. If you find the string, it means that the IUD is in place and working. However, if the string feels longer or shorter than before, it may be that the IUD has moved and needs to be repositioned by a clinician. Be sure to use another form of birth control until it is repositioned.

- Do not pull on the string. Pulling might make the IUD move out of place or even come out. Remember, your IUD was carefully positioned during insertion; it shouldn't be disturbed.

Warnings that Something Is Wrong with Your IUD

Tell your clinician immediately if you are not able to find and feel the string; if you think you might be pregnant; or if you have:

- severe cramping or increasing pain in the lower abdomen
- feeling faint
- pain or bleeding during sex
- unexplained fever and/or chills
- increased or bad-smelling discharge
- a missed, late, or unusually light period
- unexplained vaginal bleeding after the usual adjustment phase.

If you can't feel the IUD string, your uterus might have pushed out the IUD without your knowing it. It's also possible, although rare, that the IUD may have worked through your uterus into your abdomen. This could result in an internal injury. In either case, medical attention is required.

If you feel the hard plastic bottom of the "T" of the IUD against the cervix, it is not in the correct position and is not protecting you against pregnancy. Tell your clinician immediately.

If your periods last much longer than usual or the flow is much heavier than usual, you may become anemic. In that case, it may be necessary to have the IUD removed.

If you have severe pain or cramps in the abdomen, pain while having sex, or an abnormal discharge or fever, you may have a pelvic infection. Medical treatment may be necessary. The longer you wait to find out, the worse the infection may become.

Removal

Having an IUD removed or replaced is usually a simple matter. The clinician carefully tugs on the string ends at a certain angle, the IUD "arms" fold up, and the IUD slides through the opening of the cervix. Replacing the IUD with a new one can be done immediately after removal in most circumstances. Women should never try to remove IUDs themselves or ask non-professionals to do it for them. Serious damage could result.

In rare cases, IUDs become embedded in the uterus and cannot be easily pulled free. In these cases, the cervix may have to be dilated and a surgical tool—forceps—may be used to free the IUD. A local anesthetic is used for such removals.

In very rare cases, surgery becomes necessary. Women may have to be hospitalized for removals that require incision.

Sexually Transmitted Infection and the IUD

Like the Pill, the IUD does not offer protection against sexually transmitted infections (STIs). An STI can permanently damage the reproductive system. If you think you have been exposed to an STI, see your clinician for an examination as soon as possible. Treatment may be necessary. The longer you wait, the greater the risk of developing a serious pelvic infection. Pelvic inflammatory disease may result in loss of fertility, ectopic pregnancy, or surgical removal of the fallopian tubes or uterus.

To protect yourself against STIs whenever you have sexual intercourse with a partner who may be infected, use a latex condom every time.

Possible Problems and Side Effects While Using IUDs

IUD use offers much less risk to a woman's life and health than pregnancy. However, there are some risks associated with any method of birth control. Serious problems connected with the use of the IUD are rare, but they do happen once in a while. Knowing what could happen is your safeguard. The sooner you report any problems to your clinician, the better your chances of avoiding serious complications.

Heavy Menstrual Flow

Spotting between periods is common with IUD use. The Copper T IUD may cause a 50 to 75 percent increase in menstrual flow. The Progestasert, on the other hand, frequently decreases the amount of bleeding—but it has been known to prolong bleeding and increase the incidence of spotting.

Menstrual Cramps

Copper T IUDs can increase menstrual cramping. The Progestasert may decrease painful periods.

Expulsion

From 1.2 to 7.1 percent of IUDs are partially or completely expelled from the uterus in the first year, especially in the first few months after insertion. If the expulsion is "silent" and the woman does not notice it, she can easily become pregnant. One out of five expulsions goes unnoticed. One-third of the pregnancies that occur during IUD use are due to "silent expulsions." Expulsion is more likely among younger women and women who have never had a baby. Strenuous physical activity, however, does not affect the position of the IUD.

Uterine Puncture

In one to three out of 1,000 insertions, the uterus is accidentally punctured. This is usually discovered and corrected right away. If not, the IUD can "migrate" through the perforation into other parts of the pelvic area. Although "perforation" sounds painful, it usually isn't. Some women discover it has happened only after becoming pregnant. If an IUD "migrates," surgery may be required to remove the IUD. The removal is usually performed with a laparoscope through a tiny incision below the navel.

Infection

Even though the inserter is sterilized before use, it can push bacteria that are naturally found in the vagina into the uterus. Women using IUDs are more likely to develop a pelvic infection during the four months following insertion. After that time, if a woman and her partner have sex only with each other, there is no greater risk of infection than for women not using birth control.

A mild infection usually clears up with antibiotics without having the IUD removed. Once in a while, more serious infection occurs, and the IUD may need to be removed. In rare cases, infection may cause sterility or the need to remove the reproductive organs. Left untreated, such an infection might become fatal.

Infertility

Because untreated infections associated with IUDs may make it difficult or impossible to become pregnant, IUDs are generally not recommended for:

- young women who haven't had any children
- women who want more children
- women who have had trouble conceiving in the past

However, some women without children choose to use the IUD anyway, because it is so highly effective.

Pregnancy

Most pregnancies happen to IUD users when their IUDs fall out without their knowing it.

Rarely, a pregnancy happens with the IUD in place. If it does, there is a 50-percent greater chance of miscarriage. However, the chance of miscarriage is lessened by 25 percent by having the IUD taken out as soon as possible. If a pregnancy continues with an IUD in the uterus, there is a risk to the woman of serious, perhaps life-threatening, infection. There is less danger if the IUD is taken out. If the IUD cannot be located and removed, abortion may be considered.

Leaving an IUD in place during pregnancy also increases the risk of premature rupture of the membranes. This will cause premature loss of amniotic fluid and could lead to the birth of immature or premature babies.

There is no association between IUD use and increased risk of congenital abnormalities. Although cases of fetal deformity in women with IUDs in place have been reported, the occurrence is no greater than for women who are not using birth control. IUD users are less than half as likely to have an ectopic pregnancy as women who use no contraceptive. But if pregnancy does occur during IUD use, there is an increased chance that the fertilized egg may develop in the tube instead of the uterus. Ectopic pregnancies are more likely among Progestasert users—about half of the pregnancies that occur are ectopic. Surgery may be required to remove an ectopic pregnancy.

If a woman with an IUD suspects she is pregnant, she should contact her clinician immediately. If she is pregnant and chooses to complete the pregnancy, she must have close medical supervision throughout her pregnancy.

How to Get IUDs and What They Cost

Visit your local Planned Parenthood health center, your HMO, or a private doctor. At this time in the United States, the variety of available IUDs is limited to the ParaGard and Progestasert. Consult your clinician for more information.

Before insertion, discuss with your clinician how to watch for possible side effects or other problems. Be sure to read the package insert that comes with the IUD before you decide to have one inserted. Your clinician also will provide you with a consent form containing detailed information about the risks and benefits of the IUD you are considering. You need to read, understand, and sign this form before your clinician inserts the IUD.

The cost of the exam, insertion, and follow-up visit ranges from $250 to $450. These services are priced according to income at some family planning clinics and are covered by Medicaid.

The one-time insertion cost of $400 and up for a copper IUD that lasts 10 years works out to less per year than the cost of most other forms of reversible birth control. The longer you use the IUD, the cheaper it becomes. In contrast, other methods must be replaced and paid for more frequently. Even the annual bill for the spermicides used with barrier methods can add up.

Part Seven:

Permanent Methods of Contraception (Sterilization)

Chapter 31

Sterilization as Permanent Birth Control: His or Hers?

If you have completed your family—or if you've chosen not to have children—you and your partner may have concluded that surgical sterilization is your best option for permanent birth control. It can be difficult, however, for a couple to decide who should have the procedure. Vasectomy is the only surgical method of permanent sterilization for men, while tubal ligation is by far the most common method of female sterilization. Most medical experts agree that vasectomy is generally the safer and easier procedure, but you should discuss your situation with your doctor or a counselor before making a decision.

Here are some of the relative advantages and disadvantages of vasectomy and tubal ligation.

What's Involved?

Vasectomy—The doctor injects a local anesthetic into the scrotum, then makes two small incisions. The tubes (vas deferens) that carry sperm to the penis are severed and sealed, either with sutures or surgical clips on each end of the severed tubes.

Tubal ligation—Tubal ligation prevents contraception by closing off and sealing the fallopian tubes so that egg and sperm cannot meet.

Mayo Clinic Health Oasis, September 11, 1997; © 2000 Mayo Foundation for Medical Education and Research; available at http://www.mayohealth.org/mayo/9709/htm/steril.htm; reprinted with permission.

The procedure may be done either laparoscopically (in which viewing and operating instruments are inserted into the abdomen), or by minilaparotomy (where the doctor uses a small incision to open the abdomen and seal the tubes). The tubes are sealed by cauterizing with electric current (electrocoagulation), by using specially designed clips, or by cutting out a portion of the tubes.

Where Will the Procedure Be Done?

Vasectomy—Usually done on an outpatient basis, in a room designed for minor surgical procedures at a clinic or doctor's office.

Tubal ligation—Performed in a hospital or clinic surgical unit, usually as day surgery.

What Kind of Anesthetic Is Used?

Vasectomy—Requires only a local anesthetic. You are awake during the procedure.

Tubal ligation—Depending on the procedure used, tubal ligation may be done with either local or general anesthetic. With general anesthesia, you are unconscious during the operation. If a local is used, you will probably also receive a sedative.

How Long Does It Take to Recover?

Vasectomy—The procedure is brief (about 30 minutes) and you can go home within a few hours. You will be told to refrain from strenuous activity for 48 hours. If your work does not involve hard physical labor, you may return to the job as soon as you feel able.

Tubal ligation—You will probably be up and around within eight hours. For most women, recovery takes only a day or two, but you should refrain from heavy lifting for at least a week.

Are There Potential Complications?

Vasectomy—The rate of complications is low. You may have some swelling and pain in the scrotum for a few days to several weeks.

Sperm granulomas—small, hard inflamed nodules—sometimes develop at the severed ends of the vas deferens. These usually resolve on their own, but surgery may be necessary to eliminate them. Infection and bleeding are infrequent complications.

Tubal ligation—Risks are low, with infection and bleeding the most likely complications. Bleeding is usually the result of injury to a blood vessel during surgery. General anesthesia, if used, carries higher risks than a local anesthetic.

Are There Long-term Health Risks?

Vasectomy—Although the relationships between vasectomy and atherosclerosis (buildup of plaque on artery walls), heart disease, and testicular cancer have been a concern in the past, studies now suggest these fears are unfounded. Another concern is increased risk of prostate cancer. Studies to date have been inconclusive. Some research has shown a weak but statistically significant relationship between vasectomy and prostate cancer, but most does not. In 1993, the National Institutes of Health convened a panel of experts to review the published reports. The committee recommended that further research should be conducted, but that changes in current vasectomy practices were not warranted.

Tubal ligation—The long-term effects of sterilization on the menstrual cycle, pelvic pain, and later pelvic surgery are controversial. Although menstrual disturbance had been considered a possible effect of sterilization, recent studies show little or no difference in menstrual cycles in women before and after sterilization, or between sterilized and unsterilized women, according to the American College of Obstetricians and Gynecologists (ACOG). ACOG notes that women sterilized before age 30 are more likely to have a hysterectomy later on.

Sterilization may have a slight protective effect for ovarian cancer and pelvic inflammatory disease. A study that monitored some 77,000 women for 12 years found a reduced rate of ovarian cancer in women who had had tubal occlusion or hysterectomy.

How Often Does Sterilization Fail?

Vasectomy—The failure rate is less than 1 percent. Most failures are due to having unprotected sex too soon after the procedure. It takes about three months or 20 ejaculations to flush all viable sperm from the system and your semen must be tested to determine when that has occurred. Failure may also be due to the unlikely occurrence of spontaneous rejoining of the vas deferens or from failure to cut the correct structures in the scrotum.

Tubal ligation—While the failure rate for tubal ligation was long thought to be about the same as vasectomy, a recent Centers for Disease Control and Prevention (CDC) study indicated that over a ten-year period, the failure rate was slightly higher (about 2 percent) and that the risks of ectopic pregnancy are greater for women with tubal ligation. This is a concern because ectopic pregnancy (in which an embryo implants and develops outside the uterus) can be life-threatening. The risk is highest for women who are sterilized before age 30 or whose sterilization was with bipolar coagulation in which electric current cauterizes (burns) the tubes.

Does Sterilization Affect Sexual Desire or Function?

Vasectomy—Sexual function and desire are not affected. The ability to achieve and maintain erections and have orgasms with ejaculation is unchanged.

Tubal ligation—Sexual function and desire are not affected. In fact, both men and women frequently report increased pleasure because they are no longer worried about unwanted pregnancy.

How Expensive Is Sterilization?

Vasectomy—The cost may range from $250 to $1,000.

Tubal ligation—The cost may range from $1,000 to $2,500.

Can the Procedures Be Reversed?

Vasectomy—Should be considered permanent. Surgical reversal of a vasectomy is possible, but the outcome is very uncertain and expensive.

Tubal ligation—Should be considered permanent, but may be reversed. An attempt at reversal involves major surgery with about a 70 percent success rate.

Chapter 32

Female Sterilization

Chapter Contents

Section 32.1

All about Tubal Sterilization

Tubal sterilization is a permanent method of birth control. More and more women today choose sterilization. They know that this single procedure can provide highly effective protection against pregnancy for the remainder of their reproductive years. They also know that there is an increased chance of failure with many temporary methods, that some temporary methods have side effects, and that some may be inconvenient.

Sterilization does not decrease a woman's sexual pleasure. It is often the answer for women who have completed their families and for women who do not want children.

How Tubal Sterilization Works

Tubal sterilization is a surgical operation. It closes off the fallopian tubes, where eggs are fertilized by sperm. When the tubes are closed, sperm cannot reach the egg, and pregnancy cannot happen.

Sterilization does not affect femininity. It is very unlikely that sterilization will affect your sexual organs, or your sexuality. No glands or organs will be removed or changed. All of your hormones will still be produced. Your ovaries will release an egg every month. Your menstrual cycles will most likely follow their regular pattern.

Sterilization is more than 99 percent effective in the first year. In following years, there is a limited possibility that tubes may reconnect by themselves. Up to one out of 100 women become pregnant each year after sterilization. About one out of three of these pregnancies are ectopic (developing in the fallopian tubes) and may require emergency surgery.

What Are the Signs of Ectopic Pregnancy?

The signs of ectopic pregnancy include:

- severe pain on one or both sides of the lower abdomen
- abdominal pain and spotting, especially after a missed menstrual period or a very light one
- faint or dizzy feeling

If you think you have an ectopic pregnancy and can't reach your clinician, go to a hospital emergency room quickly.

You Must Consider the Operation Permanent

You and your partner will need no other birth control method after a successful tubal sterilization. It is possible to reverse it in some cases, but your decision not to have a child in the future must be firm. You must be absolutely sure you will never change your mind or regret your choice—no matter how your life changes.

Sterilization will not cause symptoms of menopause (change of life) or make menopause happen earlier.

Reasons for Considering Sterilization:

- You want to enjoy having sex without causing pregnancy.
- You don't want to have a child in the future.
- You and your partner agree that your family is complete, and no more children are wanted.
- You and your partner have concerns about the side effects of other methods.
- Other methods are unacceptable.
- Your health would be threatened by a future pregnancy.
- You don't want to pass on a hereditary illness or disability.

Reasons against Considering Sterilization:

- You may want to have a child in the future.

- You are being pressured by your partner, friends, or family. *You must want the operation.*

- You have problems that may be temporary—marriage or sexual problems, short-term mental or physical illnesses, financial worries, or being out of work. Sterilization is not a good solution for problems such as these.

- You have not considered possible changes in your life, such as divorce, remarriage, or death of children.

- You have not discussed it fully with your partner.

Thinking It Over

Consider **all** other methods before you choose sterilization. Birth control pills, Norplant® (implanted under the skin), Depo-Provera® (injection), and IUDs (intrauterine devices) can be similarly effective. Most women can use them with little risk of serious complications. Other methods, such as diaphragms, cervical caps, periodic abstinence, withdrawal, male or female condoms, spermicide foams, creams, jellies, and suppositories, are not as effective as sterilization. But they have very few serious side effects, if any.

Your partner also may want to consider sterilization. Sterilization for men is called vasectomy. Vasectomy is simpler, costs less, and has fewer risks than tubal sterilization. But vasectomy must also be considered permanent. So, think carefully about what sterilization will mean for both of you before you make your decision.

Sterilization Methods

Sterilizations are done in hospitals or in clinics with surgical units. They are done under local (patient awake) or general (patient asleep) anesthesia. Closing the tubes for sterilization can be done in several ways. Sometimes the tubes are closed off by tying and cutting (tubal ligation), sealing (cautery), or applying clips, clamps, or rings. Sometimes, a small piece of the tube is removed.

A woman's health condition may indicate which procedure is better suited for her. Previous surgery and body weight are two factors to consider when choosing the best and safest method. Women who have had certain types of abdominal surgery may not be able to have tubal sterilization. Consult your health care provider if you have any questions.

More than half of all sterilizations are performed shortly after child-birth or abortion. (The decision to combine sterilization with other procedures needs to be made in advance.)

Abdominal Procedures

Laparoscopy

Laparoscopy is one of the two most common methods of steriliza-tion. First the abdomen is inflated with an injection of harmless gas (carbon dioxide). This allows the organs to be seen clearly. Then the surgeon makes a small incision near the navel and inserts a laparo-scope (a rod-like instrument with a light and a viewing lens) for lo-cating the tubes. The surgeon also may insert an instrument for closing the tubes, usually through a second small opening. Sometimes only one incision and one instrument are used. The procedure can be per-formed in outpatient surgical clinics. It takes 20 to 30 minutes. Very little scarring occurs. Women often go home the same day. They may have sexual intercourse as soon as they feel comfortable about it. In-jury to the bowel or bleeding inside the abdomen occurs in five out of 1,000 cases. Major surgery may be required to resolve such complica-tions.

Mini-laparotomy

Mini-laparotomy is another common method of sterilization. It is often performed after childbirth. No gas or visualizing instrument is used in mini-laparotomy. A small incision is made in the lower abdo men, just above the pubic hair. (If the operation takes place within 48 hours of delivery, the incision is made just below the navel.) The sur-geon locates the tubes, then ties, clips, or uses electrocautery to block them off. The incision is then closed. Women usually recover in a few days. Doctors will advise when sexual intercourse can be resumed.

Laparotomy

Laparotomy is major surgery. It is less commonly used than mini-laparotomy and laparoscopy. The surgeon makes a two-to-five-inch incision in the abdomen. The surgeon locates and closes off the tubes. The operation requires general or spinal anesthesia. A woman may need to be hospitalized for two to four days. It may take several weeks at home to completely recover. If the procedure is done after delivery, the woman's hospital stay may be extended by one or two days. When to resume sexual intercourse depends on the rate of recovery.

Vaginal Procedures

Vaginal procedures are not performed very frequently. Fewer and fewer U.S. surgeons are trained in the procedure.

Culdoscopy

The surgeon makes an incision in the vagina. Then the surgeon inserts a culdoscope (an instrument with a light on the end) through the incision. The tubes are located, brought into view, closed off, and returned to their normal position.

Colpotomy

The surgeon makes an incision in the vagina. No visualizing instrument is used. The tubes are located, brought into view, closed off, and returned to their normal position.

Culdoscopy and **colpotomy** take 15 to 30 minutes. Women usually go home the same day. It may take a few days at home to recuperate. Sexual intercourse is usually postponed until the incision is completely healed, as advised by the doctor. This may take several weeks. There are no visible scars. However, there may be more risk of serious infection than with other procedures. Also, the failure rate (about 2 percent) is higher than for abdominal procedures.

Tubal Sterilization Is Low-Risk Surgery

Complications can occur with any kind of surgery. The complications that can occur during or after sterilization are:

- bleeding
- infection
- reaction to the anesthetic

Infection is rare, but it occurs more frequently after sterilization performed through the vagina. Infections are treated with antibiotics. Very rarely, the bowel or blood vessels are injured. Major surgery may be required to repair this.

Complications may develop in 1 to 4 percent of sterilizations performed through the abdomen. They may develop in 2 to 13 percent of sterilizations performed through the vagina. Deaths resulting from tubal sterilization are extremely rare—the rate is about four per 100,000.

Higher Risk Surgery: Hysterectomy

Hysterectomy is the removal of the uterus (womb). It is major surgery and is not usually used for sterilization. It is used to correct significant medical conditions. Hysterectomy ends menstruation as well as the possibility of pregnancy. It does not necessarily affect the fallopian tubes. However, some medical conditions also call for the removal of a tube and/or ovary, on one side or both.

Hysterectomy is performed through the abdomen or vagina. Sometimes a combined approach is used. Women need to spend several days in the hospital. They usually spend several weeks at home recuperating. They should abstain from sexual intercourse for four to six weeks, until the doctor advises it is all right.

Complications after hysterectomy occur in 10 to 20 percent of cases. Because hysterectomy is usually performed in conjunction with a significant medical condition, the risk of death is much greater than it is for tubal sterilization—300 to 500 per 100,000 cases. The cost is also considerably greater.

Questions and Answers about Tubal Sterilization

Will Sterilization End an Existing Pregnancy?

No. Sterilization will not be performed if you are pregnant.

Will It Cause Menopause?

No. Sterilization does not cause menopause or any of its symptoms.

Will It Prevent Menopause?

No. You will still experience menopause later in life.

Will It Prevent Sexually Transmitted Infections?

No.

Will I Still Have a Period?

Yes. Most menstrual cycles and flow are the same after the operation as they were before. However, women who have had their tubes cauterized may have more menstrual disturbances. Also, if you were using birth control pills before the surgery, it may take a while for your cycle to get back to normal.

What Happens to the Eggs?

An egg is released each month. It dissolves and is absorbed by the body. Other dead and unused cells are absorbed naturally by the body throughout life.

Will I Be as Feminine?

Yes. The hormones that affect hair, voice, sex drive, muscle tone, breast size, etc., are still made in your ovaries. They will still flow throughout the body in the bloodstream.

Will I Gain Weight or Develop Facial Hair?

No. Sterilization does not cause weight gain or facial hair.

Will It Hurt?

A general or local anesthetic will be used. The choice depends on your physical condition and the method of sterilization being used. Local anesthesia is much safer than general anesthesia. There is less risk of serious complications, including death.

General anesthesia is entirely painless. When a local anesthetic is injected, you may feel some discomfort. The pain is relieved with medications and sedatives. You will remain conscious but sleepy. You will feel little or no discomfort during the procedure.

How Will I Feel After?

The discomfort you feel after the operation depends on your general health, the type of operation, and your tolerance of pain. You may feel tired and have slight abdominal pain. You may occasionally feel dizzy, nauseous, bloated, gassy, pain in the shoulder, or abdominal cramping. Most or all of such symptoms will last one to three days.

Contact your doctor immediately if you:

- develop a fever
- bleed from an incision
- have severe, continuous abdominal pain
- have fainting spells

How Soon Can I Have Sexual Intercourse Again?

Ask your doctor's advice. Do not have intercourse until you feel comfortable about it. It usually takes about a week after abdominal sterilization. You will have to wait at least four weeks after a vaginal sterilization or sterilization after childbirth.

Will Sterilization Decrease My Sexual Pleasure?

No. In fact, many women and men report that they have less tension about unwanted pregnancy after sterilization. They feel that the lack of tension increases their sexual pleasure.

Can Sterilization Be Reversed?

If you are thinking about reversal, don't have a tubal sterilization. Reversal procedures require complicated surgery and cost thousands of dollars. Even though tubes can sometimes be rejoined, pregnancy cannot be guaranteed. Many women cannot even attempt reversals because there is not enough of their tubes left in the reproductive tract.

How Soon Can I Go Back to Work after Sterilization?

That depends on your general health, attitude, job, and the method of sterilization that you have. With the most common methods—mini-laparotomy and laparoscopy—recovery is usually complete in a day or two. You may want to take it easy for the next week or so. In any case, you should avoid heavy lifting for about one week.

How Much Does a Tubal Sterilization Cost?

For the most common procedures, the cost is about $1,000 to $2,500. Some clinics and doctors adjust fees on a sliding scale according to income. Procedures that require hospitalization are more expensive.

Is Help with Payment Available?

Private health insurance policies may pay some or most of the cost. In about 35 states, Medicaid pays but puts some restrictions on patient eligibility. A 30-day waiting period is required from the signing of the consent form to the time that federally funded operations are performed. Federally funded sterilizations may not be performed on anyone under 21 or anyone incapable of legal consent. Check with your local welfare department to see if you are covered.

Is It Legal to Sterilize Anyone Who Doesn't Want It?

No. Sterilization is legal for mentally competent, adult women and men in all 50 states **only if it is voluntary**. No mentally competent person can be forced to have the operation. It is also illegal to deny, or threaten to deny, welfare benefits to women and men who choose to remain fertile.

Can Anyone Become Sterilized?

Under some circumstances—if a person is single or childless—sterilization may be difficult to arrange. Policies and practices vary with individual doctors and hospitals, and from place to place.

Do I Need My Husband or Partner's Consent?

No. However, discussing the operation beforehand is usually best for most relationships.

How Can I Get a Sterilization?

For assistance, contact any of the following:

- your family health care provider
- your local hospital
- your local public health department
- your local Planned Parenthood health center. Call toll-free 1-800-230-PLAN for the Planned Parenthood center nearest you.
- you may also contact:

  AVSC (Access to Voluntary and Safe Contraception International)
  440 Ninth Avenue
  New York, NY 10001
  (212) 561-8000
  www.avsc.org
  info@avsc.org

Section 32.2

Does Female Sterilization Affect Menstrual Patterns?

Female sterilization procedures, particularly laparoscopy and minilaparotomy, are both safe and effective. Most evaluations of the safety of sterilization have focused on the short-term complications and complaints associated with the procedures, but some researchers have looked at long-term effects. Concern has been expressed that sterilization may be related to subsequent disturbance of menstrual patterns to such a degree that hysterectomy or other surgical treatment is required.

Family Health International (FHI) collected data on menstrual patterns during clinical trials at 45 hospitals in 23 countries. Menstrual pattern changes were examined for 1,550 interval women (more than 42 days postpartum or post abortion) who sought sterilization for contraceptive purposes, who were aged 25–34 years old and who had between two and six live births. Women were asked at the time of the sterilization procedures about the characteristics of their three most recent menstrual cycles. These questions were repeated at all follow-up visits.

Four variables of the menstrual cycle were studied: regularity (regular or irregular); length of cycle (in days); duration of bleeding (in days); and dysmenorrhea (none, mild, moderate, severe).

Research has shown that use of certain contraceptives before sterilization can influence post-sterilization menstrual patterns:

- Former pill users have an increase in flow and in dysmenorrhea (menstrual pain) and irregularity, usually caused by stopping the pill and not by the operation.

- Former IUD users experience decreased flow and dysmenorrhea; and again, these changes are probably caused by the termination of IUD use, not by the sterilization procedure.

- Users of barrier methods report minimal disruption of menstrual patterns.

Because previous contraceptive use can influence pre-sterilization menstrual patterns, none of the women selected for this study were using hormonal or intrauterine contraception in the three months immediately before the sterilization.

Results

The majority of the women in the FHI study experienced no change in the 12 months following sterilization, and among those who did, changes in one direction were counterbalanced by changes in another direction. Specifically:

- 87 percent of the women had no change in regularity of cycles; more women became regular than became irregular.

- 61 percent of the women had no change in cycle length of more than two days; 20 percent reported shorter cycles; and 19 percent reported longer cycles.

- 52 percent of the women had no more than one day's change in duration of menstrual bleeding; 26 percent reported shorter menstrual periods; and 22 percent reported longer menstrual periods.

- 70 percent reported no change in dysmenorrhea; 17 percent reported less pain; and 13 percent reported more pain.

Women were separated according to whether their menstrual cycles were "normal" or "abnormal" at admission. This was done to see whether women with abnormal menstrual patterns were more or less likely to experience change. Normal was defined rather broadly: regular cycles with a length of 28 plus or minus seven days, duration of bleeding of two to seven days, and no more than mild dysmenorrhea. Women outside one or more of these parameters at the time of the sterilization procedures were defined as having an abnormal menstrual pattern; 21 percent were so defined.

Abnormality was the best predictor of change when all women were considered. Women with abnormal menstrual patterns at the time of sterilization were more likely to experience change in their menstrual patterns than women with normal patterns.

Percentage distribution of the number of menstrual pattern changes experienced at 12 months after sterilization for women with normal and abnormal menstrual patterns at admission.

No. of Changes	Normal at admission (%)	Abnormal at admission (%)	All women %	N
No change	61.9	20.4	53.3	830
One change	29.3	51.0	33.8	525
Two changes	8.2	24.2	11.5	179
Three changes	0.6	4.4	1.4	21
Total (%)	100.0	100.0	100.0	
N	1,237	318		1,555

Other findings:

- Both tubal rings and spring-loaded clips were associated with less change than the other methods of tubal occlusion, and ligation with excision was associated with more change. However, this difference was small and of little clinical significance.

- Surgical difficulties in performing the procedure had no demonstrable effect on change in the menstrual pattern.
- Complications during surgery or in the postoperative period did not appear to affect change in menstrual pattern.
- Although none of these women was scheduled to have concurrent surgery, a number underwent surgery in addition to tubal sterilization to treat conditions discovered at the time of the procedure. Concurrent surgery neither increased nor decreased the likelihood of change in the menstrual pattern.

Conclusion

Among women using neither hormonal nor intrauterine contraception before the sterilization, slightly more than half reported no change in their menstrual patterns a year after their sterilization operation. A substantial minority (47 percent) did report change. The changes included improvements in some parameters as well as changes for the worse. For example, more women reported that dysmenorrhea had decreased than reported that it increased. More women reported their menstrual patterns became regular than irregular.

In general, women whose menstrual patterns are abnormal at the time of the sterilization procedure are more likely to experience change than women with more average menstrual patterns.

Chapter 33

Male Sterilization

Chapter Contents

Section 33.1

All about Vasectomy

Vasectomy is permanent birth control for men. It is a surgical operation that causes sterility. About 500,000 men in the United States choose vasectomy every year. It is chosen by men who have completed their families or by men who want no children. These men want birth control that will last for as long as their partners are fertile. They prefer vasectomy because most reversible methods are less reliable, sometimes inconvenient, and may have unpleasant side effects for the women in their lives.

Vasectomy is nearly 100 percent effective. It is intended to be permanent. It is safe. It doesn't limit sexual pleasure.

How Vasectomy Works

Vasectomy is a simple operation. It makes men sterile by keeping sperm out of the fluid that spurts from the penis during sex. Sperm are the reproductive cells in men. Pregnancy can happen if a sperm joins with a woman's egg.

Sperm are produced in the testicles. They pass through tubes, the vas deferens, to other glands and mix with seminal fluids to form semen. Vasectomy blocks the vas deferens and keeps sperm out of the seminal fluid. The sperm are absorbed by the body instead of being ejaculated. Without sperm, your "cum" (ejaculate) cannot cause pregnancy.

Vasectomy does not affect masculinity. And it will not affect your ability to get hard and stay hard. The same is true for your sex organs, sexuality, and sexual pleasure. No glands or organs are removed or altered. Your hormones and sperm continue being produced. Your ejaculate will look just like it always did. And there will be about as much of it as before.

Vasectomy is not immediately effective. Sperm remains in the system beyond the blocked tubes. You must use other birth control until the sperm are used up. It usually takes from 15–20 ejaculations. A simple test—semen analysis—shows when there is no more sperm in the seminal fluid.

Very rarely, tubes grow back together again and pregnancy may occur. This happens in one out of 1,000 cases in the first year.

To Prevent Unintended Pregnancy: Vasectomy is the most effective birth control for sexually active men. You and your partner will need no other contraceptive after a successful vasectomy. You must regard sterilization as permanent, even though it may be reversible in some cases. Your decision to have no biological children in the future must be firm. You must be absolutely sure you will never change your mind or regret your choice no matter how your life changes.

Reasons for Considering Vasectomy:

- You want to enjoy having sex without causing pregnancy.
- You don't want to have a child in the future.
- Your partner agrees that your family is complete, and no more children are wanted.
- You and your partner have concerns about the side effects of other methods.
- Other methods are unacceptable.
- Your partner's health would be threatened by a future pregnancy.
- You don't want to pass on a hereditary illness or disability.
- You want to spare your partner the surgery and expense of tubal sterilization for women, which is more complicated and costly.

Do Not Consider Vasectomy if:

- You want to have a child in the future.
- You are being pressured by your partner, friends, or family—you must want the operation.
- You have marriage or sexual problems, short-term mental or physical illnesses, financial worries, or you are out of work—vasectomy is not a good solution for temporary problems.
- You have not considered possible changes in your life, such as divorce, remarriage, or death of children.
- You have not discussed it fully with your partner.

- You plan to bank sperm in case you change your mind—sperm banks collect, freeze, and thaw sperm for artificial insemination. However, some men's sperm does not survive freezing. And after six months, frozen sperm may begin to lose the ability to fertilize an egg.

Other Options: Consider all other methods before you choose vasectomy. The Pill, Norplant®, Depo-Provera®, and IUDs are more than 97 percent effective. Most women can use them with little risk of serious complications. Other methods that have little or no side effects are diaphragms, cervical caps, condoms, vaginal pouches, periodic abstinence, and contraceptive foams, jellies, and suppositories.

Your partner also may want to consider sterilization. There are new sterilization procedures for women that reduce the cost, recovery time, and extent of the surgery. But vasectomy is simpler, costs less, and has fewer risks. In all cases, the results must be considered permanent.

So, think carefully about what sterilization will mean for both of you and your futures.

Vasectomy Is Low-Risk Surgery

Complications can occur with any kind of surgery. Major complications with vasectomy are rare and are usually associated with infection. Warning signals include:

- a fever over 100.4 F
- blood or pus oozing from the cite of the incision
- excessive pain or swelling.

Other potential problems:

- Bleeding into the skin during surgery may cause bruises that will clear up by themselves. Swellings containing blood hematomas occur in fewer than two out of 100 cases. They usually clear up by themselves, or with bed rest or ice packs. Surgical drainage is rarely needed.
- Swellings containing fluid hydrocels and tenderness near the testicles occur in less than one out of 100 cases. This usually clears up in about a week. Applying heat and wearing an athletic support helps. Surgical drainage is rarely needed.

- Sperm leak from the tubes can cause a small lump granuloma under the skin near the site of the operation in about 18 out of 100 cases. Sperm granuloma usually clear up by themselves. Surgical treatment is sometimes required.
- Mild infections occur in up to seven out of 100 cases. Rarely, an abscess may develop. Treatment with antibiotics is successful.
- Very rarely, the cut ends of the vas deferens grow back together (recanalization). This most often happens within four months of the operation and may allow pregnancy to happen.
- Decreased sexual desire or inability to become erect occur in four out of 1,000 cases. The most likely cause is emotional ... there is no physical cause for sexual dysfunction associated with vasectomy.

There has been no proven association between vasectomy and prostate cancer. However, all men between 50 and 70 years old should be screened for prostate cancer every year whether or not they have had vasectomies.

Some Questions and Answers

Can the Operation Fail?

Yes, but in fewer than two in 1,000 cases.

How Soon Can I Have Sex Again?

That depends on you. Most men start again within a week. Others have sex sooner. Some wait longer. But remember, it takes about 15–20 ejaculations to clear sperm out of your system. Use another form of birth control for vaginal intercourse until a semen analysis shows there are no longer sperm in your seminal fluid.

How Is Semen Analysis Done?

You will provide a sample of your semen by masturbating or by using a special condom during sexual intercourse. The fluid will be examined under a microscope to see if there are any sperm in your seminal fluid.

Will Vasectomy Affect My Sexual Pleasure?

Your erections, orgasms, and ejaculations will very likely be the same. Most men say they have greater sexual pleasure because they don't have to worry about an unwanted pregnancy. Many say there is no change.

Rarely, men lose some sexual desire. More rarely, men lose the ability to become hard. Often, such losses have to do with their emotional condition before the operation.

Will I Be as Masculine?

Yes. Vasectomy is not castration. Sterility is not impotence. The hormones that affect masculinity, beard, voice, sex drive, etc., are still made in testicles. They still flow throughout the body in the blood stream.

Will There Be "Cum" when I "Come"?

Yes. But there will be no sperm in the ejaculate. Your semen is between 2 and 5 percent sperm. The rest is seminal fluid from the prostate and other glands. The change in the amount of fluid is too little to notice.

After Vasectomy Where Do the Sperm Go?

They dissolve and are absorbed into the body. Dead and unused cells are absorbed by the body throughout life. Antibodies to sperm develop in 50 percent of men who have vasectomies. Normally, antibodies protect the body against viruses and bacteria. Sperm antibodies will not affect your general health. But they may lessen the chance of restoring fertility if vasectomy is reversed.

How Much Time Will I Have to Take Off Work?

That depends on your general health, attitude, and your job. Most men lose little or no time from work. A few need a day or two to rest. You will have to avoid strenuous labor or exercise for three to five days.

Rare complications may require more days at home. However, prompt medical attention should clear up any problems.

How Long Will the Operation Take?

The surgery takes about 20 minutes.

Who Will Do It?

A doctor urologist does it in an office, hospital, or clinic.

How Is Vasectomy Done?

Usually, a local anesthetic is injected into the area. Then, to reach the tubes, the doctor makes an incision on each side of the scrotum. Sometimes a single incision is made in the center. Each tube is blocked. In most procedures, a small section of each tube is removed. Tubes may be tied off, cauterized, or blocked with surgical clips.

With the no-scalpel method the skin of the scrotum is not cut. One tiny puncture is made to reach both tubes. The tubes are then tied off, cauterized, or blocked. The tiny puncture heals quickly. No stitches are needed, and no scarring takes place.

The no-scalpel method reduces bleeding and decreases the possibility of infection, bruising, and other complications.

Will It Hurt?

You and your doctor will discuss which type of anesthetic to use. Local anesthetic is most usual. Sometimes a general anesthetic is called for. No pain is felt under general anesthesia because you are asleep. Some discomfort may be felt when the local anesthetic is injected or when the tubes are brought into the incision.

As with any surgery, there's some discomfort after the operation. It will be different for each man. However, most men say the pain is "slight" or "moderate" as opposed to "excessive." An athletic support, ice bag, and aspirin may help relieve the pain. Avoid strenuous physical labor or exercise for three to five days, There seems to be less pain associated with no-scalpel procedures.

Does Vasectomy Protect against Sexually Transmitted Infections?

No. Sexually transmitted infections can be carried in ejaculate, whether or not it contains sperm.

Can Vasectomy Be Reversed?

Sometimes it is possible to reverse the operation, but there are no guarantees. Reversal costs from $1,600 to $5,000 and involves intricate surgery. Success in restoring fertility is uncertain. From 16 to 79 percent of men with reversed vasectomies are able to cause pregnancy. The factors in this wide range include:

- the length of time since the vasectomy was performed
- whether or not antisperm antibodies have developed
- age of the woman partner
- the method used for vasectomy and the length and location of segment of vas that was removed or blocked.

Is Pregnancy Possible after Vasectomy?

Some sperm will remain in your system for a short time after the operation. They can cause pregnancy. Your ejaculate will be tested after 15–20 orgasms following the operation. The test will be repeated until no sperm are seen. Only then should you stop using other birth control.

Are There Laws Covering Vasectomy?

Mentally competent adults can legally choose sterilization in all 50 states. No one who is mentally competent can be forced to have the operation. You cannot be denied welfare benefits if you do not want to have a vasectomy. Even threats to do so are against federal law.

Policies and practices vary with individual doctors, hospitals, and health centers. Sterilization may be difficult to arrange under some circumstances; for instance, if a person is single or childless.

How Much Does a Vasectomy Cost?

Fees range between $240–$1,000 for an interview, counseling, examination, operation, and follow-up sperm count. (Sterilization for women costs up to four times as much.) Some clinics and doctors use a sliding scale according to income.

Is Help with Payment Available?

Blue Cross and Blue Shield and some private health insurance policies may pay some or most of the cost. In about 35 states, Medicaid pays but puts some restrictions on patient eligibility. Check with your local department of social services to see if you are covered.

Are There Special Requirements?

You are not required to have the consent of your wife or partner, but you should discuss the operation with her beforehand. Sometimes waiting periods are required to allow more time for thought before the operation. For federally funded vasectomies, you must:

- be at least 21 years old
- observe a 30-day waiting period after signing a statement of informed consent
- be free of the influence of alcohol or other drugs at the time of consent
- reapply if the procedure is postponed for more than 180 days.

How Can I Get a Vasectomy?

Contact any of the following:

- Your family doctor.
- Your local hospital.
- Your local public health department.
- Your local Planned Parenthood health center. To make an appointment with the Planned Parenthood health center nearest you, call toll-free 1-800-230-PLAN.
- Or contact:

  AVSC (Access to Voluntary and Safe Contraception)
  440 Ninth Avenue
  New York, NY 10001
  (212) 561-8000
  www.avsc.org
  info@avsc.org

Section 33.2

No-Scalpel Vasectomy

Excerpted from "No-Scalpel Vasectomy: Good News for Men Considering Vasectomy," © 2000 AVSC International; available at http://www.avsc.org/contraception/cnsv.html; reprinted with permission.

Advantages of No-Scalpel Vasectomy

- No incision
- No stitches
- Faster procedure
- Faster recovery
- Less chance of bleeding and other complications
- Less discomfort
- Just as effective

What Is Different about a No-Scalpel Vasectomy?

No-scalpel vasectomy is different from a conventional vasectomy in the way the doctor gets to the tubes. In addition, an improved method of anesthesia helps make the procedure less painful.

In a conventional vasectomy, after the scrotum has been numbed with a local anesthetic, the doctor makes one or two small cuts in the skin and lifts out each tube in turn, cutting and blocking them so the sperm cannot reach the semen. Then the doctor stitches the cuts closed.

In a no-scalpel vasectomy, the doctor feels for the tubes under the skin and holds them in place with a small clamp. Instead of making two incisions, the doctor makes one tiny puncture with a special instrument. The same instrument is used to gently stretch the opening so the tubes can be reached. The tubes are then blocked using the same meth-

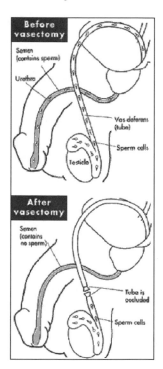

ods as conventional vasectomy. There is very little bleeding with the no-scalpel technique. No stitches are needed to close the tiny opening, which heals quickly, with no scar. The no-scalpel vasectomy was invented by a Chinese surgeon, and is used throughout China. It was introduced in the United States in 1988, and many doctors in this country have now mastered the technique.

Is No-Scalpel Vasectomy Safe?

Vasectomy in general is safe and simple. Vasectomy is an operation, and all surgery has some risks, such as bleeding, bruising, and infection. But serious problems usually do not happen.

Does No-Scalpel Vasectomy Work?

It is as effective as any other vasectomy method. There is a less than 1 percent chance that a man's partner will become pregnant.

How Long Will a No-Scalpel Vasectomy Take?

It depends upon the doctor, but on average, about ten minutes. Most vasectomies are done right in the doctor's office, or in a clinic.

Will It Hurt?

Before the vasectomy, the doctor may give you a mild sedative to relax you. When the local anesthetic is injected into the skin of the scrotum, you will feel some discomfort. But as soon as it takes effect, you should feel no pain. Afterwards, you will be sore for a couple of days, and you might want to take a mild painkiller. But the discomfort is usually less with the no-scalpel technique, because there is less injury to the tissues. Also, there are no stitches. Your doctor or nurse will provide you with complete instructions about what to do after surgery.

How Soon Can I Go Back to Work?

You should not do heavy physical labor for at least 48 hours after your vasectomy. If your job doesn't involve this kind of work, you can go back sooner. Many men have their vasectomies on Friday so they can take it easy over the weekend and go back to work on Monday.

Can a No-Scalpel Vasectomy be Reversed?

No more than any other vasectomy procedure. All vasectomies should be considered permanent. Reversal operations are expensive and not always successful. If you are thinking about reversal, perhaps vasectomy is not right for you.

Where Can I Find a Doctor Who Does No-Scalpel Vasectomy?

AVSC provides an up-to-date listing of U.S. and Canadian doctors who have reported that they have received training in no-scalpel vasectomy. You can also request a more complete list of doctors in your state who do this procedure from AVSC International. Send e-mail stating your request to: info@avsc.org. The list cannot be sent via e-mail, so be sure to include your mailing address.

You can also check with your doctor, family planning clinic, or local medical society to get information about doctors in your area who use this technique.

Chapter 34

Sterilization Reversal

Most men and women who have chosen voluntary sterilization as a permanent method of family planning remain happy with the choice. However, a few of the people who have had sterilizations change their minds. Some do because of major changes in their lives; they want to be able to have children again because they have remarried after divorce or the death of a partner or because one or more of their children have died. Others have trouble adjusting to no longer being able to have children. These people often seek to have their sterilizations reversed.

What Is Sterilization Reversal?

Sterilization reversal is the surgical attempt to restore an individual's ability to have children by reconnecting the tubes that have been blocked by sterilization. These tubes are the vasa deferentia in men and the fallopian tubes in women. Reversal surgery is a major operation.

How Successful Is It?

New techniques have made reversal surgery more successful than ever, but success reports have to be weighed carefully.

Most people think about reversal because they want another child. Thus, the only way to judge success is whether a couple has a baby after the reversal operation has been performed. Unfortunately, not all reports use this definition of success.

Also, success reports do not count those men and women who have asked for reversal but have been screened out because it is unlikely that their reversal surgery will be successful. For example, one report claims that, when everything seems right for reversal, 60 percent of women and 50 percent of men who have reversal surgery will be able to have another child. However, these success rates do not include those who were rejected for the operation.

How Do I Know if I'm a Good Candidate for Reversal?

You may be a good candidate for reversal if:

- You are in your late thirties or younger (if you are a woman).
- You are in your forties or younger (if you are a man).
- You are in good health.
- Your partner is fertile (and, if you are a woman, you ovulate regularly).
- Fewer than ten years have passed since your sterilization operation.
- Only small sections of your tubes were damaged by sterilization.

How Will I Be Screened?

The screening process will probably consist of:

- A physical examination
- A medical history
- A series of laboratory tests
- A review of the medical reports of your sterilization
- An evaluation of your partner's fertility

Women will usually undergo a diagnostic laparoscopy, a surgical procedure that is done to examine the condition of their tubes. Some physicians will require a special test be performed after the couple resumes sexual relations.

How Does the Sterilization Method Used Affect Success of Reversal?

How Does the Sterilization Method Used to Block the Fallopian Tubes Affect the Success of Reversal?

The success of reversal surgery depends upon the damage done to the tubes by the sterilization operation. Some sterilization methods destroy more tissue than others. Clips do the least damage, followed by rings and tying methods. Electrocoagulation does the most damage and is the least reversible.

Although sterilization methods that destroy the most tissue are the least reversible, they are believed to be the most effective means of sterilization. This is why electrocoagulation has been widely used in the United States as a method of blocking the tubes.

What Factors in the Original Vasectomy Will Influence the Reversal Success?

Successful reversal of vasectomy also depends upon the amount of undamaged tube left after sterilization. Ligation damages less tissue than electrocoagulation. In addition, the chance of reversal success is greater if the vasectomy was done on the straight sections of the vas, and if the pieces to be joined are of equal size. Unfortunately, the surgeon can judge whether the conditions are good for successful male reversal only at the time of the reversal surgery.

Does the Reversal Technique Used Affect Success?

The use of an operating microscope or surgical loupe to magnify the surgical area during the operation is important. It is even more important in male reversal procedures than in female procedures, since the thin vas deferens is more difficult to reconnect than the larger fallopian tube.

The reports of greater success using microsurgical techniques may also be due to the increased training and experience of most microsurgeons. The skill and experience of the surgeon strongly influence the outcome of reversal surgery.

How Long Will I Have to Stay in the Hospital?

A reversal operation is major surgery and is usually performed under general anesthesia which puts you to sleep.

Female reversal surgery requires three to six hours of surgery, up to one week in the hospital, and two to three weeks of recovery at home. Most male reversal surgery takes one to two hours in the operating room, several days in the hospital, and several days of recovery at home. Some physicians and clinics do male reversal surgery on an outpatient basis.

What Are the Risks of Reversal Surgery?

For women, reversal surgery carries with it the risks usually associated with major surgery of the abdomen or pelvis and the risks associated with anesthesia. In addition, after a reversal that leads to a pregnancy, there is increased likelihood of ectopic (tubal) pregnancy. In an ectopic pregnancy, the fertilized egg attaches outside the uterus, usually in the fallopian tube. Ectopic pregnancy is dangerous and requires immediate medical attention. This risk may be greater if a more destructive method, like electrocoagulation, was used for the sterilization.

For men, hematoma (a collection of blood under the skin) and infection are more common after reversal surgery than after vasectomy. There are also risks associated with anesthesia.

How Much Does Reversal Surgery Cost?

As with most medical procedures, costs vary according to the doctor and part of the country, but reversal surgery is expensive. First, you will be charged for the screening tests that will help the surgeon decide whether you are a good candidate for reversal. If you go ahead with the operation, the surgeon's fee for female reversal can be $5,000 or more; male procedures are very close to that figure. Added to this are the costs of the operating room, the assistant surgeon, the anesthesiologist, and the hospital stay.

You will want to ask your surgeon for an estimate of the total cost of the procedure before you decide to go ahead with it.

Will My Medical Insurance Pay for a Sterilization Reversal?

At the present time, most insurance plans do not cover reversal surgery. Assistance from Medicaid is available in some states. You should check with your source of medical insurance to find out just how much financial help you will have.

I've Had a Sterilization and Am Thinking about Reversal. What Should I Do?

First, you might want to explore your reasons for thinking about reversal with a family planning counselor. Many people have had sterilizations because they have not been satisfied with other kinds of birth control. If you are one of these people, you should think about what form of family planning you will use if the reversal operation is successful.

Then, if you decide you are still interested, contact a surgeon who specializes in reversals to discuss your chances for success. You should be able to get the name of such a physician from your urologist or gynecologist, your family doctor, a family planning clinic, or the nearest large medical center. You will want to know about the physician's experience, success rate (in terms of babies born), and surgical techniques.

I Haven't Had a Sterilization but Am Planning One and Am Interested In Reversal. What Should I Do?

Because the success of reversal cannot be guaranteed, sterilization should be considered permanent. If you are considering a sterilization and are also thinking about reversal, perhaps sterilization is not for you. Think about the step carefully. Discuss it with your partner and with your doctor or family planning counselor. Explore temporary methods of birth control, which may better suit your needs at this time. No one should have a sterilization as a temporary measure. It is intended to be permanent. If you have further questions or want additional information, please send e-mail at info@avsc.org or write or call:

AVSC International
440 Ninth Avenue
New York, NY 10001
(212) 561-8000

Note: AVSC does not make referrals to individual physicians.

Part Eight:

Emergency Contraception

Chapter 35

Emergency Contraception Backgrounder

In the United States, 28.8 million women age 15 to 44 have had at least one unintended pregnancy, according to the Centers for Disease Control and Prevention. Each year, contraceptive failure causes approximately half of the 2.7 million unintended pregnancies in the United States. About 1.35 million unintended pregnancies end in abortion annually. According to researchers, on the average night in America, over 700,000 women of childbearing age do not use any birth control at all. Each night, approximately 27,000 condoms break or slip.

These are startling statistics, and public education efforts aimed at curbing unintended pregnancy have to a large degree overlooked the important role emergency contraception (EC) can play in reducing the number of unintended pregnancies and abortions across America.

Emergency contraception is not new. In the mid-1960s, a Dutch family planning pioneer, Dr. Ary Haspels, first administered high doses of postcoital estrogen to a 13-year-old rape victim. His regimen became the first standard use of steroidal hormones as emergency contraception to prevent pregnancy. Further research, primarily that of Canadian physician Dr. Albert Yuzpe in the 1970s, led to a standard regimen utilizing oral contraceptives ("the pill").

For years, the U.S. Food and Drug Administration invited pharmaceutical companies to submit applications for approval of emergency contraceptives but no manufacturer responded. In 1997 the FDA declared the Yuzpe regimen to be safe and effective in a further effort to encourage the development of dedicated EC products. One company did answer the FDA's challenge, Gynetics Inc. (Belle Mead, NJ), and in September 1998, the FDA approved the PREVEN™ Emergency Contraceptive Kit, which to date is the only product packaged and marketed exclusively for use as an emergency contraceptive.

What Is Emergency Contraception?

The most common emergency contraception regimen uses progestin and estrogen (levonorgestrel and ethinyl estradiol), the same hormones found in birth control pills. Emergency contraception, started as soon as possible within 72 hours, can prevent pregnancy after sex without birth control or sex with known or suspected birth control failure. The sooner emergency contraception is started, the more effective it will be. EC (combination levonorgestrel and ethinyl estradiol) works the same way birth control pills do to prevent pregnancy, in that it can delay or prevent the release of an egg (ovulation).

Emergency contraception is sometimes called the "morning-after pill." Actually, it can be taken up to 72 hours (three days) after sex to prevent pregnancy.

Emergency contraception should not be confused with RU-486, the European "abortion pill," which interrupts an existing pregnancy. Emergency contraception is not an "abortion pill" and will not harm an existing pregnancy.

Another reason emergency contraception is a preferred term is that EC is not a replacement for the responsible use of regular contraception. It is an important "back-up" method for use when contraception fails or was not used. Further, as with all oral contraceptives, EC does not protect against infection with HIV, the virus that causes AIDS, and other sexually transmitted diseases.

How Does Emergency Contraception Work?

Emergency contraception works the same way birth control pills do to prevent pregnancy, in that it can delay or prevent the release of an egg (ovulation). For a pregnancy to happen, an egg must be released, fertilized in the fallopian tube, and then travel to the uterus where it implants. Thus, fertilization is an important step toward pregnancy, but it is not synonymous with pregnancy.

Not everyone understands the basic facts of life regarding pregnancy and the many steps involved between intercourse and a successful pregnancy. A pregnancy begins with implantation in the uterus, not fertilization. A woman can only become pregnant during a specific time frame during her menstrual cycle. Researchers have estimated this as approximately the five days before ovulation and the day of ovulation (when the chance of getting pregnant is highest—30 percent). Some research indicates that fertilization might also occur in the 12 to 24 hours after ovulation, but the latest research indicates that this would be extremely rare if it occurs at all.

The roles of ovulation and fertilization as steps toward pregnancy help explain why emergency contraception, which can delay or prevent ovulation, and thus fertilization, can prevent pregnancy. It has been theorized that birth control pills may also prevent fertilization or implantation but no definitive evidence of this has been demonstrated.

Is Emergency Contraception Safe?

The FDA based its support of emergency contraception on a meta-analysis of ten studies with special doses of regular birth control pills that showed a favorable safety profile. No published studies using evidence-based criteria have reported contraindications to the use of the most common—and most studied—EC regimen, combination levonorgestrel and ethinyl estradiol.

While the regular use of birth control pills is associated with both health benefits and slightly increased risks for cardiovascular and other uncommon side effects, it is not known whether this would also apply to their use as emergency contraception. As with all oral contraceptives, studies indicate that interactions between ethinyl estradiol and other drugs may occur, decreasing the effectiveness of ethinyl estradiol. EC side effects are similar to those of birth control pills. The most commonly reported side effects were nausea and/or vomiting. Other more serious side effects, although infrequent, can occur.

Additional Background Facts about Pregnancy and Abortion

In 1995, there were 2.7 million unintended pregnancies, about half (48 percent) of all pregnancies. When surveyed, 48 percent of women aged 15 to 44 reported that they have had at least one unintended pregnancy. More than half of the women who have an unintended pregnancy (53 percent) reported that they were using contraception when they got pregnant.

Unintended pregnancies have a severe impact on society and women's health. Nearly half (47 percent) of all unintended pregnancies end in abortion and 13 percent in miscarriage. Among women using contraception, 51 percent of unintended pregnancies end in abortion, and among women who are not using contraception, 43 percent end in abortion.

For unintended pregnancies carried to term (40 percent), the mother is at greater risk of depression, abuse, and not achieving her educational, financial, and career goals. Relationships that she may be in are at three times a greater risk of ending.

Other Methods of Emergency Contraception

While combined oral contraceptives are the most common form of emergency contraception, two others are progestin-only pills and the Copper T IUD. Research has been conducted in the use of progestin-only pills ("mini-pills") for emergency contraception. Treatment must be initiated within 72 hours (three days) after unprotected intercourse and requires two doses taken 12 hours apart. Published data suggest progestin-only pills are as effective as the Yuzpe regimen and may cause fewer side effects. As currently used in the United States, a large number of pills (20) is required for each dose.

Insertion of a Copper T IUD (intrauterine device) within five days after unprotected intercourse also can prevent pregnancy. Although not a common method, use of a Copper T IUD offers a wider time interval for administration, a favorably low failure rate, and leaves an ongoing contraceptive method in place. The IUD is generally not recommended for women at risk of sexually transmitted diseases.

Chpater 36

Combined Emergency Contraceptive Pills

Combined emergency contraceptive pills are ordinary birth control pills containing the hormones estrogen and progestin. Although this therapy is commonly known as the "morning-after" pill, this term is misleading; ECPs may be used immediately after unprotected intercourse, and up to 72 hours beyond. The treatment schedule is one dose within 72 hours after unprotected intercourse, and a second dose 12 hours after the first dose.

The hormones that have been studied in clinical trials of postcoital hormonal contraception are found in:

- Preven (one dose is 2 blue pills)
- Ovral (one dose is 2 white pills)
- Alesse (one dose is 5 pink pills)
- Levlite (one dose is 5 pink pills)
- Nordette (one dose is 4 light-orange pills)
- Levlen (one dose is 4 light-orange pills)
- Levora (one dose is 4 white pills)
- Lo/Ovral (one dose is 4 white pills)
- Triphasil (one dose is 4 yellow pills)

"Combined Emergency Contraceptive Pills" and "Instructions for Using Combined Emergency Contraceptive Pills," undated documents produced by the Office of Population Research at Princeton University; available at http://opr.princeton.edu/ec/ecp.html; reprinted with permission.

- Tri-Levlen (one dose is 4 yellow pills)
- Trivora (one dose is 4 pink pills)

Use of combined ECPs reduces the risk of pregnancy by about 75 percent. This does not mean that 25 percent of women will become pregnant. Rather, if 100 women have unprotected intercourse once during the second or third week of their menstrual cycle, about eight will become pregnant. If those same women had used combined emergency contraceptive pills, only two would have become pregnant (a 75 percent reduction). Therapy is more effective the earlier it is initiated within the 72-hour window.

About 50 percent of women who use combined ECPs experience nausea and 20 percent vomit. If vomiting occurs within two hours after taking a dose, the dose may need to be repeated. The long-acting non-prescription anti-nausea medicine meclizine (sold as a generic or under the brand names Dramamine II and Bonine) can reduce the risk of nausea when taken an hour before ECPs.

Almost all women can safely use combined ECPs. Although some women at risk of stroke, heart disease, blood clots, or other cardiovascular problems should not use birth control pills on a regular basis, medical experts believe that one-time emergency use of birth control pills by active women (women who are not bed-ridden) does not carry the same risks. Among women who definitely need to avoid estrogen, most could use one of the other two emergency contraceptive methods (progestin-only emergency contraceptive pills or the Copper-T IUD.

Emergency contraceptive pills require a prescription. Do not attempt to use them except under the supervision of a licensed clinician authorized to prescribe.

Instructions for Using Combined Emergency Contraceptive Pills

There are several choices for combined ECPs listed below. You need to take only one type of pill, not all of them. For example, if you use Ovral, you do not need Nordette. If you are getting your ECPs from a regular pack of birth control pills containing 28 pills (one for every day), remember that the last seven pills do not contain any hormones. In a 28-pill pack of Ovral, Alesse, Levlite, Lo/Ovral, Nordette, Levlen, or Levora, any of the first 21 pills can be used as ECPs. If you are using Triphasil or Tri-Levlen, the first 21 pills have three different colors, but only the yellow pills can be used as ECPs. If you are using Trivora, the first 21 pills have three different colors, but only the pink pills can be used as ECPs.

Brand of Pill

- Preven (blue pills)
  - — Swallow 2 pills as soon as possible
  - — Swallow 2 more pills 12 hours later
- Ovral (white pills only)
  - — Swallow 2 pills as soon as possible
  - — Swallow 2 more pills 12 hours later
- Lo/Ovral (white pills only), Nordette (yellow pills only), Levlen (orange pills only), Levora (white pills only), Triphasil (yellow pills only), Tri-Levlen (yellow pills only), or Trivora (pink pills only)
  - — Swallow 4 pills as soon as possible
  - — Swallow 4 more pills 12 hours later
- Alesse (pink pills only), Levlite (pink pills only)
  - — Swallow 5 pills as soon as possible
  - — Swallow 5 more pills 12 hours later

1. Swallow the first dose no later than 72 hours after having unprotected sex. The non-prescription anti-nausea medicine meclizine (Dramamine II or Bonine) may reduce the risk of nausea when taken an hour before the first ECP dose.

2. Swallow the second dose 12 hours after taking the first dose.

   Do not swallow any extra ECPs. More pills will probably not decrease the risk of pregnancy any further. More pills will increase the risk of nausea.

   About half of women have temporary nausea. It is usually mild and should stop in a day or so. If you vomit within two hours after taking a dose, call your clinician. You may need to repeat a dose. You may need some anti-nausea medicine.

   Watch for pill danger signals for the next couple of weeks. See your clinician at once if you have:

— severe pain in your leg (calf or thigh)

— severe abdominal pain

— chest pain or cough or shortness of breath

— severe headaches, dizziness, weakness, or numbness

— blurred vision, loss of vision, or trouble speaking

— yellow jaundice

3. Your next period may start a few days earlier or later than usual. If your period doesn't start within three weeks, see your clinician for an exam and pregnancy test. If you think that you may be pregnant, see your clinician at once, whether or not you plan to continue the pregnancy. ECPs may not prevent an ectopic pregnancy (in the tubes or abdomen). Ectopic pregnancy is a medical emergency.

4. Get started as soon as you possibly can with a method of birth control you will be able to use every time you have sex. ECPs are meant for one-time, emergency protection. ECPs are not as effective as other forms of birth control. If you want to resume use of birth control pills after taking ECPs, consult your clinician. Protect yourself from AIDS and other sexual infections as well as pregnancy. Use condoms every time you have sex if you think you may be at risk.

Preven has been approved by the U.S. Food and Drug Administration (FDA) for use for emergency contraception. Ovral, Lo/Ovral, Nordette, Levlen, Levlite, Triphasil, Tri-Levlin, Levora, Trivora, and Alesse have been approved by the FDA as regular birth control pills. These products have not been submitted to the FDA for use as ECPs, but clinical research studies have shown that ECPs are safe and effective. The FDA has explicitly declared all brands of birth control pills listed above to be safe and effective for use as emergency contraceptives.

Chpater 37

Progestin-only Emergency Contraceptive Pills

Progestin-only emergency contraceptive pills contain only progestin (and no estrogen). These not-commonly-used birth control pills are called mini-pills because they contain no estrogen and even less progestin than is found in ordinary oral contraceptives containing both estrogen and progestin. The treatment schedule is one dose within 72 hours after unprotected intercourse, and a second dose 12 hours after the first dose. In the United States, each dose is 20 Ovrette tablets. In other countries a single pill contains the amount of progestin needed for a single dose. Several companies are planning to introduce a dedicated progestin-only ECP in the United States.

Use of progestin-only ECPs reduces the risk of pregnancy by about 88 percent. This does not mean that 12 percent of women will become pregnant. Rather, if 100 women have unprotected intercourse once during the second or third week of their menstrual cycle, about eight will become pregnant. If those same women had used progestin-only ECPs, only one would have become pregnant (an 88 percent reduction). Therapy is more effective the earlier it is initiated within the 72-hour window.

Progestin-only ECPs are more effective than combined ECPs, and nausea and vomiting are far less common. Progestin-only ECPs are an excellent alternative for most women who cannot use combined ECPs, which contain estrogen.

"Progestin-only Emergency Contraceptive Pills" and "Instructions for Using Progestin-only Emergency Contraceptive Pills," undated documents produced by the Office of Population Research at Princeton University; available at http://opr.princeton.edu/ec/ecminip.html; reprinted with permission.

Emergency contraceptive pills require a prescription. Do not attempt to use them except under the supervision of a licensed clinician authorized to prescribe.

Instructions for Using Progestin-only Emergency Contraceptive Pills

There is currently only one choice in the United States for progestin-only pills. While no dedicated product exists in the United States, several companies are planning on introducing a dedicated progestin-only emergency contraceptive in the near future. In other countries, dedicated progestin-only products are available.

- Ovrette (yellow pills)
  - Swallow 20 pills as soon as possible
  - Swallow 20 more pills 12 hours later

1. Swallow the first dose no later than 72 hours after having unprotected sex.

2. Swallow the second dose 12 hours after taking the first dose.

   Do not swallow any extra ECPs. More pills will probably not decrease the risk of pregnancy any further. More pills will increase the risk of nausea.

   Nausea and vomiting occur less frequently with progestin-only ECPs than with combined ECPs. However, if you vomit within two hours after taking a dose, call your clinician. You may need to repeat a dose. You may need some anti -nausea medicine.

3. Your next period may start a few days earlier or later than usual. If your period doesn't start within three weeks, see your clinician for an exam and pregnancy test. If you think that you may be pregnant, see your clinician at once, whether or not you plan to continue the pregnancy. ECPs may not prevent an ectopic pregnancy (in the tubes or abdomen). Ectopic pregnancy is a medical emergency.

4. Get started as soon as you possibly can with a method of birth control you will be able to use every time you have sex. ECPs

are meant for one-time, emergency protection. ECPs are not as effective as other forms of birth control. If you want to resume use of birth control pills after taking ECPs, consult your clinician. Protect yourself from AIDS and other sexual infections as well as pregnancy. Use condoms every time you have sex if you think you may be at risk.

Chapter 38

Brands of Oral Contraceptives That Can Be Used for Emergency Contraception in the United States

Brands of Oral Contraceptives That Can Be Used for Emergency Contraception in the United States

Brand	Manufacturer	Pills per Dose	Ethinyl Estradiol per Dose (µg)	Levonor-gestrel per Dose (mg)
Preven	Gynétics	2 blue pills	100	0.50
Ovral	Wyeth-Ayerst	2 white pills	100	0.50
Alesse	Wyeth-Ayerst	5 pink pills	100	0.50
Levlite	Berlex	5 pink pills	100	0.50
Nordette	Wyeth-Ayerst	4 light-orange pills	120	0.60
Levlen	Berlex	4 light-orange pills	120	0.60
Levora	Watson	4 white pills	120	0.60
Lo/Ovral	Wyeth-Ayerst	4 white pills	120	0.60
Triphasil	Wyeth-Ayerst	4 yellow pills	120	0.50
Tri-Levlen	Berlex	4 yellow pills	120	0.50
Trivora	Watson	4 pink pills	120	0.50
Ovrette	Wyeth-Ayerst	20 yellow pills	0	0.75

Undated table produced by the Office of Population Research at Princeton University; available at http://opr.princeton.edu/ec/dose.html; reprinted with permission.

Chapter 39

Copper-T IUD as Emergency Contraception

The copper-T intrauterine device (IUD) can be inserted up to five days after unprotected intercourse or five days after the expected date of ovulation, whichever is later, to prevent pregnancy. Insertion of a copper-T IUD is much more effective than use of ECPs or minipills, reducing the risk of pregnancy following unprotected intercourse by more than 99 percent. And a copper-T IUD can be left in place to provide continuous effective contraception for up to ten years. But IUDs are not ideal for all women. Women at risk of sexually transmitted infections because they or their partners have other sexual partners may not be good candidates for IUDs because insertion of the IUD can lead to pelvic infection, which can cause infertility if untreated. The risk of pelvic infection from insertion of an IUD is slight among women not at risk of sexually transmitted infections.

Undated document produced by the Office of Population Research at Princeton University; available at http://opr.princeton.edu/ec/eciud.html; reprinted with permission.

Part Nine:

Abortion

Chapter 40

Abortion: Commonly Asked Questions

What Is Abortion?

Abortion ends a pregnancy before birth takes place. When an embryo or fetus dies in the womb and is expelled by the body, it is called a spontaneous abortion or "miscarriage." When a woman decides to end her pregnancy voluntarily, she has an induced abortion. When a fetus is dead at birth, it is called a "stillbirth."

When Are Abortions Performed?

More than 90 percent of all induced abortions are performed during the first trimester—the first three months of pregnancy. In fact, more than half are performed within the first two months of pregnancy. These abortions are usually performed at a clinic, health center, or in a doctor's office, and the women go home an hour or so later.

Fewer than 9 percent of abortions take place in the second trimester—14 through 24 weeks of pregnancy. Abortions in the second trimester are more complicated procedures but are safer than childbirth.

Abortion in the last three months of pregnancy is extremely rare. Only one out of 10,000 abortions takes place after 24 weeks. It is more complicated and is performed only when the pregnancy seriously threatens a woman's health or life or when the fetus is severely deformed.

Who Has Abortion?

Approximately 1.5 million U.S. women with unwanted pregnancies choose abortion each year. Most are under 25 years old and unmarried. Women who are separated from their husbands and poor women are more likely to choose abortion than other women. More than two-thirds of the women who seek abortions have jobs. Nearly one-third are in school. More than two-thirds plan to have a child in the future.

Approximately six million women in the U.S. become pregnant every year. About half of those pregnancies are unintended. Either the woman or her partner did not use contraception or the contraceptive method failed.

Why Do Women Choose Abortion?

A recent survey showed that in most cases a woman who chooses abortion has at least three reasons. The most common of these reasons are:

- She is not ready for the way becoming a parent will change her life—it would be hard to keep her job, continue her education, and/or care for her other children.
- She cannot afford a baby now.
- She doesn't want to be a single parent, she doesn't want to marry her partner, he can't or won't marry her—or she isn't in a relationship.
- She is not ready for the responsibility.
- She doesn't want anyone to know she has had sex or is pregnant.
- She is too young or too immature to have a child.
- She has all the children she wants.
- Her husband, partner, or parent wants her to have an abortion.
- She or the fetus has a health problem.
- She was a victim of rape or incest.

Whatever your situation may be, it is important to consider all of your options and make your own decision. Whatever option you choose, Planned Parenthood is ready to offer you its expertise and support.

Who Will Help Me Decide if Abortion Is Right for Me?

Abortion is not always the best solution to an unwanted pregnancy. You have to decide for yourself if abortion is your best choice. However, most women look to their husbands, partners, families, health care providers, religious leaders, and friends for support and guidance as they make their decisions.

Family planning and abortion clinics also have specially trained counselors to talk with you about your choices when you face an unwanted pregnancy. You may bring your partner or your parents to the counseling session it you wish. All options—adoption, parenting, and abortion—will be discussed.

Your counselor will describe the abortion procedure and try to make sure that you are not being pressured into having an abortion by your husband, partner, family, or friends. The counselor should not try to influence your decision.

If you want to have a child and are being pressured to have an abortion, call Planned Parenthood for help. The Planned Parenthood policy is to provide counselors who will listen objectively, provide accurate information, and support your decision—whatever it is.

If abortion is chosen, the counselor or other clinic staff person may be with you during your pelvic exam and during the abortion. Some clinics may allow a supportive partner, husband, friend, or family member to be with you during the abortion.

Does My Partner, My Husband, or a Parent Need to Know?

Up to half of all women who have abortions go to the clinic with their partners. However, you do not have to notify your partner or husband to have an abortion. The clinic will ensure complete confidentiality.

More than half of all teenagers who have abortions have already talked with at least one parent. However, telling a parent is not required in many states.

But 26 states do require a woman under 18 to tell a parent or get a parent's permission before she can have an abortion. If she cannot talk with her parents, or chooses not to, she can appear before a judge who will decide whether she is mature enough to make her own decision about abortion. If she is not mature, the judge must decide whether an abortion is in her best interests.

If you are a minor considering abortion, you must find out about the laws in your state. Your local Planned Parenthood health center can provide this information.

Is Abortion Safe?

Yes. Today, abortion is about twice as safe as having your tonsils out and is safer than childbirth. In fact, abortion is *11* times safer than giving birth up to the 18th week of pregnancy. However, the risk of rare, serious complications or death from abortion increases the longer a pregnancy goes on.

Does Abortion Hurt?

Most women say the discomfort of early abortion with local anesthetic is like menstrual cramps. For some women, abortion is very uncomfortable. Others feel very little. Abortion with local anesthetic after 24 weeks of pregnancy is about as painful as labor during birth. With a local anesthetic, a woman's pain is relieved, but she remains awake. Some clinics offer general anesthesia so the woman sleeps and feels nothing. General anesthesia, however, increases the medical risks and the length of time a woman must remain at the clinic.

What Tests, Exams, and Counseling Must I Have before I Can Have an Abortion?

You must be tested for pregnancy. You must be counseled about your pregnancy options. And you must have a physical examination before an abortion can take place.

The usual tests include:

- a urine or blood test for pregnancy
- a test for the Rh factor in your blood
- a blood test to screen for anemia
- a pelvic exam.

Sometimes a sonogram is needed to help determine how long you've been pregnant. Depending on your circumstances, testing for sexually transmitted infections such as gonorrhea or chlamydia may also be helpful.

During the physical:

- your medical history will be taken
- your weight, temperature, and blood pressure will be measured.

Depending on your circumstances, the physical exam may be more comprehensive.

Your counselor will answer any questions you have about your pregnancy and provide information about your choices, which are:

- having a baby and keeping it
- having a baby and giving it up for adoption
- abortion.

Depending on your needs, your counselor will review:

- prenatal care and where it is provided
- adoption and the location of adoption agencies
- abortion and where it is provided
- birth control and how to get it
- insurance coverage or other reimbursement for abortion, prenatal care, and delivery
- psychological counseling services available in the community.

Will I Have to Sign Anything?

You will need to sign a form requesting abortion services. This assures the clinician performing the abortion that you:

- have been informed about all your options
- have been counseled about the procedure, its risks, and how to care for yourself afterward
- have chosen abortion of your own free will.

How Is Abortion Performed?

The procedure used for an abortion depends on how long a woman has been pregnant.

How Is a Very Early Abortion Performed?

In very early abortion, the uterus is emptied with the gentle suction of a syringe. It can be done up to 49 days after the last menstrual period.

In some clinics, women can choose to use a combination of drugs to end their pregnancies. This is called medical abortion.

As we go to press, the U.S. Food and Drug Administration is expected to approve methods for medical abortion in the near future. Medical abortion uses medication prescribed by a doctor and does not require surgery. Medical abortion must take place within the first six weeks of pregnancy. Two combinations of medication are used for medical abortion:

- **The methotrexate-misoprostol method**—a woman receives an injection of methotrexate from her clinician. From five to seven days later she returns and inserts suppositories of misoprostol into her vagina. The pregnancy usually ends at home within a day or two. The embryo and other tissue that develops during pregnancy are passed out through the vagina.

- **The mifepristone-misoprostol method**—a woman swallows a dose of mifepristone under the guidance of her clinician. She returns in several days and inserts suppositories of misoprostol into her vagina. The pregnancy usually ends at home within four hours. The embryo and other tissue that develops during pregnancy are passed out through the vagina.

From 5 to 10 percent of medical abortions fail. In these cases, surgical procedures are required to end the pregnancy.

Medical abortion may not be available from all abortion providers even after it is approved.

How Is Early Abortion Performed?

The usual method of early abortion is suction curettage. It is performed from six to 14 weeks after your last period. The procedure takes about ten minutes.

- The vagina is washed with an antiseptic.
- Usually, a local anesthetic is injected into or near the cervix.

- The opening of the cervix is gradually stretched. One after the other, a series of increasingly thick rods (dilators) are inserted into the opening. The thickest may be the width of a fountain pen.

- After the opening is stretched, a tube is inserted into the uterus. This tube is attached to a suction machine.

- The suction machine is turned on. The uterus is emptied by gentle suction.

- After the suction tube has been removed, a curette (narrow metal loop) may be used to gently scrape the walls of the uterus to be sure that it has been completely emptied.

How Are Early Second-trimester Abortions Performed?

Abortions performed early in the second trimester are performed in two steps—dilation and evacuation (D&E). Second-trimester abortions are available in some clinics, as well as certain hospitals, up to the 25th week of pregnancy.

During the first step of a D&E:

- The vagina is washed with an antiseptic.

- Absorbent dilators may be put into the cervix, where they remain for several hours, often overnight. The dilators absorb fluids from the cervical area and stretch the opening of the cervix as they thicken.

- If you are to go home with the dilators in place, you will be given instructions for your care until you return for the abortion. You may be given antibiotics to prevent infection. If the dilators are left in overnight, you will also be given a 24-hour telephone number so you can contact the clinic staff should any problem arise. Gradual dilation is safer than having it done all at once. However, you may feel pressure or cramping while the dilator is in place.

During the second step of a D&E:

- You may be given intravenous medications to ease pain and/or prevent infection.

- A local anesthetic is injected into or near the cervix.

- The dilators are removed from the cervix.

- The fetus and other products of conception are removed from the uterus with instruments and suction curettage. This procedure takes about 10–20 minutes.

How Is Abortion after 24 Weeks of Pregnancy Performed?

Only one out of every 10,000 women who have abortions have them after 24 weeks. These are performed only when there is a serious threat to a woman's life or health or if the fetus is severely deformed.

One of the procedures is called the induction method. The doctor injects urea or salt solution into the uterus to induce contractions (labor) and cause a stillbirth. Or the doctor may insert prostaglandin into the vagina to induce labor and expel the fetus. Labor pains, which usually last from six to 24 hours, can be relieved with medication.

The induction method is usually done in a hospital and usually means staying overnight or longer. The chance of complications is greater than with early abortion or D&E—abortion after 24 weeks is about as risky as carrying the pregnancy to term.

Some providers use a three-step D&E procedure instead of the induction method for abortions after 24 weeks. In the first two steps, the cervix is dilated several times until it is wide enough to allow removal of the fetus with grasping instruments.

What Are the Health Risks of Abortion?

Complications can occur with any kind of medical procedure. Fewer than five out of 1,000 women who have early abortion will have serious complications. Women giving birth are much more likely than women having abortions to need major abdominal surgery, such as cesarean section, as a result of complications.

Complications from early abortion include:

- Allergic reactions to specific anesthetics or other medications. Women taking medications or drugs, including street drugs, may experience serious reactions to anesthesia. Be sure to tell your clinician what medications or recreational drugs you take. What you say will be strictly confidential.
- Incomplete abortion. This occurs in fewer than one out of 100 abortions. Incomplete D&E abortion occurs in one out of 200 of those performed. In such cases it may be necessary to repeat the suction and remove the tissue. Incomplete abortion may lead to

infection, heavy bleeding, or both. In rare instances, more surgery is required.

- Blood clots in the uterus. Clots that may cause severe cramping occur in about one out of 100 abortions. The clots are usually removed by a repeated suction curettage.

- Infection by germs from the vagina or cervix that get into the uterus. In many cases, the infection is a flare-up of a preexisting sexually transmitted infection. Fewer than one out of 100 women who have abortion become infected. Usually antibiotics clear up the infection. In rare cases, a repeat suction, hospitalization, or surgery is needed.

- Heavy bleeding that requires medical treatment. This is rare. Such bleeding may require medication, a repeat suction or dilation and curettage, or, rarely, surgery. Fewer than one in 1,000 cases require blood transfusions.

- A cut or torn cervix. This occurs in fewer than one out of 100 early abortions. Stitches are rarely needed to repair the injury.

- Perforation of the wall of the uterus. In about one of 1,000 early abortions, an instrument goes through the wall of the uterus. In even fewer cases, perforation leads to infection, heavy vaginal or abdominal bleeding, or both. In D&E the number of perforations rises to three in 1,000 abortions. Surgery may be necessary to repair the uterine tissue. Very rarely, hysterectomy is required.

- Very rarely, in about six out of one million cases, a woman dies of complications from legal abortion.

Is Abortion Always 100 Percent Effective?

Abortion is almost always effective. It fails to end the pregnancy in only two out of 1,000 cases. This usually happens if there is more than one embryo or fetus or if an ectopic pregnancy has developed outside the uterus where suction curettage does not reach. Ectopic pregnancy threatens the life of the woman and requires surgery.

In cases when abortion fails, curettage is usually repeated. Otherwise, the pregnancy may develop abnormally.

What Happens after an Abortion?

After an abortion up to the 25th week, you will rest in a medically supervised recovery room for as long as necessary, usually about an hour. You will be able to rest until you feel ready to leave. During that time, you will be observed to make sure there are no complications.

If you have an Rh negative blood type, you will receive an injection to prevent the development of antibodies that could endanger any future pregnancy.

The clinic will give you written instructions for after-care and a 24-hour emergency phone number to use if complications arise. You will be able to discuss birth control with your counselor, and an appointment will be made for a follow-up examination in two to four weeks.

Can I Leave the Clinic Alone?

You may need to have a companion with you when you leave the clinic. Depending on which procedure you have, you may be weak or disoriented from the medication or anesthetic. Your health care providers will tell you what to do. They want to be sure you get home safely. You should not drive after general anesthesia or sedation.

How Long Will It Take to Recover from an Abortion?

Usually you can return to work or your normal activities the day after early abortion—depending on how strenuous your normal activities are. The day of the abortion, you may want to relax for the rest of the day. You may shower as soon as you wish. Do not take tub baths, douche, use vaginal medications, or have vaginal intercourse until after your follow-up exam—from two to four weeks after the abortion. Recovery after later abortions may take longer.

Will I Bleed after Abortion?

Very often there is a dark, menstrual-like flow that occurs off and on for a couple of weeks after the abortion. Some women will have cramps and pass a few large clots of blood up to ten days after the abortion. Some will have little or no bleeding. After an abortion, use sanitary pads—do not use tampons—until bleeding stops.

Your next regular period may come at any time within six weeks after the abortion. Be sure to contact your clinician if you do not have a period in six weeks.

Are Heavy Bleeding, Pain, and Fever Normal after an Abortion?

No. If you experience any of these after an abortion, contact your clinician immediately.

How Soon May I Have Intercourse after Abortion?

Wait until after your follow-up exam or until three weeks after bleeding has stopped. Abstaining from vaginal intercourse will allow time for the cervix to close and protect you from infection. If you choose not to abstain, use a condom to reduce your risk of infection, but having vaginal intercourse before the cervix has closed is not a good idea.

How Soon Might I Get Pregnant Again after an Abortion?

It is possible to get pregnant again within two weeks after an abortion. That is why it is important to use birth control when you begin to have sexual intercourse again.

How Soon Should I See a Health Care Provider after an Abortion?

Follow-up should take place within two to four weeks after a suction curettage. After a D&E, see your clinician within four weeks.

What Are the Emotional Effects of Abortion?

The emotion most women experience after an abortion is relief. Because of the abrupt hormonal changes caused by abortion, some women experience short-term anger, regret, guilt, or sadness. After abortion most women who feel a brief sadness or other negative feeling recover very quickly.

Serious, long-term emotional problems after abortion are rare and less frequent than those following childbirth. They are more likely if:

- the pregnancy was wanted but the health of the fetus or the woman was jeopardized by its continuation

- having an abortion is related to serious problems in a relationship or other disturbing life events.

In spite of these facts, some people who are opposed to abortion claim that most women who have an abortion suffer severe and long-lasting emotional problems. They call these problems "post-abortion syndrome." This "syndrome" is not recognized by the American Psychological Association, the American Psychiatric Association, or the National Association of Social Workers.

If a woman does have prolonged feelings of sadness, guilt, or depression it is important for her to talk about her feelings with a counselor. Her abortion provider may be able to offer follow-up counseling or refer her to a counselor in the community.

What about Future Pregnancies?

- **Will an early abortion affect my ability to have a child?**

  No. Safe, uncomplicated, legal abortion should not affect fertility.

- **Does an early abortion make miscarriage more likely in future pregnancies?**

  No.

- **Does an early abortion make ectopic pregnancy more likely in the future?**

  Not unless infection occurs after an abortion. Ectopic pregnancies usually result from sexually transmitted infections. Infection occurs in only one out of 100 first-trimester abortions.

- **Does an early abortion cause premature birth in future pregnancies?**

  No.

- **Does an early abortion cause birth defects in future pregnancies?**

  No.

- **Does an early abortion lead to low infant birthweight in the future?**

  No.

- **Does an early abortion increase the chance of infant death in the future?**

  No.

- **Does having several abortions affect future pregnancies?**

  Early abortions done by experienced clinicians that are not followed by complications like infection do not cause infertility. Neither do they make it more difficult to carry a later pregnancy to term. It is unclear whether several abortions in later pregnancy result in a greater risk of miscarriage or premature birth.

- **Does abortion cause breast cancer?**

  No, but abortion does not offer the protection against breast cancer that having several full-term pregnancies does.

How Much Does Abortion Cost?

Fees vary depending on how long you've been pregnant and where you go for the abortion. In most cases, the fees cover one examination and laboratory tests, the anesthetic, the procedure, the follow-up exam, and a birth control method. At clinics the cost ranges from about $250 to $450 for abortion in the first trimester. Costs at hospitals will be higher, depending on how long you stay and what anesthetics are used. There may be additional charges if extra tests or medications are needed.

Ask beforehand about payment. Some places want to be paid in advance. Some accept credit cards. An installment plan or other special arrangement can sometimes be worked out. Some health insurance policies will cover some or all of the cost. In all states, Medicaid will pay for an abortion when the life of the woman is in danger. In some states, Medicaid will pay for abortions under other circumstances as well. Check with your local Planned Parenthood health center or your state or local health or welfare department for the kind of Medicaid coverage in your state.

How Can I Find an Abortion Provider?

Some providers perform abortions during the first 12 weeks of pregnancy in their offices. Abortions are also available in many Planned Parenthood health centers, in many other reproductive health clinics, and in hospitals. Most large cities and many smaller communities have abortion providers. Look under "abortion" in the Yellow Pages.

Be aware that hundreds of so-called "crisis pregnancy centers" have been established across the country to frighten women away from choosing abortion. Instead of offering accurate information about all available options, these centers show pregnant women shocking and deceptive films or slide shows. They give frightening misinformation about the medical and emotional effects of abortion. Most often, they perform pregnancy tests without professional medical supervision. And they discourage sexually active women from using the most common and effective methods of birth control.

If you need help choosing a reputable clinic that will not try to influence your decision, call your local Planned Parenthood health center. For the Planned Parenthood health center nearest you, call toll-free: 800-230-PLAN. Or, you can call the National Abortion Federation hot line: 800-772-9100.

You can get abortion information and assistance at Planned Parenthood health centers, other family planning clinics, women's centers, youth centers, and departments of health or social services. Some doctors and hospitals do not perform abortions, but they can tell you where you can get one.

Chapter 41

Medical Abortion

Mifepristone and Misoprostol: How the Drug Works

What Is Mifepristone?

Mifepristone is an antiprogestin. One of its actions is to interrupt pregnancy in its early stages. It does this by blocking the action of the natural hormone, progesterone, which prepares the lining of the uterus for a fertilized egg and then maintains the pregnancy. Without the effect of progesterone, the lining of the uterus softens and breaks down, and bleeding begins.

What Is Misoprostol?

Misoprostol is a drug approved in the United States as an ulcer medicine. It belongs to the class of drugs known as prostaglandins. When used for abortion, prostaglandins work by causing contractions of the uterus, helping to expel the fertilized egg. The small dosage of oral prostaglandin taken following use of mifepristone is less than the dosage taken daily by those who use the medication for long-term care of ulcers.

Excerpted from "Medical Abortion: Frequently Asked Questions," a document produced by the Population Council, May 24, 2000; available at http://www.popcouncil.org/faqs/abortion.html; reprinted with permission.

Why Combine Mifepristone with Another Drug?

Studies have shown that, by itself, mifepristone is an effective abortifacient 65 to 80 percent of the time when used by women within 49 days since the beginning of their last menses. When combined with a small dose of prostaglandin, however the regimen is effective in approximately 95 percent of women when used within 49 days since the beginning of their last menstrual period.

How Are These Drugs Used?

The regimen used in both the French and the Council-sponsored U.S. clinical trials required at least three visits to the clinic, beginning with thorough counseling, a physical examination, and determination of length of pregnancy. At the first visit, the woman swallows three 200 microgram (mcg) tablets of mifepristone (a total of 600 mcg) and remains under observation for 30 minutes. At the second visit—two days later—the woman swallows two 200 mcg tablets of misoprostol (oral prostaglandin) under supervision and remains at the clinic for up to four hours. After two weeks the woman returns for a follow-up visit to confirm that the abortion is complete. If the abortion is not complete at this time, a surgical method of abortion, generally vacuum aspiration, is used. About half of the women have their abortions during their second visit to the clinic, and roughly 75 percent abort within 24 hours after taking misoprostol.

Why Would a Woman Choose Medical Abortion instead of Surgical Abortion?

A woman might choose medical abortion over surgical abortion because:

- It can be used in the earliest weeks following fertilization;
- It requires no invasive procedure or surgery;
- It requires no anesthesia;
- Side effects other than bleeding tend to be short-lived;
- It does not carry risk of uterine perforation or injury to the cervix;
- It has the potential for greater privacy;
- Some women feel it gives them greater control over their bodies.

Why Would a Woman Choose Surgical Abortion over Medical Abortion?

A woman might choose surgical abortion over medical abortion because:

- It requires one fewer office visit;
- It is performed quickly;
- It is slightly more effective than medical abortion, where five of every 100 women require surgical abortion;
- The woman notices less blood loss and is unaware of the passing of the products of conception.

Are There Any Long-term Health Effects from This Regimen?

In ten years of clinical use, there is little evidence of risk with mifepristone. It is believed risks are unlikely because the drug causes very few side effects; exposure is so brief; the dosage is small; and most of the drug is eliminated from the body within two or three days. The oral prostaglandin has been used safely at much higher doses for gastric ulcers in many thousands of patients for many years. The dosage taken in conjunction with mifepristone for medical abortion is low.

What Is the Effect of Mifepristone on a Woman's Future Fertility?

There are no indications that use of mifepristone to end a pregnancy has affected a woman's ability to have a baby when she was ready. Women who have taken mifepristone have been able to conceive and subsequently bear healthy children. Having an early medical or surgical abortion does not make future miscarriage more likely.

How Soon Can a Woman Have a Medical Abortion?

A woman can choose medical abortion with mifepristone as soon as she suspects she is pregnant and the pregnancy can be confirmed.

Why Is Mifepristone Effective Only in the Earliest Weeks of Pregnancy?

In the first few weeks following fertilization and implantation, the ovaries produce progesterone. By the ninth and tenth weeks, the placenta itself produces progesterone and does so in larger amounts, so that antiprogestins are unable to compete with the naturally produced hormone.

How Is the Age of a Pregnancy Determined?

Pregnancies are dated from the first day of the woman's last menstrual period (LMP). However, those concerned with the actual age of the embryo should realize that there are usually two weeks between the time a woman's menstrual period starts and the time she ovulates.

How Large Is the Embryo at 49 Days?

At 49 days the actual embryo inside the amniotic sac measures one-fifth of an inch, about the size of an aspirin tablet.

Does Mifepristone Cause Fetal Deformities?

Little is known about the effect of mifepristone on a developing embryo. Only a few instances are known where women decided to continue with their pregnancies after taking mifepristone to produce an abortion. In most cases a normal baby was delivered, but in several cases abnormalities have occurred. It is not clear whether these resulted from mifepristone, from misoprostol, from neither, or from both. Women whose medical abortion fails should have the pregnancy terminated surgically.

What Happens if the Drugs Fail to End a Pregnancy?

The mifepristone/oral prostaglandin combination fails in about five of every 100 cases when used up to 49 days LMP. Failures include not only ongoing pregnancies (1 in 100) and incomplete abortions (3 in 100), but also surgical termination done at the patient's request or for medical reasons (11 in 100). When drug failure happens, the abortion should be completed through surgical means, generally vacuum aspiration.

Can a Woman Change Her Mind after Taking the First Drug, and before Taking the Second?

Good counseling will make sure that a woman knows that she may risk birth abnormalities if she continues her pregnancy after taking mifepristone. Although the informed consent signed by each patient makes it clear that she should not continue her pregnancy after taking mifepristone, no one can or will force a woman to have a surgical abortion.

Side Effects

What Are the Side Effects from Mifepristone and Oral Prostaglandin Use?

Some women do not experience any physical discomfort after taking mifepristone; others have slight nausea. Most women experience uterine bleeding in the two days before taking the prostaglandin. The side effects of mifepristone appear to be similar to the side effects of "morning sickness" during a normal pregnancy—nausea, headache, weakness, and fatigue. Side effects are more common after taking the oral prostaglandin. They include:

- Cramps and abdominal pain similar to those associated with a menstrual period or a natural miscarriage. They are a normal, expected part of the abortion process and most women get them;
- Nausea and vomiting, sometimes requiring medication;
- Diarrhea (can occur, but is rare);
- Uterine bleeding, similar to a heavy period and lasting at least one week, or bleeding and spotting that is not heavy but can last for one to three weeks. In rare cases, if uterine bleeding is extremely heavy, the woman may require surgical abortion and/or blood transfusion.

What Is the Risk of Bleeding Requiring Blood Transfusion?

Heavy uterine bleeding is rare. These cases of excessive bleeding can necessitate a blood transfusion. Some bleeding or spotting can continue for more than two weeks.

Has the Regimen Caused Any Deaths?

One fatal heart attack occurred in France during a medical abortion following injection of an older form of prostaglandin (sulprostone), which is no longer used in France and is not used in the United States. Beginning in May 1992, France replaced the injectable prostaglandin with misoprostol. There have been no deaths since. There is no evidence that the oral prostaglandin—a different class of prostaglandin widely prescribed for long-term use in the prevention and treatment of peptic ulcer disease—is associated with any cardiovascular side effects. There have been no serious complications in the women using the mifepristone/oral prostaglandin combination of drugs for pregnancy termination.

Mifepristone in the United States

What Is the Population Council's Role?

The rights to mifepristone in the United States were donated without recompense to the Population Council in May 1994. The Council's mission was to conduct a U.S. clinical trial, file a New Drug Application (NDA), and arrange for a new manufacturer and distributor.

The 164-volume NDA, which was submitted to the U.S. Food and Drug Administration (FDA) in March 1996, was based on data from the French pivotal studies. In July 1996, after a public hearing, an FDA advisory committee recommended that the FDA approve use of mifepristone in combination with misoprostol for medical abortion. The FDA issued an approvable letter in September 1996, saying that mifepristone was safe and effective, but that the Council needed to provide additional information on labeling and manufacturing.

The United States clinical trials, which included 2,121 women at 17 clinics throughout the country, started in September 1994 and concluded a year later. Two articles—one on safety and efficacy, the other on acceptability—were published: "Early Pregnancy Termination with Mifepristone and Misoprostol in the United States" on April 30, 1998 in the *New England Journal of Medicine,* and "Acceptability and Feasibility of Early Pregnancy Termination by Mifepristone-Misoprostol: Results of a Large Multicenter Trial in the United States," in July/August, 1998 by *Archives of Family Medicine.*

When Will Mifepristone Be Available?

The Council's distributor for mifepristone, The Danco Group, has said it will give the FDA all the information needed to permit approval in 2000. [**Note:** *the FDA approved mifepristone in September 2000.*]

Were Any U.S. Government Funds Used for the Project?

No.

Mifepristone in Europe

Where Has Mifepristone Been Used?

Since 1981, women in 20 countries (including the United States) have used mifepristone and a prostaglandin as a medical method of pregnancy interruption. Studies have shown mifepristone to be safe and effective. Government regulatory agencies in France, Great Britain, China, and Sweden have approved the drug for marketing, following clinical studies like the one conducted in the United States. In Europe, an estimated 500,000 women have used mifepristone as a medical abortifacient in combination with various prostaglandins: injectable, vaginal suppository, or oral. In 1999, mifepristone was approved for marketing in Austria, Belgium, Denmark, Finland, Germany, Greece, the Netherlands, and Spain.

Do All Countries Use the Same Prostaglandin?

No. French women now use mifepristone together with misoprostol and have used this combination since May 1992. British and Swedish women currently use gemeprost, a suppository form of prostaglandin.

What Is the European Experience?

France has the most extensive experience with the mifepristone/prostaglandin combination. Mifepristone has been marketed in France since September 1989 as a medical alternative to surgical abortion. A study of French data published in the *New England Journal of Medicine* in May 1993 showed the combination of mifepristone and oral prostaglandin to be effective "for the termination of early pregnancy in terms of success, tolerance, safety, and practicality." About 70 percent of eligible women—those with pregnancy duration of less than 49 days—have selected medical abortion over surgical abortion. Overall, this means that over one-third of all abortions in France are medical abortions. There has been no increase in the total number of abortions in France since the method was introduced in 1989. The main impact of availability of medical abortion has been that more women have sought abortions earlier in their pregnancies. Medical abortion is generally available in public hospitals.

In the United Kingdom, where mifepristone was introduced in 1991, it can be used up to 9 weeks gestation in combination with gemeprost, a vaginal suppository that is not available in the United States. Medical abortion is administered under medical supervision in approximately 200 hospitals and clinics, mostly within the National Health Service sector. Mifepristone is not sold through pharmacies. Since it went on the market, medical abortion has accounted for about 20 percent of all abortions under nine weeks.

In Sweden mifepristone has been used in hospitals since 1992. By 1995 it accounted for 16 percent of the 31,000 abortions performed that year.

U.S. Mifepristone Clinical Trial Summary of Findings

Highlights

- The method was provided safely and effectively within the diverse U.S. healthcare system.

- The efficacy in providing abortions up to 49 days was comparable to the European experience.

- Nearly all of the women in the study reported they would recommend medical abortion to others and that they would choose it again, if necessary.

- Almost three-quarters of the women who had had a previous surgical abortion said medical abortion was more satisfactory.

- Providers' feedback suggests that efficacy increases as physicians, nurses, and counselors gain experience and familiarity with the method. This finding reinforces the need for extensive physician information and education.

Chapter 42

Facts in Brief: Induced Abortion

Incidence of Abortion

- 49% of pregnancies among American women are unintended; 1/2 of these are terminated by abortion.
- In 1996, 1.37 million abortions took place, down from an estimated 1.61 million in 1990. From 1973 through 1996, more than 34 million legal abortions occurred.
- Each year, 2 out of every 100 women aged 15–44 have an abortion; 47% of them have had at least one previous abortion and 55% have had a previous birth.
- An estimated 43% of women will have at least 1 abortion by the time they are 45 years old.
- Each year, an estimated 50 million abortions occur worldwide. Of these, 30 million procedures are obtained legally, 20 million illegally.

Who Has Abortions

- 52% of U.S. women obtaining abortions are younger than 25: Women aged 20–24 obtain 32% of all abortions, and teenagers obtain 20%.
- 2/3 of women having abortions intend to have children in the future.
- While white women obtain 60% of all abortions, their abortion rate is well below that of minority women. Black women are more than 3 times as likely as white women to have an abortion, and Hispanic women are roughly 2 times as likely.
- Women who report no religious affiliation are about 4 times as likely as women who report some affiliation to have an abortion.
- Catholic women are 29% more likely than Protestants to have an abortion, but are about as likely as all women nationally to do so.
- 2/3 of all abortions are obtained by never-married women.
- On average, women give at least 3 reasons for choosing abortion: 3/4 say that having a baby would interfere with work, school or other responsibilities; about 2/3 say they cannot afford a child; and 1/2 say they do not want to be a single parent or are having problems with their husband or partner.
- About 14,000 women have abortions each year because they became pregnant after rape or incest.

The number of abortions per 1,000 women aged 15–44, by year

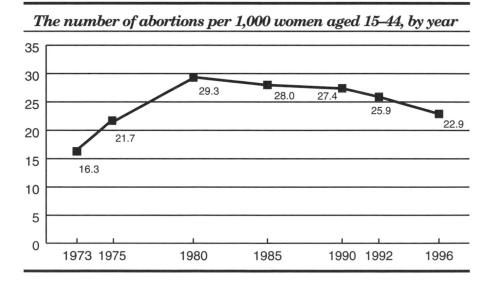

Contraceptive Use

- 58% of women having abortions in the mid-1990s had used a contraceptive method during the month they became pregnant, compared with 51% in the late 1980s.
- 11% of women having abortions have never used a method of birth control; nonuse is greatest among those who arc young, unmarried, poor, black, Hispanic, or poorly educated.
- 9 in 10 women at risk of unintended pregnancy are using a contraceptive method.
- 49% of the 6.3 million pregnancies that occur each year are unplanned; 53% of these occur among the small portion of women at risk of unintended pregnancy who do not practice contraception.

Providers and Coverage

- 93% of U.S. abortions are performed in clinics or doctors' offices.
- The number of abortion providers declined by 14% between 1992 and 1996 (from 2,380 to 2,042). 86% of all U.S. counties

When Women Have Abortions (in weeks)

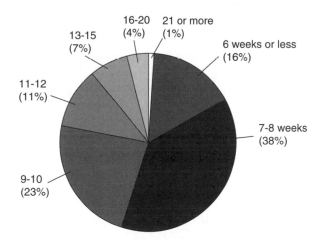

Eighty-eight percent of abortions occur in the first 12 weeks of pregnancy

lacked an abortion provider in 1996. These counties were home to 32% of all 15–44-year-old women.

- 52% of all abortion facilities provide services only through the 12th week of pregnancy.

- In 1993, the cost of a nonhospital abortion at 10 weeks ranged from $140 to more than $1,700, and the average amount paid was $296.

- 9 in 10 managed care plans routinely cover abortion or provide limited coverage.

Safety of Abortion

- The risk of abortion complications is minimal; less than 1% of all abortion patients experience a major complication, such as serious pelvic infection, hemorrhage requiring a blood transfusion, or unintended major surgery.

- The risk of death associated with abortion increases with the length of pregnancy, from 1 death for every 530,000 abortions at 8 or fewer weeks to 1 per 17,000 at 16–20 weeks and 1 per 6,000 at 21 or more weeks.

- 1 death occurs in every 150,000 legal abortions, compared with 1 in every 34,000 in 1974.

- The risk of death associated with childbirth is about 10 times as high as that associated with abortion.

- The main reason women give for delaying abortion is that they had not recognized earlier that they were pregnant. Almost half of the women having abortions beyond 15 weeks of gestation say they were delayed because of problems in obtaining abortion services—either in affording the cost or in finding or getting to a provider.

- Teens are more likely than older women to delay having an abortion until after 16 weeks of pregnancy, when medical risks associated with abortion increase significantly.

- There is no evidence of childbearing problems among women who have had a vacuum aspiration abortion, the most common type, within the first 12 weeks of pregnancy.

Law and Policy

- In the 1973 *Roe v. Wade* decision, the Supreme Court ruled that women, in consultation with their physician, have a constitutionally protected right to have an abortion in the early stages of pregnancy—that is, before viability—free from government interference.
- In 1992, the Court upheld the right to abortion in *Planned Parenthood v. Casey*. However, the ruling significantly weakened the legal protections previously afforded women and physicians by giving states the right to enact restrictions that do not create an "undue burden" for women seeking abortion.
- The most common restrictions in effect are parental involvement requirements, mandatory counseling and waiting periods, and limitations on public funding.
- 30 states currently enforce parental consent or notification laws for minors seeking an abortion: AL, AR, CO, DE, GA, IA, ID, IN, KS, KY, LA, MA, MD, MI, MN, MO, MS, NC, ND, NE, OH, PA, RI, SC, SD, UT, VA,WI, WV, and WY. The Supreme Court ruled that in states that require parental involvement, minors must have the alternative of seeking a court order authorizing the procedure.
- 45% of minors who have abortions tell their parents, and 61% undergo the procedure with at least one parent's knowledge. The great majority of parents support their daughter's decision to have an abortion.

Public Funding

- The U.S. Congress has barred the use of federal Medicaid funds to pay for abortions, except when the woman's life would be endangered by a full-term pregnancy or in cases of rape or incest.
- About 14% of all abortions in the United States are paid for with public funds, virtually all of which are state funds. Sixteen states (CA, CT, HI, ID, IL, MA, MD, MN, MT, NJ, NM, NY, OR, VT, WA, and WV) pay for abortions for some poor women.
- Without publicly funded family planning services, an estimated 1.3 million additional unplanned pregnancies would occur annu-

ally; approximately 632,300 would end in induced abortion—at least a 40% increase in the incidence of abortion.

The data in this fact sheet are the most current available. Most of the data are from research conducted by The Alan Guttmacher Institute and/or published in its peer-reviewed journal, *Family Planning Perspectives*. An additional source is the Centers for Disease Control and Prevention.

Chapter 43

What Are the Long-Term Health Risks of Abortion?

—*by Candace C. Crandall*

A woman faced with the decision of whether or not to seek an abortion will ask herself many questions. The question she may least consider—until after the fact—is how an abortion will affect her future health. Will it jeopardize her ability to have other children? Will it increase her chance of developing a life-threatening disease, like breast cancer?

With tens of millions of women having undergone one or multiple abortions, these are questions for which there are still no definitive answers. Not because science is unable to provide them, but because political pressures work against objective research.

Instead, women who have had abortions are subject to an almost monthly assault of conflicting information about what risks, exactly, they may have incurred. On the cancer issue, for instance, media reports produced the following over three years: "Higher Risk of Breast Cancer Found in Young Women Who Had Abortions" (October 1994); "Strong Abortion–Breast Cancer Link Revealed" (October 1996); "New Study Questions Abortion–Cancer Link" (December 1996); "Study Finds No Link between Abortion and Breast Cancer" (1997). Reports have raised the specter of other potentially serious long-term health effects—among them infertility, miscarriage, and ectopic pregnan-

"None of Our Business?," *The Women's Quarterly*, No. 12, Summer 1997; reprinted with permission.

cies—only to have them refuted by one study, and then raised again by another. Which is right?

Journalists often have their own ax to grind on this issue, of course, but even the few who attempt to interpret the research objectively run into a wall of half-truths and distortions. Try to obtain unbiased information on abortion-related health risks and here are some of the "experts" one encounters:

At one end of the spectrum is Joel Brind, professor of endocrinology at the City University of New York and a celebrity in the pro-life camp, who publishes a newsletter called the *Abortion-Breast Cancer Quarterly*. Brind is often quoted by journalists on the abortion issue, but his publication sounds less than scientific, fond as he is of words like "cover-up," "crisis pregnancy," "desperate mothers," and "mainstream denial" of "a woman's right to know." "Is it worth $45 a year," he asks in his advertisements, "to spare even *one woman* the life-threatening agony of *breast cancer?*" [Emphasis his.] Subscribe now and he'll throw in a free, autographed copy of his latest analysis.

But are those in the pro-choice camp any more reliable? And should federal agencies responsible for monitoring the nation's health be disseminating these advocates' research as the last word in objectivity? Carol Rowland Hogue, a feminist academic who holds an endowed chair at Emory University in Atlanta, reviews research papers on the effect of abortion on future reproduction. Her conclusions are cited and distributed by the federal Centers for Disease Control. But get her on the telephone and it becomes clear that she prefers lengthy harangues against the pro-life movement to any boring discussion of health risks. And when she does discuss such risks, her views sound disturbingly tainted by personal politics.

Hogue notes approvingly, for example, that "many feminists now recommend barrier devices, backed up by abortion" as the "safest" contraceptive strategy for women. When asked if that wouldn't encourage multiple abortions, she replies that multiple abortions are not a problem. After all, she says, in Eastern Europe under the communists, it was not uncommon for women to have as many as 25 abortions and feel no ill effects at all. Besides, women who have multiple abortions really can't help it. Such women, Hogue insists, are simply "more fertile" than other women. And how does she know? Because studies comparing women one month after an abortion with women one month after childbirth show that the abortion group have much higher rates of repeat pregnancy during that period.

That such a remark might sound idiotic to some women—particularly those who know firsthand just how sexy they feel within a month of having a baby—apparently never occurs to Hogue. But don't ask her to elaborate. When I did she bristled: "It's apparent that I'm not talking to someone with an open mind on this issue!"

The effect is to leave those of us trying to sort out the facts caught somewhere between "The sky is falling!" and "What, me worry?" Anecdotal reports of risks related to abortion, particularly miscarriage, are troubling. Of the six women I know who have had abortions, five later experienced multiple miscarriages and were unable to carry a pregnancy to term. But this kind of evidence can be misleading too.

The problem—and this is true for epidemiological research as well—is that it is impossible for an observer to know all of the other risk factors such women may have incurred. Genetic predisposition, for example, may present the clearest risk for developing breast cancer, but other studies have implicated fatty diets, alcohol consumption, oral contraceptives, pesticides, a late first pregnancy, smoking, failure to breast-feed, age at the onset of menstruation, and even a woman's weight at birth! Similarly, a woman's ability to become pregnant and successfully carry a pregnancy to term may be adversely affected by age, a history of IUD use, sexually transmitted disease, pelvic inflammatory disease, inherited physiological disorders, and even psychological problems.

Epidemiologists trying to credibly establish, or disprove, a connection between abortion and disease or dysfunction have to try to eliminate or in some way account for these other risk factors. Certainly many women experience infertility, miscarriage, and breast cancer, with no previous history of abortion; others who have had abortions may have no problems at all.

What is worse, getting sound health information to the public is hampered by the fact that we live in an era of grant-driven research, where vague conclusions and poorly designed studies are nevertheless used to grab headlines, whip up public hysteria, underpin absurd government policies on everything from radon exposure to secondhand smoke—and get more grants. In the *New York Times* in 1995, Dr. Charles H. Hennekens of the Harvard School of Public Health characterized the situation with surprising honesty: "Epidemiology is a crude and inexact science. Eighty percent of the cases are almost all hypothesis. We tend to overstate findings, either because we want attention or more grant money."

Those of us who follow this degradation of science tend to take a cynical view of new research results, particularly those announced with great fanfare at press conferences. But here are the troubling facts we do know: the incidence of breast cancer among women took a big jump after 1980, particularly among black women under 50, a group that also shows a high rate of abortion. Breast cancer among men, a more rare condition, increased not at all. What is more, the possibility that undergoing an induced abortion can increase a woman's risk of developing breast cancer—or lead to problems with infertility and miscarriage—is biologically plausible, and that is the first test of whether a risk factor should be taken seriously or not.

What may link abortion to breast cancer is this: in pregnancy, a woman's body experiences a huge surge in the hormone estrogen—as much as twenty-fold—resulting in dramatic increases in the number of new breast cells. Because of the known link between estrogen and cancer, these rapidly dividing new cells are thought to be particularly susceptible to malignancy. But then something interesting happens. While estrogen begins the process of rapid cell division and tissue growth, a second hormone released during the last trimester shuts it down, allowing the cells to mature and differentiate into specialized cells that can produce milk. This hormone also sorts out and eliminates cells growing out of control, making the woman's breast tissue actually less susceptible to cancer. An abortion, whether performed in a clinic or induced chemically—with RU-486, for example—would interrupt the release of this protective second hormone.

Evidence purporting to show a positive association between induced abortion and breast cancer was first published in 1957 in Japan in a comprehensive study examining risk factors for cancer. Since then, more than 40 studies have looked at induced abortion as a possible risk factor for breast cancer but, like the Japanese study, the overwhelming majority were not designed to examine solely the breast cancer/induced abortion relationship. Instead, they combined induced abortion with spontaneous abortion (miscarriage), oral contraceptive use, environmental factors, and other risks, which tended to confuse conclusions about any effect attributable solely to abortion. Moreover, many studies did not control for age, family history, or other contributing factors such as diet, alcohol consumption, and income, which affects a woman's access to health care. When a positive association was found, it was often dismissed as largely due to "recall bias"—the notion that when women are asked to recollect risk factors, those stricken with breast cancer are more likely to reveal a past abortion than those free of disease.

As a result, little public attention was paid to a possible breast cancer/abortion link until 1994, when Janet Daling, of the Fred Hutchinson Cancer Research Center in Seattle, published a paper in the *Journal of the National Cancer Institute*. She concluded that women who had undergone an induced abortion incurred a 50 percent greater risk of developing breast cancer before age 45, with even higher risks for women under 18 or over 30 at the time of their abortions, or for those who had aborted a pregnancy after the eighth week. For the women aged 17 or younger who aborted a first pregnancy after the eighth week—a small subset of Daling's study—the risk went up an alarming 800 percent.

Interestingly, Daling found that a miscarriage did not elevate a woman's risk of breast cancer. She speculated that, with miscarriage, the fetus may have died days earlier than when it was actually expelled or that the woman may not have experienced a sufficient hormonal surge to sustain the pregnancy to begin with. Even more intriguing, Daling tested for "recall bias" by conducting a concurrent study of induced abortion and cervical cancer. Experts agree there is no relationship between abortion and cervical cancer, but if "recall bias" was a factor, this study should have turned up a similar elevated risk; it did not.

Daling, who is pro-choice (in the current climate, scientists must now state their politics along with their results), was unprepared for the furor her report touched off. Pro-choice activists sought to discredit her conclusions; even some of her own colleagues implied that she had somehow cooked her results to impede a woman's legal right to abortion. Editors at the *Journal of the National Cancer Institute* got so testy, they took the unusual step of publishing an editorial disclaimer in the same issue as Daling's report.

But since 1994, seven additional studies have been published, honing in on the breast cancer/induced abortion relationship. Results have been mixed. Daling also published a study of abortion and breast cancer among young white women in August 1996; she found a 90 percent increased risk. In December 1996, the *Journal of the National Cancer Institute* published a Dutch study that also found a 90 percent increased risk, but the editors—and the authors themselves—then went to great lengths to explain why the results were irrelevant, including a claim of reporting bias among Catholic women.

Then, in January 1997, a retrospective look at the medical records of 1.5 million Danish women was published in the *New England Journal of Medicine*. The authors concluded that induced abortion posed no increased risk of breast cancer and only a tiny risk for those having late-trimester abortions; indeed, an editorial in the same issue stated flatly that now "a woman need not worry."

Unfortunately, the Danish study has since been shown to have serious flaws. The authors admitted in their report that they "might have obtained an incomplete history of induced abortions for some of the oldest women" in the group, an error that likely misclassified tens of thousands of women with breast cancer as having had no abortions. In addition, many of the younger women studied—those who'd had the most abortions—had not yet reached an age where most breast cancers begin to develop.

So what are women to make of the cancer risk? To begin with, the association between induced abortion and an overall increase in the risk of breast cancer is still weak. Even Joel Brind concedes this. Claims by some pro-life activists that thousands of breast cancer deaths are attributable solely to induced abortion cannot be credibly substantiated, and allegations of a "cover-up" are needlessly inflammatory. But neither can we confidently insist—as some in the pro-choice movement do—that there is no risk. Scattered throughout these studies are unsettling results among certain subsets of women: Daling's teenagers in her 1994 paper, for example; women who have undergone second- and third-trimester abortions (also heavily represented among teenagers); or women who aborted a first pregnancy after age 40.

It would be premature to draw any conclusions from the incidence of breast cancer in these women, because the smaller the group studied the larger the margin for error. But researchers are getting better at identifying high-risk populations. What is needed now is to locate such women at the time of their abortions and to track them over time. That is a costly process that yields no quick answers, but it could yield some conclusive ones.

For many women, however, risks to future pregnancies are a much greater and more immediate concern than cancer, especially since environmentalists in recent years have repeatedly promoted various bogus cancer scares, even as life expectancy has gone up and up. Surveys by the Alan Guttmacher Institute show that just over 70 percent of the women undergoing abortion do intend, at some point, to have other children. And here, some noteworthy developments have taken place. The Family Growth Survey of the National Center for Health reports that women who have never had a child, who once accounted for just 17 percent of all women experiencing infertility and miscarriage, now account for half, with married black women showing higher rates than married white women.

In fact, women have been flooding into fertility clinics in recent years, and physician visits to treat infertility have more than tripled in the last three decades. Researchers peg this change to a greater prevalence of sexually transmitted diseases and pelvic inflammatory disease and, perhaps more important, baby boomers delaying marriage and childbearing until their late 30s or early 40s. But how much of that delay is due to abortion, no one seems to know.

Abortion and Women's Health, a publication of the Alan Guttmacher Institute—which is partly funded by the Planned Parenthood Federation of America, an abortion provider—reassures women about future fertility, citing "an extensive review of the worldwide literature," conducted by researchers from the federal Centers for Disease Control (CDC) and the Population Council—*i.e.*, Carol Hogue and colleagues. It concludes that a single, first-trimester abortion by vacuum aspiration entails no increased risk of subsequent infertility, ectopic pregnancy, or miscarriage. But it is only by reading the footnotes that one learns that this review was published way back in 1982. Moreover, Hogue's review hedges on the effect of multiple abortions or abortions after the first trimester, saying only that additional research is needed.

Susan Tew, deputy communications director for Guttmacher, concedes that its data on long-term risks are old and "pretty poor." The National Abortion Federation should have this information "but they don't because the providers don't follow up on their patients." Also, she says, pregnancy risks can be difficult to measure because the primary cause may be STDs or infection.

Ay, and there's the rub. Aside from those instances where an abortion turns out badly and the woman ends up with a hysterectomy, only a handful of infertility cases have been attributed solely to induced abortion—such as cases where fetal bone fragments have been left in the uterus where they act, researchers believe, in much the same way as an IUD. But several studies have now shown an association between induced abortion in women with untreated sexually transmitted disease—largely chlamydia—and infertility and miscarriage. Chlamydia, it must be noted, has reached epidemic proportions in the United States, with nearly half a million cases diagnosed each year.

421

In 1992, a Danish study found that 20 percent of the women harboring chlamydia at the time of their abortions progressed to pelvic inflammatory disease, a serious chronic infection which can result in miscarriage and/or scarring of the fallopian tubes. Of those, 10 percent became infertile and 22 percent miscarried a subsequent pregnancy. The researchers advised that women seeking abortion be examined for chlamydia and treated with appropriate antibiotics no later than at the time of their abortion. Another Danish study, published in Germany in 1994, found that 72 percent of the women studied whose chlamydia was not treated at the time of their abortions, progressed to pelvic inflammatory disease within two years. Debates over whether pregnancy problems that may arise from this effect are truly "abortion-related" hinge on whether the STD is considered the primary cause, even if the abortion was the mechanism for introducing infection into the uterus.

Meanwhile, each year some 700,000 American women undergo at least their second abortion, some 300,000 at least their third. According to the CDC, about 15 percent of all abortions in the United States will be performed in the second trimester or later. Yet incredibly, there is little research being done on the effect of multiple and late-term abortions on women's future reproduction. In the dozen or so states that have Supreme Court-sanctioned informed consent laws, women are told that multiple abortions may make it difficult to have children later in life. Some infertility support groups also list two or more abortions as a risk factor for infertility and miscarriage.

But an updated review of the literature published in 1990, again by Carol Hogue and colleagues, still focused only on single, vacuum-aspiration abortions performed during the first trimester. The report concluded that there were generally no long-term risks, except in those abortions complicated by infection, but noted that "a variety of conditions"—among them sterility, miscarriage, tubal pregnancies, stillbirths, premature births, birth defects, and emotional disorders—had been "ascribed anecdotally to induced abortion."

So what we have at this point are some associations between induced abortion and long-term health risks that are biologically plausible, and some evidence along the lines of what we might expect to see if indeed there were a cause-and-effect relationship. What we don't see (and unfortunately the definitive studies are not being done) is conclusive statistical evidence linking the two.

This controversy, however, should provoke caution. Political pressures—as demonstrated by the editorial disclaimers accompanying abortion studies published in scientific journals—work against the funding of abortion research. Moreover, because breast cancer in women usually develops after age 40, if there is any increased risk to certain subgroups—*i.e.*, women who aborted a first pregnancy before age 18—the first of these cancers would only just now be showing up 25 years after *Roe v. Wade*.

It cannot be stressed enough that having an abortion, whether chemically or surgically induced, can carry certain risks. As Susan Tew of the Alan Guttmacher Institute puts it, the magnitude of these risks may "depend on how well the patient chooses to inform herself." In the current political climate, obtaining accurate information is almost impossible. And as deliberately misleading as some pro-life activists can be, much of the blame for this situation must fall on those who have made abortion an unassailable shibboleth.

The bottom line is that women seeking abortions would do well to identify factors that may put them into one of the groups thought to be at a higher risk for breast cancer, and take that into consideration when making their decision. They should certainly ensure that any sexually transmitted disease is diagnosed and treated before undergoing an abortion. And, given the uncertainties, women should regard the idea that multiple abortion is a reasonable contraception strategy as the obvious nonsense that it is. There are many debatable points about this issue. Health should not be one of them.

Candace C. Crandall writes on women's health issues for The Science & Enviromental Policy Project in Fairfax, Virginia.

Part Ten:

Future Methods of Contraception

Chapter 44

Future Birth Control Methods for Women

Most of the contraceptive products that will soon be available for women are refinements of similar products that are already on the market.

Potential Barrier Methods for Women

FemCap®—The FemCap® is made of soft silicone and looks like a tiny white sailor's cap. The dome covers the cervix. Designed to last for at least three years, FemCap will be available in three sizes and is expected to cost about $60 for a package of two.

Vaginal Sponge—A new vaginal sponge made of polyurethane foam is also under development. It contains a combination of chemicals that serve as spermicide and microbicide to protect against sexually transmitted infections. Other sponges include Protectaide®, which is available in Canada and Hong Kong, and the Today® Sponge, which is already FDA-approved and expected to return to the U.S. market in 2001.

PPFA Web Site © 1999, Planned Parenthood® Federation of America, Inc.; available at http://www.plannedparenthood.org/articles/bcfuture_w.html; reprinted with permission.

Potential Contraceptive Pills, Patches, and Rings for Women

A new birth control pill—B-Oval® is expected to be available at the turn of the century. A synthetic version of melatonin, a hormone found naturally in the body, is used instead of estrogen in this combination pill.

Transdermal patches—Worn like Band-Aids®, transdermal patches gradually release a hormone into the body. The method works like the Pill, but women only need to remember to use it twice a month, not every day.

Soft silicone vaginal rings—Placed in the vagina, soft silicone vaginal rings, like the combination pill, will include both estrogen and progestin. A progestin-only vaginal ring is also being developed.

Potential Contraceptive Injections and Vaccines for Women

Injectables—Timed-release microspheres that gradually release progestin to protect against unintended pregnancy for 90 days are being developed for injection. The World Health Organization has approved two injectables containing estrogen and progestin.

Oral or injectable vaccines—Oral or injectable vaccines to immunize women against pregnancy are being developed. In the future, it may be possible to use antibodies that attack eggs or sperm. Another vaccine would stimulate the immune system to create antibodies to a crucial type of protein molecule found on the head of sperm.

Potential Contraceptive Implants for Women

Implanon®—Designed to work for two or three years, this single capsule contains a progestin called 3-ketodesogestrel, which is more potent than levonorgestrel.

Norplant II®—Norplant II is the second generation of Norplant. Only two implants are necessary.

Biodegradable implants—Biodegradable implants containing progestin are implanted under the skin of the arm or hip. The hormone is released gradually into the body for 12 to 18 months.

Intrauterine Devices (IUDs)

Levonorgestrel IUD—Levonorgestrel IUD is shaped like a 'T" and contains a progestin, levonorgestrel, that is released steadily into the uterus for up to seven years. The LNg-20 is made and sold in Finland.

"Frameless IUDs"—Two "frameless" IUDs are being used in European clinical trials. It is hoped that they will cause less cramping because there is no rigid frame to press against the uterus.

Potential Ovulation Predictors

Computerized fertility monitors—Under the sympto-thermal method, a computer device, the Fertility Monitor®, predicts "safe" days for sexual intercourse by measuring daily changes in body temperature and cervical mucus. Another method, under the brand name Persona®, uses a computer to monitor hormonal levels in urine. The Bioself 110® measures basal body temperature to determine fertility. Other methods include the brand names, PFT 1-2-3 Kit®, Cycle View®, Maybe Baby®, and Ovu-Tech®, which are saliva-based "fertility testers."

Potential Methods for Tubal Sterilization

Chemical Scarring—Two chemical combinations are used for tubal sterilization in China. One is phenol (carbolic acid), combined with a thickening agent. The other is phenol, combined with quinacrine. The chemicals are used to damage the fallopian tubes. The scar tissue that forms eventually blocks the tube.

Chemical Plugs—Canada and the Netherlands have approved permanent non-surgical tubal sterilization through the introduction of chemicals into the fallopian tubes such as methylcyanoacrylate (MCA)—Krazy Glue®.

Silicone Plugs—A reversible, non-surgical method of tubal sterilization, liquid silicone is injected into the fallopian tubes. The silicone hardens and blocks the tube with a rubbery plug that can be removed.

Cryosurgery—Liquid nitrogen is used to freeze the connection between each fallopian tube and the uterus (the cornu). The resulting scar tissue blocks the tubes and prevents fertilization of the egg.

Unisex Contraception

One of the methods of reversible contraception being developed may be appropriate for both women and men. A new group of drugs known as gonadotropin-releasing hormone (GnRH) agonists can be used to prevent the release of FSH and LH from the pituitary gland. The release of FSH and LH triggers ovulation and spermatogenesis—the development of sperm. Blocking the release of these hormones will temporarily suppress fertility for women and men.

Chapter 45

Future Birth Control Methods for Men

The challenge to develop reversible methods of contraception for men is a complicated one. Healthy men are always producing sperm. The continuous fertility of men does not offer the opportunities for reversible intervention that are offered by women's cycles of fertility. Developing effective contraceptive methods for men without permanently impairing their fertility has proved to be very elusive, but progress is being made.

Potential Oral Contraceptive Methods for Men

Oral contraception for men reduces sperm counts to levels that are unlikely to cause pregnancy. In Italy, a contraceptive pill containing synthetic hormones is being used by men in a clinical study. The men also receive testosterone injections to boost the effectiveness of the pill.

Potential Contraceptive Injections, Implants, and Vaccines for Men

World Health Organization studies have shown greatly reduced sperm counts in men injected once a week with testosterone enanthate

(TE), a synthetic hormone. Research continues with a combination of TE and depot-medroxyprogesterone acetate (DMPA), the progestin used in Depo-Provera. The combination injection may be needed only once a month.

A potential three-month injection using testosterone buciclate is in preliminary development.

Subdermal Implants—Two rods are inserted under the skin. One of the rods contains a synthetic version of gonadotropin-releasing hormone (GnRH). The other contains an androgen. The androgen, 7-alpha methyl-19-nortestosterone (MENT), is 10 times stronger than natural testosterone.

Battery-powered capsules—Capsules implanted into each vas deferens emit low-level electrical currents that immobilizes sperm as they flow by.

Potential Methods for Vasectomy

Chemical Compounds—Phenol mixed with alcohol is injected into each vas deferens.

Silicone Plugs—Tiny silicone cylinders are inserted into each vas deferens. The cylinders physically block the tubes.

Reversible Vasectomy—Chemicals inserted into the vas derens block the movement of sperm.

Unisex Contraception

One of the methods of reversible contraception being developed may be appropriate for both women and men. A new group of drugs known as gonadotropin-releasing hormone (GnRH) agonists can be used to prevent the release of FSH and LH from the pituitary gland. The release of FSH and LH triggers ovulation and spermatogenesis—the development of sperm. Blocking the release of these hormones will temporarily suppress fertility for women and men.

Part Eleven:

Additional Help and Information

Chapter 46

Family Planning Terms

This glossary contains many of the terms used throughout this volume of the Health Reference Series. Some words have many meanings; the definitions given are those most applicable to pregnancy, contraception, and infertility. The use of brand names is for identification purposes only; it does not constitute an endorsement.

A

Abortifacient: A drug, herb, or device that can cause an abortion.

Abortion: The premature termination of a pregnancy; may be induced or spontaneous (miscarriage).

Abstinence: Not having sexual intercourse.

Adoption: When a birth mother and a birth father legally give up the rights to take care of a child and another person assumes responsibility for raising the child. The laws governing adoption differ for every state.

AIDS (acquired immune deficiency syndrome): A progressive, usually fatal condition (syndrome) that reduces the body's ability to fight certain infections. Caused by infection with HIV (human immunodeficiency virus).

Alveoli: Sacs inside the breast that produce milk.

Amenorrhea: Absence of menstrual periods.

Amniocentesis: The aspiration of amniotic fluid from the uterus, usually performed at three to three and one-half months of pregnancy, to test the fetus for genetic abnormalities.

Androgens: Certain hormones that stimulate male sexual development and secondary male sex characteristics. They are most abundantly produced in the testicles of men but are also produced in small amounts in women's ovaries. The most common androgen is testosterone.

ART (assisted reproductive technology): All treatments or procedures that involve the handling of human eggs and sperm for the purpose of establishing a pregnancy. Types of ART include IVF, GIFT, ZIFT, embryo cryopreservation, egg or embryo donation, and surrogate birth.

Artificial insemination (AI): Placement of a sperm sample inside the female reproductive tract.

B

Backup method: A family planning method such as condoms or spermicide that can be used temporarily for extra protection against pregnancy when needed.

Barrier method: A birth control method that provides a physical barrier between the sperm and the egg. Examples of barrier contraceptive methods include condoms, diaphragms, foam, sponges, and cervical caps.

Bartholin's glands: Glands in the labia minora on each side of the opening to the vagina that provide lubrication during sexual excitement.

Basal body temperature (BBT): The temperature of the body at rest. Because it rises slightly after ovulation, basal body temperature can indicate when ovulation has occurred. To obtain the basal body temperature chart, the woman records her temperature every day in the morning before beginning any activity. The temperature may be taken orally, rectally, or vaginally, but it must be taken in the same body location throughout any single menstrual cycle.

Basal body temperature method: A method of natural family planning that uses the woman's basal body temperature to identify the infertile phase of the menstrual cycle after ovulation has occurred. This information is used to plan intercourse and abstinence so as to achieve or to avoid pregnancy.

Billings method. *See* cervical mucus method.

Birth control method: Also known as contraceptive method. An effective, safe, comfortable method used to prevent pregnancy. Birth control can be temporary, meaning one can stop using the method and possibly become pregnant. Temporary methods are birth control pills, Depo-Provera®, Norplant®, IUD, diaphragm, cervical cap, condoms, spermicidal foam and cream. Birth control can be permanent, meaning it cannot be reversed if one decides to become pregnant. Permanent methods are tubal ligation for women and vasectomy for men.

Birth control pills: Often called the Pill, this method of birth control uses certain female hormones called estrogen and progestin to prevent pregnancy. A woman must take one pill at the same time each day. The pill prevents pregnancy by stopping the release of an egg and thickening the cervical mucus.

Breakthrough bleeding: Vaginal bleeding between menstrual periods.

Breastfeeding: The process by which the mother nourishes her infant with her breast milk.

Breasts: Two glands on the chests of women. Men also have breast tissue. Breasts are considered sex organs because they are often sexually sensitive and may inspire sexual desire. They produce milk during and after pregnancy.

C

Calendar method (rhythm method): A traditional method of natural family planning. The fertile phase of the menstrual cycle is determined by calcuating the length of at least six previous menstrual cycles. The beginning of the fertile phase is determined by subtracting 18 to 20 from the length of the shortest menstrual cycle. The end of the fertile phase is determined by subtracting 10 or 11 from the longest menstrual cycle.

Cervical cap: A firm rubber cap intended to fit securely on the cervix. Used with contraceptive jelly, the cervical cap is a barrier method of birth control that is reversible and available only by prescription.

Cervical mucus: A thick fluid plugging the opening of the cervix. Most of the time the cervical mucus is thick enough to prevent sperm from entering the uterus. At midcycle, however, under the influence of estrogen, the mucus becomes thin and watery, and sperm can more easily pass into the uterus.

Cervical mucus method (Billings method; ovulation method): A method of natural family planning developed by Drs. John and Evelyn Billings. A woman determines her days of infertility, possible fertility, and greatest fertility by observing changes in her cervical mucus and sensations at the vulva. To avoid pregnancy, abstinence is practiced during the fertile period. The Billings method refers to the "authentic" method as outlined and modified by Drs. Billings. Several adaptations of this method, and the rules for observing the mucus and practicing this method, have been developed. These modified, generic methods are referred to as cervical mucus methods.

Cervix: The lower portion of the uterus that extends into the upper vagina.

Chlamydia: A common sexually transmitted organism that can cause sterility in women and men.

Circumcision: An operation to remove the foreskin of the penis.

Clinician: A qualified health care professional, such as a doctor, nurse practitioner, or physician assistant.

Clitoral hood: A small flap of skin that covers and protects the clitoris.

Clitoris: The female sex organ that is very sensitive to the touch; located between the labia at the top of the vulva.

Coitus interruptus (withdrawal): Sexual intercourse in which the penis is deliberately withdrawn from the vagina so that ejaculation occurs outside the vagina; commonly called withdrawal.

Colposcopy: Examination of the cervix through a magnifying telescope (colposcope) to detect abnormal cells.

Combined oral contraceptives: Birth control pills that contain the hormones estrogen and progestin.

Conception. *See* fertilization.

Condom, male: A sheath (a case or cover that protects) of thin latex, plastic, or animal tissue that covers a man's penis. It prevents sperm from reaching the egg and is most effective when used with spermicide. Condoms prevent the spread of most sexually transmitted diseases (STDs). They can be bought over the counter in a drug store.

Condom, female. *See* vaginal pouch.

Contraception: The conscious use by sexually active people of chemicals (spermicides), drugs (hormones), devices (condoms, diaphragms, intrauterine devices), surgery, or withdrawal to prevent pregnancy.

Contraceptive creams and jellies: Substances containing spermicide, which immobilizes sperm, preventing it from joining with an egg; used with diaphragms or cervical caps. These are over-the-counter, reversible barrier methods of birth control.

Contraceptive film: Inserted deep into the vagina, a square of tissue that melts into a thick liquid and blocks the entrance to the uterus with a spermicide to immobilize sperm, preventing it from joining with an egg; an over-the-counter, reversible barrier method of birth control. Most effective when used with a condom.

Contraceptive foam: Inserted deep into the vagina, a substance that blocks the entrance to the uterus with bubbles and contains a spermicide to immobilize sperm, preventing it from joining with an egg; an over-the-counter, reversible barrier method of birth control. Most effective when used with a condom.

Contraceptive suppository capsule: Inserted deep into the vagina, a solid that melts into a fluid liquid to immobilize sperm, preventing it from joining with an egg; an over-the-counter, reversible barrier method of birth control. Most effective when used with a condom.

Corpus luteum: A small yellow gland that develops in the ovarian follicle after ovulation. It secretes the hormone progesterone.

Cowper's glands: The glands beneath the prostate gland that are attached to the urethra. They produce a substance that makes seminal fluid sticky.

D

Depo-Provera®: Also called the Shot or Depo, Depo-Provera® is a hormone shot that is injected by a doctor or clinician every 12 weeks. Like the Pill, it prevents pregnancy by stopping the release of an egg and thickening the cervical mucus.

Diaphragm: A soft rubber dome intended to fit securely over the cervix. Used with contraceptive cream or jelly, the diaphragm is a reversible barrier method of birth control available only by prescription.

Dilation and curettage (D&C): An operation that involves stretching the cervical opening to scrape out the uterus.

Donor embryo: An embryo formed from the egg of a woman who has donated it for transfer to a woman who is unable to conceive with her own eggs (the recipient). The donor relinquishes all parental rights to any resulting offspring.

Douche: A spray of water or solution of medication into the vagina.

E

Ectopic pregnancy: A pregnancy in which the fertilized egg implants in a location outside the uterus—usually in the fallopian tube, the ovary, or the abdominal cavity. Ectopic pregnancy is a dangerous condition that must receive prompt treatment.

Effectiveness rate. *See* method-effectiveness and use-effectiveness.

Egg: A female reproductive cell, also called an oocyte or ovum.

Egg retrieval (oocyte retrieval): A procedure to collect the eggs contained in the ovarian follicles.

Egg transfer (oocyte transfer): The transfer of retrieved eggs into a woman's fallopian tubes through laparoscopy. This procedure is used only in GIFT (see definition).

Ejaculation: The release of semen from the penis.

Embryo: The organism that develops from the pre-embryo and begins to share the woman's blood supply about nine days after fertilization.

Embryo transfer: Placement of embryos into a woman's uterus through the cervix after IVF (see definition) or, in the case of ZIFT (see definition), into her fallopian tubes.

Emergency contraception: The use of oral contraceptives or IUDs to prevent pregnancy after unprotected intercourse.

Emergency hormonal contraception: The use of oral contraceptives to prevent pregnancy after unprotected intercourse.

Endometriosis: The presence of tissue similar to the uterine lining in locations outside the uterus, such as the ovaries, fallopian tubes, and abdominal cavity.

Endometrium: The inner lining of the uterus composed mostly of functioning tissue, mucus, and blood that develops during each menstrual cycle in response to female sex hormones. In pregnancy the early embryo implants in the endometrium. If no pregnancy occurs, part of the endometrium is shed during menstruation.

Epididymis: The tube in which sperm mature. It is tightly coiled on top of and behind each testis. The plural of epididymis is epididymides.

Erectile dysfunction: The inability to become erect or maintain an erection with a partner.

Erection: A "hard" penis when it becomes full of blood and stiffens.

Estrogen: Female sex hormones produced mainly by the ovaries. Estrogen stimulates the development and function of the female reproductive system, including the growth of the endometrium after menstruation and the production of fertile-type mucus in the cervix.

F

Fallopian tube: Either of a pair of slender ducts that connect the uterus to the region of each ovary. It carries the ovum (egg) from the ovary to the uterus, and carries the sperm from the uterus toward the ovary. Fertilization usually takes place in the fallopian tube.

Family planning: Methods used by sexually active people to prevent, space, or achieve pregnancy in order to attain the desired family size.

Fertile phase: The days of the menstrual cycle when sexual intercourse or genital contact are most likely to result in pregnancy. A woman is normally fertile for several days around the time of ovulation.

Fertility: The ability to reproduce: the ability of a man to father a child and of a woman to conceive and carry a pregnancy to live birth.

Fertility awareness (also called natural family planning or periodic abstinence): This method of birth control requires a woman (with help from her partner) to pay attention to and keep notes on the changes in three areas of the body: cervical mucus, basal body temperature, and cervix changes. Many women use fertility awareness in combination with a barrier method during their fertile time of each menstrual cycle.

Fertilization: The penetration of the egg by the sperm and the resulting fusion of genetic material that develops into an embryo. Also known as conception.

Fetus: The developing baby from the second month of pregnancy until birth.

Follicle: A structure in the ovaries that contains a developing egg.

Follicle stimulating hormone (FSH): The pituitary hormone that stimulates follicle growth in women and sperm formation in men.

Foreplay: Physical and sexual stimulation—kissing, touching, stroking, and massaging—that often happens in the excitement stage of sexual response; often occurs before intercourse, but can lead to orgasm without intercourse, in which case it can be called outercourse.

Foreskin: A retractable tube of skin that covers and protects the glans of the penis.

Fully breastfeeding: Giving a baby no food or liquid other than breast milk. To nearly fully breastfeed signifies that the baby is given some additional food or liquid, but at least 85% of the baby's feedings are breast milk.

G

Gamete: A reproductive cell, either a sperm or an egg.

Genitals: External sex and reproductive organs—the penis and scrotum in men, the vulva in women. Sometimes the internal reproductive organs are also called genitals.

Gestation: The period of development of the new organism from conception to the end of pregnancy and birth.

Gestational sac: A fluid-filled structure that develops within the uterus early in pregnancy.

GIFT (gamete intrafallopian transfer): An ART procedure that involves removing eggs from the woman's ovary, combining them with sperm, and using a laparoscope to place the unfertilized eggs and the sperm into the woman's fallopian tubes through a small incision into her abdomen.

Glans: The soft, highly sensitive tip of the clitoris or penis. In men, the urethral opening is located in the glans.

Gonadotropins: Hormones secreted by the pituitary gland that trigger puberty by stimulating the gonads.

Gonads: The organs that produce reproductive cells—the ovaries of women, the testes of men.

Gonorrhea: A sexually transmitted bacterium that can cause sterility, arthritis, and heart problems.

Gynecology: Sexual and reproductive health care for women.

Gynecological exam: An exam that checks a woman's reproductive system, performed by a doctor or clinician. It may include a breast exam and a pelvic exam. The pelvic exam includes a speculum exam, a Pap smear, testing for STDs, and a bimanual exam. During a bimanual exam, the clinician inserts one or two gloved fingers into the vagina and presses on the woman's stomach with the other hand to feel the uterus, fallopian tubes, and ovaries to make sure they feel normal.

H

HIV (human immunodeficiency virus): An infection that weakens the body's ability to fight disease and can cause AIDS.

Hormonal contraceptives: Prescription methods of birth control that use hormones to prevent pregnancy. These include the Pill, implants, and injectables.

Hormone: A chemical substance that is usually produced and released by a gland. Hormones circulate in the blood and affect different body functions.

Hymen: A thin fleshy tissue that stretches across part of the opening to the vagina.

I

ICSI (intracytoplasmic sperm injection): A procedure in which a single sperm is injected directly into an egg; this procedure is most commonly used to overcome male infertility problems.

Implantation: The imbedding of the embryo into tissue so it can establish contact with the mother's blood supply for nourishment. Implantation usually occurs in the endometrium (the membrane lining the inner surface of the uterus); however, in an ectopic pregnancy it may occur elsewhere in the body.

Induced or therapeutic abortion: An operative procedure used to end a pregnancy.

Infertility: Inability of a couple to achieve a pregnancy or to carry a pregnancy to term after one year of unprotected intercourse.

Intercourse: Sexual activity between two people in which insertion of the penis occurs. This includes vaginal intercourse, oral intercourse, and anal intercourse.

IUD (intrauterine device): A small piece of plastic, which may contain copper or hormones, that is inserted into the uterus by a clinician. Although doctors are not entirely sure how the IUD works, they think it makes it hard for the sperm to swim through the uterus to reach the egg and it prevents a fertilized egg from implanting.

IVF (in vitro fertilization): An ART procedure that involves removing eggs from a woman's ovaries and fertilizing them in the laboratory. The resulting embryos are then transferred into the woman's uterus through the cervix.

L

Labia: Two folds of skin that cover and protect the clitoris, urethra, and vaginal opening.

Lactational Amenorrhea Method (LAM): A family planning method that relies on breastfeeding as natural protection against pregnancy for up to six months after childbirth. Women who use LAM must fully breastfeed or nearly fully breastfeed to protect themselves from pregnancy.

Laparoscopy: A surgical procedure in which a fiber-optic instrument (a laparoscope) is inserted into the pelvic area through a small incision in the abdomen.

Levonorgestrel: A synthetic progestin similar to the hormone progesterone, which is produced by the body to regulate the menstrual cycle; the active ingredient in Norplant.

LMP: Shorthand for Last Menstrual Period. In the world of family planning and gynecology, the start date of the last menstrual period is important and a woman will be asked for the date every time she sees her clinician.

M

Masturbation: Touching one's sex organs for pleasure.

Menarche: The time when a woman has her first menstrual period.

Menopause: The time in a woman's life when menstrual periods (menses) stop. Occurs when a woman's ovaries stop producing eggs and monthly bleeding from the uterus stops.

Menstrual cycle: A repeating series of changes in the ovaries and endometrium that includes ovulation and about two weeks later the beginning of menstrual bleeding. In most women the cycle averages 28 days, but it may be shorter or longer.

Menstruation (menses): The cyclic discharge of the lining of the endometrium (menstrual blood, cellular debris, and mucus) that occurs about two weeks after ovulation if the woman is not pregnant. Also called menses or period.

Method-effectiveness: The reliability of a contraceptive method itself—when it is always used consistently and correctly.

Milk ducts: The passages in women's breasts through which milk flows from the alveoli to the nipple.

Mini-pills: Birth control pills that contain only the hormone progestin.

Miscarriage. *See* spontaneous abortion.

"Morning-after" pills: Emergency hormonal contraception that is taken within 72 hours of unprotected intercourse.

Mucus. *See* cervical mucus.

N

Natural family planning. *See* fertility awareness.

Nipple: The dark tissue in the center of the areola of each breast in women and men that can stand erect when stimulated by touch or cold. In a woman's breast, the nipple may release milk that is produced by the breast.

Norplant®: A birth control method involving the placement of six small capsules under the skin of the upper arm by a trained clinician. The capsules constantly release small amounts of hormones that prevent pregnancy by stopping the release of an egg and thickening the cervical mucus.

O

Obstetrician-gynecologist (Ob-gyn): A physician who specializes in the treatment of female disorders and pregnancy.

Oocyte: The female reproductive cell, also called an egg or ovum.

Oral contraceptives: Birth control pills.

Oral sex: Sex play involving the mouth and sex organs.

Outercourse: Sex play that does not include inserting the penis in the vagina or anus.

Ovaries: The female gonads above the uterus that produce ova (eggs) and hormones that control female reproduction and secondary sexual characteristics.

Over-the-counter: Available without a prescription.

Ovulation: The release of an ovum (egg cell) from an ovary.

Ovulation method. *See* cervical mucus method.

Ovum: The female reproductive cell, also called an egg or oocyte.

P

Pap smear: A procedure where cells are scraped from the surface of the cervix and examined in a laboratory, under a microscope. It is used for the early detection of cervical cancer and some infections.

ParaGard® (Copper T 380A): An IUD that contains copper and can be left in place for ten years.

Pelvic exam: *See* gynecological exam.

Pelvic inflammatory disease (PID): An infection of a woman's internal reproductive system that can lead to sterility, ectopic pregnancy, and chronic pain. It is often caused by sexually transmitted infections such as gonorrhea and chlamydia.

Penis: A man's reproductive and sex organ that is formed of spongy tissue and fills with blood during sexual excitement, a process known as erection. Urine and seminal fluid pass through the penis.

Perfect use: The contraceptive effectiveness for women and men whose use is consistent and always correct.

Perimenopause: The period of change leading to menopause.

Period: The days during menstruation.

Periodic abstinence: Intentional avoidance of vaginal intercourse on fertile days to prevent pregnancy.

Pill, The: Common expression for oral hormonal contraception. *See* birth control pills.

Postpartum: The first six weeks after childbirth.

Pre-ejaculate: The liquid that oozes out of the penis during sexual excitement before ejaculation; produced by the Cowper's glands.

Pre-embryo: The ball of cells that develops from the fertilized egg until after about nine days, when it attaches to the lining of the uterus and the embryo is formed.

Pregnancy: The state of a female after she has conceived until she gives birth.

Pregnancy, Chemical: Pregnancy documented by a blood or urine test that shows a rise in the level of the human chorionic gonadotropin (hCG) hormone.

Pregnancy, Clinical: Pregnancy documented by the presence of a gestational sac on ultrasound.

Pregnancy test: A blood or urine test that determines the level of the human chorionic gonadotropin (hCG) hormone. Elevated levels of this hormone are chemical evidence of a pregnancy.

Premenstrual syndrome (PMS): Undesirable physical and emotional symptoms experienced by some women before menstruation occurs. PMS symptoms include irritability, tension, breast tenderness, fatigue, anxiety, and depression.

Prenatal care: The care a pregnant woman should receive during her pregnancy to assure a healthy baby.

Progestasert®: An IUD containing natural hormones that must be replaced every year.

Progesterone: A hormone secreted chiefly by the corpus luteum, which develops in a ruptured ovarian follicle (small round structure in the ovary that contains an ovum) during the luteal phase of the menstrual cycle (after ovulation). Progesterone prepares the endometrium for possible implantation by a fertilized ovum. It also protects the embryo, enhances development of the placenta, and aids in preparing the breasts for nursing the new infant.

Progestin: A word used to cover a large group of synthetic drugs that have an effect similar to that of progesterone.

Prolactin: A hormone produced by the pituitary gland that causes the breasts to produce milk.

Prophylactic: A device used to prevent infection; the condom.

Prostate: A gland that produces the milky fluid that, along with the sperm, makes up the semen.

Puberty: A time in life when a girl is becoming a woman and a boy is becoming a man. Puberty is marked by physical changes of the body such as breast development and menstruation in girls and facial hair growth and ejaculation in boys.

R

Reproductive cell: The unique cell—egg in women, sperm in men—that can join with its opposite to make reproduction possible.

Rhythm method. *See* calendar method.

S

Safer sex: Ways in which people reduce the risk of getting sexually transmitted infections, including HIV.

Scrotum: A sac of skin, divided into two parts, enclosing the testes, epididymides, and a part of the vasa deferentia.

Semen: The fluid containing sperm and secretions from the testicles, prostate, and seminal vesicles that is expelled during ejaculation.

Seminal fluid: A fluid that nourishes and helps sperm to move. Seminal fluid is made in the seminal vesicles.

Seminal vesicles: The paired glands at the base of the bladder that produce seminal fluid and fructose.

Seminiferous tubules: A network of tiny tubules in the testes that constantly produce sperm. Seminiferous tubules also produce androgens, the male sex hormones.

Sex cell: A reproductive cell.

Sexual intercourse: *See* intercourse.

Sexually transmitted disease (STD): A sexually transmitted infection that has developed symptoms.

Sexually transmitted infections (STIs): Infections that are often or usually passed from one person to another during sexual or intimate contact.

Shaft: A part of the penis and clitoris.

Speculum: A plastic or metal instrument used to separate the walls of the vagina so the clinician can examine the vagina and cervix.

Sperm: The male reproductive cell.

Sperm bank: A place where sperm are kept frozen in liquid nitrogen for later use in artificial insemination.

Sperm count: The number of sperm in the ejaculate (when given as the number of sperm per milliliter it is more accurately known as the sperm concentration or sperm density).

Spermarche: The time when sperm is first produced by the testes of a boy.

Spermicides: Chemicals used to immobilize sperm and protect against certain sexually transmitted infections.

Spontaneous abortion (miscarriage): A pregnancy ending in the spontaneous loss of the embryo or fetus before 20 weeks of gestation.

Sterilization: Surgical methods of birth control that are intended to be permanent—blocking of the fallopian tubes for women or the vasa deferentia for men.

Sterilization reversal: A surgical procedure used to undo a previous sterilization operation and restore fertility.

Surrogate: A woman who carries an embryo that was formed from the egg of another woman, or a woman who becomes artificially inseminated with a man's sperm and carries the pregnancy for an infertile couple, who adopt the baby after its birth.

Sympto-thermal method: A method of natural family planning. Fertile and infertile days are identified by observing and interpreting cervical mucus, basal body temperature, and other signs and symptoms of ovulation, which include intermenstrual bleeding, breast tenderness, abdominal pain, cervical changes, and calendar calculations.

Syphilis: A sexually transmitted organism that can lead to disorders, or death.

T

Testes: Two ball-like glands inside the scrotum that produce sperm.

Testicles: The testes.

Testosterone: The primary male hormone produced mainly by the testes. It influences the development of male sexual characteristics and reproductive organs.

Toxic shock syndrome: A rare but very dangerous overgrowth of bacteria in the vagina. Symptoms include vomiting, high fever, diarrhea, and a sunburn-type rash. May occur if a tampon or diaphragm is left in the vagina for too long.

Traditional methods: Family planning methods that have been practiced by couples for many generations; examples include coitus interruptus (withdrawal) and abstinence for varying periods of time.

Tubal ligation: Surgical sterilization of a woman by obstructing or "tying" the fallopian tubes.

Typical use: Contraceptive effectiveness for women and men whose use is not consistent or always correct.

U

Ultrasound: A noninvasive technique for visualizing the follicles in the ovaries and the gestational sac or fetus in the uterus.

Uncircumcised: Description of a penis that has a foreskin.

Urethra: The tube and opening from which women and men urinate. The urethra empties the bladder and carries urine to the urethral opening. In men, the urethra runs though the penis and also carries ejaculate and pre-ejaculate during sex play.

Urinary tract infection (UTI): A bacterial infection of the bladder (also called cystitis), the ureters, or the urethra; can be sexually transmitted.

Urologist: A physician who specializes in the surgical treatment of disorders of the urinary tract and male reproductive tract.

Use-effectiveness: The reliability of a contraceptive method as it is usually used—when it is not always used consistently or correctly.

Uterus: The pear-shaped, muscular reproductive organ from which women menstruate and where normal pregnancy develops; the womb.

V

Vagina: The stretchable passage that connects a woman's outer sex organs—the vulva—with the cervix and uterus; also known as the birth canal.

Vaginal pouch (female condom): A polyurethane sheath with flexible rings at each end that is inserted deep into the vagina like a diaphragm. It is an over-the-counter, reversible method of birth control that may provide protection against many sexually transmitted infections.

Vas deferens: A long, narrow tube that carries sperm from each epididymis to the seminal vesicles. The plural of vas deferens is vasa deferentia.

Vasectomy: Known as male sterilization, a vasectomy is a surgical procedure in which a segment of the vas deferens is removed and the ends tied, or burned to prevent the sperm from leaving the scrotum. This is a permanent way to prevent pregnancy.

Virginity: Never having had sexual intercourse.

Vulva: A woman's external sex organs, including the clitoris, the labia (majora and minora), the opening to the vagina (introitus), and two Bartholin's glands.

W

Withdrawal. *See* coitus interruptus.

Z

ZIFT (zygote intrafallopian transfer): An ART procedure in which eggs are collected from a woman's ovary and fertilized in the laboratory. A laparoscope is then used to place the resulting zygote (fertilized egg) into the woman's fallopian tubes through a small incision in her abdomen.

Zygote: An egg that has been fertilized but not yet divided.

This chapter includes terms excerpted from the following sources: *1995 Assisted Reproductive Technology Success Rates: National Summary and Fertility Clinic Reports, Vol. 2—Central United States*, U.S. Department of Health and Human Services, December 1997; Planned Parenthood website, http://www.plannedparenthood.org; Natural Family Planning Inc. New Zealand website, http://www.natfamplan.co.nz; Family Planning Council website, http://www.familyplanning.org; Fertilitext: Fertility and Infertility Information website, http:// www.fertilitext.org; and Reproductive Health Outlook website, http:// www.rho.org. Selected terms reprinted with permission.

Chapter 47

Family Planning Information Resources

Additional information on family planning can be obtained from the organizations, websites, and hotlines listed below.

The Alan Guttmacher Institute (AGI)
120 Wall Street
New York, NY 10005
(212) 248-1111
Fax: (212) 248-1951
E-mail: info@agi-usa.org
Washington office:
1120 Connecticut Avenue, NW, Suite 460
Washington, DC 20036
(202) 296-4012
Fax: (202) 223-5756
E-mail: policyinfo@agi-usa.org
http://www.agi-usa.org

The mission of AGI is to protect the reproductive choices of all women and men in the United States and throughout the world, and to support their ability to obtain information and services needed to achieve their full human rights, safeguard their health, and exercise their individual responsibilities in regard to sexual behavior, reproduction, and family formation. Its website provides information on sexual behavior, pregnancy and birth, prevention and contraception, abortion, sexually transmitted diseases, youth, and law and public policy. AGI publishes *Family Plan-*

ning Perspectives, a bimonthly research journal, and *International Family Planning Perspectives*, a quarterly research journal. Both cover such topics as contraceptive practice and research; fertility levels, trends, and determinants; adolescent pregnancy; abortion; public policies and legal issues affecting family planning and childbearing; program operation, development, and evaluation; information, education, and communication activities; sexually transmitted diseases; and reproductive, maternal, and child health.

American Academy of Family Physicians (AAFP)
11400 Tomahawk Creek Parkway
Leawood, KS 66211-2672
(913) 906-6000
(800) 274-2237
E-mail: fp@aafp.org
http://www.aafp.org

The AAFP was founded to promote and maintain high quality standards for family doctors who are providing continuing comprehensive health care to the public. Its website includes patient information on family planning.

American Academy of Natural Family Planning (AANFP)
3680 Grant Drive, Suite O
Reno, NV 89509
(775) 827-5408
http://www.aanfp.org

Comprised of individuals who participate in natural family planning instruction, the AANFP disseminates information on natural family planning in order to promote public recognition and acceptance. Natural family planning methods require abstinence from genital contact during the days of possible fertility (to avoid pregnancy), and they do not involve drug taking or the use of any appliances.

The American Academy of Pediatrics (AAP)
141 Northwest Point Boulevard
Elk Grove Village, IL 60007-1098
(847) 434-4000
Fax: (847) 434-8000
E-mail: kidsdocs@aap.org
http://www.aap.org

The AAP is an organization of primary care pediatricians, pediatric medical subspecialists, and pediatric surgical specialists dedicated to the health, safety, and well-being of infants, children, adolescents, and young adults.

American College of Nurse-Midwives (ACNM)
818 Connecticut Avenue NW, Suite 900
Washington, DC 20006
(202) 728-9860
Fax: (202) 728-9897
E-mail: info@acnm.org
http://www.midwife.org

The mission of ACNM is to promote the health and well-being of women and infants within their families and communities through the development and support of the profession of nurse-midwifery.

American College of Obstetricians and Gynecologists (ACOG)
409 12th Street, SW
P.O. Box 96920
Washington, DC 20090-6920
(202) 863-2518 (ACOG Resource Center)
http://www.acog.org

The nation's leading group of professionals providing health care for women, ACOG serves as a strong advocate for quality health care for women, promotes patient education and patient involvement in medical care, and increases awareness among its members and the public of the changing issues facing women's health care. Patient education pamphlets on various methods of contraception may be ordered from the ACOG Resource Center. ACOG's official journal, *Obstetrics & Gynecology*, popularly known as "The Green Journal," is published monthly and contains original articles and research studies on scientific advances, new medical and surgical techniques, obstetric management, and clinical evaluation of drugs and instruments.

American Medical Women's Association (AMWA)
801 North Fairfax Street, Suite 400
Alexandria, VA 22314
(703) 838-0500
Fax: (703) 549-3864
E-mail: info@amwa-doc.org
http://www.amwa-doc.org

A national organization of women physicians and medical students, AMWA is dedicated to promoting women's health and has worked to improve reproductive health, among other issues. JAMWA, *Journal of the American Medical Women's Association*, is a quarterly medical journal that focuses on women's health.

American Public Health Association (APHA)
800 I Street, NW
Washington, DC 20001-3710
(202) 777-2742
Fax: (202) 777-2534
E-mail: comments@apha.org
http://www.apha.org

The APHA is the oldest and largest organization of public health professionals in the world. It is concerned with a broad set of issues affecting personal and environmental health.

American Society for Reproductive Medicine (ASRM)
(formerly The American Fertility Society)
1209 Montgomery Highway
Birmingham, AL 35216-2809
(205) 978-5000
Fax: (205) 978-5005
E-mail: asrm@asrm.org
http://www.asrm.org

The ASRM is devoted to advancing knowledge and expertise in reproductive medicine and biology.

Ann Rose's Ultimate Birth Control Links
E-mail: annrose@annrose.com
http://gynpages.com/ultimate

The goal of Ann Rose's website is to provide extensive links to as much information as possible for individuals of all ages to make informed decisions about sexual activity and potential childbearing. Each birth control method or topic includes numerous links to material from a variety of sources.

Association of Reproductive Health Professionals (ARHP)
2401 Pennsylvania Avenue, NW, Suite 350
Washington, DC 20037
(202) 466-3825
Fax: (202) 466-3826
E-mail: arhp@arhp.org
http://www.arhp.org

The ARHP is an interdisciplinary association composed of professionals who provide reproductive health services or education, conduct reproductive health research, or influence reproductive health policy. It has a mission to educate health care professionals, public policy makers, and the public, fostering research and advocacy to promote reproductive health. Published monthly, *Contraception* is the official journal of the ARHP and provides a medium for the rapid communication of advances and new knowledge in all areas of contraception.

AVSC International
440 Ninth Avenue
New York, NY 10001
(212) 561-8000
Fax: (212) 561-8067
E-mail: info@avsc.org
http://www.avsc.org

AVSC International works worldwide to improve the lives of individuals by making reproductive health services safe, available, and sustainable. Its website includes information on temporary and permanent contraception.

BabyCenter
163 Freelon Street
San Francisco, CA 94107
(415) 537-0900
Fax: (415) 537-0909
http://www.babycenter.com

An Internet site for new and expectant parents, BabyCenter provides information, support, and products related to pregnancy, babies, and toddlers.

BabyZone
http://babyzone.com

The BabyZone website provides information on family planning, pregnancy, and parenting.

Billings Family Life Centre
27, Alexandra Parade
Fitzroy North
Victoria, 3068
Australia
(03) 9481-1722
Fax: (+613)-9482-4208
E-mail: billings@ozemail.com.au
Canada:
The Calgary Billings Centre
Fax: (403) 252-3929
http://www.billings-centre.ab.ca
http://www.billingsmethod.com

The Billings Family Life Centre was founded by Drs. Evelyn and John Billings, who developed the Billings Ovulation Method (BOM), a natural method of family planning that can help couples achieve, avoid, or postpone pregnancy.

Billings Ovulation Method Association of the United States (BOMA-USA)
316 North 7th Avenue
St. Cloud, MN 56303
(320) 252-7719
(888) 637-6371
Fax: (320) 252-2877
E-mail: dek@cloudnet.com

Teachers of the Billings Ovulation Method of natural family planning comprise the membership of BOMA-USA. The association coordinates the continuing education and recertification of teachers.

CancerNet
National Cancer Institute
NCI Public Inquiries Office
Building 31, Room 10A03
31 Center Drive, MSC 2580
Bethesda, MD 20892-2580
(301) 435-3848
(800) 4-CANCER
http://cancernet.nci.nih.gov

CancerNet was created to meet the need for up-to-date, accurate cancer information from the National Cancer Institute's Office of Cancer Information, Communication, and Education. It is updated monthly and provides easy access to the most current information on cancer.

CDC's Reproductive Health Information Source
Division of Reproductive Health
National Center for Chronic Disease Prevention and Health Promotion
Centers for Disease Control and Prevention
4770 Buford Highway, NE, Mail Stop K-20
Atlanta, GA 30341-3717
(770) 488-5200 (general information)
(770) 488-5372 (automated information)
Fax: (770) 488-5374
E-mail: ccdinfo@cdc.gov
http://www.cdc.gov/nccdphp/drh

CDC's Reproductive Health Information Source website provides information on assisted reproductive technology, unintended pregnancy, maternal health, women's reproductive health, infant health, men's reproductive health, and racial and ethnic minorities, among other topics.

Center for Population, Health, and Nutrition, USAID
1300 Pennsylvania Avenue
Washington, DC 20523
(202) 712-4810
Fax: (202) 216-3404
http://www.info.usaid.gov/pop_health

The U.S. Agency for International Development's goals in the population, health, and nutrition sector are to stabilize world population growth and to protect human health. In order to achieve these goals, the agency has adopted a strategy based on four objectives: reducing unintended pregnancies; reducing maternal morbidity; reducing infant and child mortality; and reducing STD transmission with a focus on HIV/AIDS.

Contraceptive Research and Development (CONRAD) Program

Eastern Virginia Medical School
1611 North Kent Street, Suite 806
Arlington, VA 22209
(703) 524-4744
Fax: (703) 524-4770
E-mail: info@conrad.org
http://www.conrad.org

CONRAD has as its primary objective the development of new or improved contraceptive methods that are safe, effective, acceptable, and suitable for use in the United States and developing countries.

Couple to Couple League, International (CCLI)

P.O. Box 111184
Cincinnati, OH 45211-1184
(513) 471-2000
(800) 745-8252 (catalog orders)
Fax: (513) 557-2449
E-mail: ccli@ccli.org
http://www.ccli.org

CCLI's mission is to build healthy marriages through natural family planning. It teaches the Sympto-Thermal Method which utilizes all the fertility signs.

Emergency Contraception Hotlines

(800) 584-9911
(888) NOT-2-LATE

Open 24 hours a day, these hotlines provide women with information about emergency contraceptives (EC) and offer a list of health care providers who can prescribe them. All current forms of EC work by interrupting the process of an egg becoming fertilized and implanting in the uterus, and all reduce a woman's risk of pregnancy by at least 75 percent. The "morning after pill" EC pills are ordinary birth control pills containing the hormones estrogen and progestin; the treatment involves taking a specific dose within 72 hours of unprotected intercourse, and a second dose 12 hours after the first. Less commonly used methods of EC include a specific combination of minipills (progestin-only) taken up to 48 hours after unprotected sex, or insertion of the copper-T IUD up to seven days after unprotected intercourse.

Emergency Contraception Website
Office of Population Research, Princeton University
E-mail: ec@opr.princeton.edu
http://ec.princeton.edu

The Emergency Contraception (EC) Website is designed to provide accurate information about EC derived from the medical literature and a directory of clinicians willing to provide emergency contraceptives in the individual's local area. All forms of EC described on this server require a prescription. Emergency contraceptives are methods of preventing pregnancy after unprotected sexual intercourse. EC can be used when a condom breaks, after a sexual assault, or any time unprotected intercourse occurs, but it should not be used as ongoing birth control.

Emory University School of Medicine
c/o Dr. Robert Hatcher
69 Butler Street, SE
Atlanta, GA 30303
Fax: (404) 521-3589
http://www.emory.edu/WHSC/MED/FAMPLAN/choices.html

This website provides information on various contraceptive choices written by Dr. Robert A. Hatcher, M.D., M.P.H., professor of gynecology and obstetrics at Emory University School of Medicine. He has been the senior author of 16 editions of *Contraceptive Technology* and is active in a number of reproductive health organizations.

Family Health International (FHI)
P.O. Box 13950
Research Triangle Park, NC 27709
(919) 544-7040
Fax: (919) 544-7261
http://www.fhi.org

FHI works to improve reproductive and family health around the world through biomedical and social science research, innovative health service delivery interventions, training, and information programs. It is committed to helping women and men have access to safe, effective, acceptable, and affordable family planning methods. Its website includes facts sheets and frequently asked questions about family planning options.

Family of the Americas
(800) 443-3395
http://www.familyplanning.net

The Family of the Americas website provides an overview of the ovulation method of natural family planning, which is based on a woman's natural fertility.

Feminist Women's Health Center (FWHC)
Cedar River Clinic
4300 Talbot Road South, #403
Renton, WA 98055
(425) 255-0471
Fax: (425) 277-3640
E-mail: info@fwhc.org
http://www.fwhc.org

The FWHC promotes and protects a woman's right to choose and receive reproductive health care. Its website includes information on women's health, birth control, abortion, and clinic sites.

Fertility UK
Clitherow House
1 Blythe Mews, Blythe Road
London, W14 ONW
England
(011) (+44) 207-371-1341
Fax: (011) (+44) 207-371-4921
http://www.fertilityuk.org

Fertility UK is the national fertility awareness and natural family planning service for the United Kingdom. The service provides comprehensive and objective information to the general public and health professionals on all aspects of fertility awareness.

Go Ask Alice!

Columbia University's Health Education Program
Lerner Hall
2920 Broadway, 7th Floor
MC 2608
New York, NY 10027
(212) 854-5453
Fax: (212) 854-8949
http://www.goaskalice.columbia.edu

The mission of Go Ask Alice!, a health question and answer Internet site, is to provide factual, in-depth, straightforward, and nonjudgmental information to assist readers' decision-making about their physical, sexual, emotional, and spiritual health.

healthfinder®

A service of the U.S. Department of Health and Human Services
http://www.healthfinder.gov

A free gateway to reliable consumer health and human services information, healthfinder® can lead to selected online publications, clearinghouses, databases, websites, and support and self-help groups, as well as the government agencies and not-for-profit organizations that produce reliable information for the public.

Healthy Devil On-Line

Duke University
http://healthydevil.stuaff.duke.edu/info/healthinfo.html

This website includes information on women's and men's health, sex, contraceptive options, STDs, and pregnancy.

The Henry J. Kaiser Family Foundation (KFF)

2400 Sand Hill Road
Menlo Park, CA 94025
(650) 854-9400
Fax: (650) 854-4800
Washington office:
1450 G Street, NW, Suite 250
Washington, DC 20005
(202) 347-5270
Fax: (202) 347-5274
http://www.kff.org

An independent philanthropy focusing on major health care issues facing the nation, the foundation is an independent voice and source of facts and analysis for policymakers, the media, the health care community, and the general public. Reproductive health is one of the four main areas of its work. The *Kaiser Daily Reproductive Health Report* provides timely news reports and editorial commentary on such topics as abortion, contraception and family planning, public health and education, and bioethics and science.

International Planned Parenthood Federation (IPPF)

Regent's College
Inner Circle, Regent's Park
London, NW1 4NS
England
(011) (+44) 207-487-7900
Fax: (011) (+44) 207-487-7950
E-mail: info@ippf.org
http://www.ippf.org

IPPF is the largest voluntary organization in the field of sexual and reproductive health including family planning, linking national autonomous family planning associations in over 150 countries worldwide. IPPF and its member associations are committed to promoting the right of women and men to decide freely the number and spacing of their children and the right to the highest possible level of sexual and reproductive health. IPPF publishes the *IPPF Medical Bulletin,* a bimonthly publication that provides up-to-date information on clinical, service delivery, and managerial aspects in family planning and sexual and reproductive health.

Jacobs Institute of Women's Health (JIWH)

409 12th Street, SW
Washington, DC 20024-2188
(202) 863-4990
Fax: (202) 488-4229 or (202) 554-0453
http://www.jiwh.org

JIWH is a nonprofit organization dedicated to advancing knowledge and practice in the field of women's health. Members of the Jacobs Institute are a multidisciplinary group of health care providers, researchers, policy makers, and advocates with the common goal of improving the health status of women. *Women's Health Issues*, the official journal of

JIWH, is devoted exclusively to women's health issues at the medical/social interface.

JAMA Women's Health Contraception Information Center

Produced by the *Journal of the American Medical Association*
E-mail: Contraception@ama-assn.org
http://www.ama-assn.org/special/contra

This website is designed as a resource for physicians and other health professionals. It is produced and maintained by *JAMA* editors and staff under the direction of an editorial review board of leading contraception authorities.

JHPIEGO Corporation

An affiliate of Johns Hopkins University
1615 Thames Street, Suite 200
Baltimore, MD 21231-3447
(410) 955-8558
Fax: (410) 955-6199
E-mail: info@jhpiego.org
http://www.jhpiego.org

Dedicated to improving the health of women and families globally, JHPIEGO's goal since its inception has been to increase the availability of high quality reproductive health services, with an emphasis on family planning services. It promotes, initiates, and supports activities that lead to increased numbers of health professionals trained in reproductive health.

Johns Hopkins Bayview Medical Center (JHBMC)

Department of Obstetrics and Gynecology
4940 Eastern Avenue
Baltimore, MD 21224
(410) 550-0335
http://www.jhbmc.jhu.edu/obgyn/ob-gyn.html

Contraceptive research is an important area of activity at JHBMC. Research projects exploring new methods of contraception include the investigation of new barrier methods of contraception, a single implant hormonal contraceptive, and an oral contraceptive with lower hormonal dosages.

La Leche League International (LLLI)
1400 North Meacham Road
Schaumburg, IL 60173-4048
(847) 519-7730
(800) 525-3243
(800) 665-4324 (Canada)
Fax: (847) 519-0035
E-mail: OrderDepartment@llli.org
http://www.lalecheleague.org

LLLI's mission is to help mothers worldwide to breastfeed through mother-to-mother support, education, encouragement, and information, and to promote a better understanding of breastfeeding as an important element in the healthy development of the baby and mother.

The Male Health Center Internet Education Site
400 West LBJ Freeway, Suite 360
Irving, TX 75063
(972) 751-6253
http://www.malehealthcenter.com

The Male Health Center provides treatment for all areas of male health, including impotence, prostate disorders, sexually transmitted diseases, vasectomy, cancer screening, and wellness. Its website provides information on men's health issues.

March of Dimes Birth Defects Foundation
1275 Mamaroneck Avenue
White Plains, NY 10605
(914) 428-7100
(888) 663-4637
Fax: (914) 997-4763
http://www.modimes.org

The March of Dimes recognizes four major problems as threatening the health of America's babies: birth defects, infant mortality, low birthweight, and lack of prenatal care. It has established goals to combat these problems: reduce birth defects by 10 percent; reduce infant mortality to 7 per 1,000 live births; reduce low birthweight to no more than 5 percent of all live births; increase the number of women who get prenatal care in the first trimester to 90 percent.

Mayo Clinic Health Oasis

200 First Street SW
Rochester, MN 55905
(507) 284-2511
http://www.mayohealth.org

This website is directed by a team of Mayo Clinic physicians, scientists, writers, and educators who update it every weekday to provide the most relevant health information. The sections on women's and men's health include information on family planning.

National Abortion Federation (NAF)

1755 Massachusetts Avenue, NW, Suite 600
Washington, DC 20036
(202) 667-5881
(800) 772-9100
(800) 424-2280 (in Canada)
http://www.prochoice.org

NAF is the professional association of abortion providers in the United States and Canada. Its mission is to preserve and enhance the quality and accessibility of abortion services. Its website includes medical information on abortion procedures.

National Adoption Information Clearinghouse (NAIC)

330 C Street, SW
Washington, DC 20447
(703) 352-3488
(888) 251-0075
Fax: (703) 385-3206
E-mail: naic@calib.com
http://www.calib.com/naic

NAIC was established by Congress to provide professionals and the general public with easily accessible information on all aspects of adoption, including infant and intercountry adoption and the adoption of children with special needs. NAIC maintains an adoption literature database; a database of adoption experts; listings of adoption agencies, crisis pregnancy centers, adoptive parent support groups, and search support groups; excerpts and full texts of state and federal laws on adoption; and other adoption-related services and publications.

National Association of Nurse Practitioners in Women's Health (NPWH)
503 Capitol Court, NE
Suite 300
Washington, DC 20002
(202) 543-9693
Fax: (202) 543-9858
E-mail: info@npwh.org
http://www.npwh.org

NPWH represents nurse practitioners who practice in obstetrics, gynecology, contraception, reproductive endocrinology, and infertility. It promotes delivery of quality reproductive health care to all Americans, in particular the underserved and adolescent population.

National Family Planning and Reproductive Health Association (NFPRHA)
1627 K Street, NW, 12th Floor
Washington, DC 20006
(202) 293-3114
Fax: (202) 293-1990
http://www.nfprha.org

NFPRHA works to assure access to voluntary, comprehensive, and culturally sensitive family planning and reproductive health care services and to support reproductive freedom for all.

National Institute of Child Health and Human Development (NICHD), NIH, OPHS, HHS
31 Center Drive, Building 31, Room 2A32, MSC 2425
Bethesda, MD 20892-2425
(800) 370-2943
Fax: (301) 402-1104
http://www.nichd.nih.gov

NICHD conducts and supports research on the reproductive, neurobiological, developmental, and behavioral processes that determine and maintain the health of children, adults, families, and populations.

National Organization on Adolescent Pregnancy, Parenting and Prevention (NOAPPP)
2401 Pennsylvania Avenue, NW
Suite 350
Washington, DC 20037
(202) 293-8370
E-mail: noappp@noappp.org
http://www.noappp.org

NOAPPP is a national, membership-based organization whose sole agenda is focused on adolescent pregnancy, parenting, and prevention issues. NOAPPP maintains a network of individuals and organizations concerned about these issues; provides information, resource-sharing opportunities, and technical assistance; and sponsors national, regional, and statewide conferences and training events.

The National Women's Health Information Center (NWHIC)
A project of the U.S. Public Health Service's Office on Women's
     Health, Department of Health and Human Services
(800) 994-WOMAN
http://www.4woman.gov

A one-stop gateway for women seeking health information, NWHIC is a free information and resource service on women's health issues designed for consumers, health care professionals, researchers, educators, and students. The site can help the user link to, read, and download a wide variety of material developed by the U.S. Department of Health and Human Services, the U.S. Department of Defense, other federal agencies, and the private sector.

Natural Family Planning Center of Washington, DC
8514 Bradmoor Drive
Bethesda, MD 20817-3810
(301) 897-9323
Fax: (301) 571-5267

The Natural Family Planning Center promotes education, research, training of teachers, and production of educational materials in natural family planning. Natural family planning methods require abstinence from genital contact during the days of possible fertility (to avoid pregnancy), and they do not involve drug taking or the use of any appliances.

Natural Family Planning Inc. New Zealand (NFP)
P.O. Box 5087
Regent
Whangarei
New Zealand
(09) 438-8031
(0800) 178-637
E-mail: nationalcoord.@natfamplan.co.nz
http://www.natfamplan.co.nz

NFP provides information and teaching about natural family planning and fertility awareness.

New York Online Access to Health (NOAH)
Ask NOAH About: Pregnancy
http://www.noah-health.org/english/pregnancy/pregnancy.html

NOAH's mission is to provide high quality full-text health information for consumers that is accurate, timely, relevant, and unbiased. The keyword "pregnancy" leads the user to information about family planning, prenatal care and birth, problems and risks, postnatal care, and pregnancy resources.

OBGYN.net
9101 Burnet Road, Suite 201
Austin, TX 78758
(512) 835-1111
Fax: (512) 835-6112
http://www.obgyn.net

Designed for the specific needs of professionals interested in obstetrics and gynecology, the medical industry, and women, OBGYN.net can be used to access reference materials, read up on new procedures and innovations, track new research projects and developments, shop for and acquire products and services, access medical and women's health associations and support groups, locate a service provider, and more.

Office of Adolescent Pregnancy Programs (OAPP), OPA, OPHS, OS, HHS

4350 East West Highway, Suite 200 West
Bethesda, MD 20814
(301) 594-4004
Fax: (301) 594-5980
http://www.hhs.gov/opa/titlexx/oapp.html

OAPP seeks to discover new approaches to providing care services for pregnant adolescents and adolescent parents. It emphasizes a primary prevention strategy based on reaching adolescents before they become sexually active and promotes the postponement of teenage sexual activity.

Office of Family Planning (OFP), OPA, OPHS, OS, HHS

4350 East West Highway, Suite 200 West
Bethesda, MD 20814
(301) 594-4011
Fax: (301) 594-5980
E-mail: opa@osophs.dhhs.gov
http://www.hhs.gov/opa/titlex/ofp.html

The OFP assists in making comprehensive voluntary family planning services readily available to all persons desiring such services and coordinates domestic population and family planning research with the present and future needs of family planning programs.

Office of Minority Health Resource Center (OMHRC), OPHS, OS, HHS

5515 Security Lane
Suite 101
Rockville, MD 20852
(800) 444-6472
Fax: (301) 443-8280
http://www.omhrc.gov

Established to serve as a national resource and referral service on minority health issues, the center collects and distributes information on a wide variety of health topics.

Office of Population Affairs (OPA), OPHS, OS, HHS
4350 East West Highway, Suite 200 West
Bethesda, MD 20814
(301) 594-4000
Fax: (301) 594-5980
E-mail: opa@osophs.dhhs.gov
http://www.hhs.gov/opa

OPA's mission is to improve the health and well-being of the nation by providing resources and policy advice on population, family planning, reproductive health, and adolescent pregnancy issues.

Office of Population Affairs Clearinghouse, OPA, OPHS, OS, HHS
P.O. Box 30686
Bethesda, MD 20824-0686
(301) 654-6190
Fax: (301) 215-7731
http://www.hhs.gov/opa/clearinghouse.html

The OPA Clearinghouse collects, develops, and distributes information on family planning, adolescent pregnancy, abstinence, adoption, reproductive health care, and sexually transmitted diseases, including HIV and AIDS.

Office of Population Research (OPR)
Princeton University
Wallace Hall
Princeton, NJ 08544
(609) 258-4870
Fax: (609) 258-1039
http://opr.princeton.edu

The OPR at Princeton is the oldest population research center in the United States. Its website includes information on activities, resources, and research.

Peer Health
Williams College
Williamstown, MA 01267
(413) 597-3140
E-mail: peerh@wso.williams.edu
http://wso.williams.edu/orgs/peerh

A student-run organization, Peer Health provides the Williams community with information about health and sexuality.

Planned Parenthood® Federation of America, Inc. (PPFA)
810 Seventh Avenue
New York, NY 10019
(212) 541-7800
(800) 230-PLAN
Fax: (212) 245-1845
E-mail: communications@ppfa.org
http://www.plannedparenthood.org

The world's largest and oldest voluntary family planning organization, PPFA is dedicated to the principles that every individual has a fundamental right to decide when or whether to have a child, and that every child should be wanted and loved. PPFA affiliates operate 900 health centers nationwide, providing medical services and sexuality education for millions of women, men, and teenagers each year. Its website includes information on birth control, sexual health, parenting and pregnancy, abortion, reproductive rights legislation, and international family planning.

Population Council, Inc.
One Dag Hammarskjold Plaza
New York, NY 10017
(212) 339-0500
Fax: (212) 755-6052
E-mail: pubinfo@popcouncil.org
http://www.popcouncil.org

The Population Council's mission is to improve the well-being and reproductive health of current and future generations and to help achieve a humane, equitable, and sustainable balance between people and resources. The council conducts a broad range of research. It publishes *Studies in Family Planning*, an international quarterly concerned with all aspects of reproductive health, fertility regulation, and family planning programs in both developing and developed countries.

Program for Appropriate Technology in Health (PATH)
4 Nickerson Street
Seattle, WA 98109-1699
(206) 285-3500
Fax: (206) 285-6619
E-mail: info@path.org
http://www.path.org

PATH's mission is to improve health, especially the health of women and children. Its programs address a wide variety of topic areas including child and maternal health, and reproductive health and family planning.

Reproductive Health and Rights Center
A project of the CARAL Pro-Choice Education Fund
http://www.choice.org

The Reproductive Health and Rights Center website is sponsored by the CARAL Pro-Choice Education Fund, an organization dedicated to grassroots activism in support of the right of all women to the full range of reproductive rights. The website contains a resources section that links the user to information from different sources on such topics as gynecology, contraception, sexuality education, and abortion.

Reproductive Health Online (ReproLine®)
A service of JHPIEGO, an affiliate of Johns Hopkins University
http://www.reproline.jhu.edu

ReproLine® is a family planning, contraception, and training website. It is an educational, nonprofit source of up-to-date information (reference materials and presentation graphics) designed for use by policymakers as well as individuals, particularly teachers and trainers, with an interest in maintaining a current knowledge of selected reproductive health information.

RESOLVE: The National Infertility Association Since 1974
1310 Broadway
Somerville, MA 02144
(617) 623-0744
E-mail: resolveinc@aol.com
http://www.resolve.org

RESOLVE's mission is to provide timely, compassionate support and information to individuals who are experiencing infertility issues through advocacy and public education.

RHO (Reproductive Health Outlook)
Published by the Program for Appropriate Technology in Health (PATH)
http://www.rho.org

The RHO website provides up-to-date summaries of research findings, program experience, and clinical guidelines related to key reproductive topics, along with analyses of the policy and program implications.

Sexuality Information and Education Council of the United States (SIECUS)
130 West 42nd Street, Suite 350
New York, NY 10036-7802
(212) 819-9770
Fax: (212) 819-9776
E-mail: siecus@siecus.org
http://www.siecus.org

SIECUS is dedicated to affirming that sexuality is a natural and healthy part of life. It develops, collects, and disseminates information, promotes comprehensive education, and advocates the right of individuals to make responsible sexual choices.

Teen Health Pages
Dalhousie Medical School
5849 University Avenue
Halifax, NS, B3H 4H7
Canada
(902) 494-6592
http://www.chebucto.ns.ca/Health/TeenHealth

With the help of teens in the Halifax and Dartmouth area, the Dalhousie Medical School compiled the information found on this website based on the needs and level of information requested by teens. Content includes the following topics: healthy sexuality, sexual orientation, sexually transmitted diseases, pregnancy, women's health, men's health, and sexual assault.

Teenwire
Planned Parenthood® Federation of America, Inc.
http://www.teenwire.com

Designed exclusively for teens, Planned Parenthood®'s Teenwire site provides information and news about teen sexuality, sexual health, and relationships.

Twin Cities Natural Family Planning Center
HealthEast
St. Joseph's Hospital
69 West Exchange Street
St. Paul, MN 55102
(651) 232-3088
E-mail: info@tcnfp.org
http://www.tcnfp.org

One of the first NFP centers in the United States, the Twin Cities Natural Family Planning Center is motivated by the philosophy that women and men should not have to sacrifice their health or values in order to successfully plan family size.

U.S. Department of Health and Human Services (HHS)
200 Independence Avenue, SW
Washington, DC 20201
(202) 619-0257
(877) 696-6775
E-mail: hhsmail@os.dhhs.gov
http://www.dhhs.gov

The Department of Health and Human Services is the U.S. government's principal agency for protecting the health of all Americans and providing essential human services, especially for those who are least able to help themselves. The department includes more than 300 programs covering a wide spectrum of activities. Among these are medical and social science research, assuring food and drug safety, and improving maternal and infant health.

U.S. Food and Drug Administration (FDA), OPHS, HHS
5600 Fishers Lane
Rockville, MD 20857
(888) 463-6332 (Office of Consumer Affairs)
Fax: (301) 443-9057
http://www.fda.gov

The FDA's mission is to protect, promote, and enhance the health of the American people. Among its many responsibilities, the FDA ensures that human drugs, biological products, and medical devices are safe and effective.

University of Chicago Primary Care Group Health InfoLine
http://uhs.bsd.uchicago.edu/uhs/infoline.htm

This website provides information on a number of health-related topics, including reproductive health care (contraception, menstrual cycle health, pregnancy, sexually transmitted infections, other infections, tests).

Woman's Diagnostic Cyber
http://www.wdxcyber.com

This website was created to provide information and education on women's health concerns, particularly reproductive diseases. The site can help users categorize symptoms into possible disease categories and then provide information about those diseases or problems; the emphasis is on diagnosis, not treatment.

World Health Organization (WHO)
Avenue Appia 20
1211 Geneva 27
Switzerland
(+00-41-22) 791-21-11
Fax: (+00-41-22) 791-3111
E-mail: info@who.int
http://www.who.int

WHO is the directing and coordinating authority on international health work. Its objective is the attainment of all peoples of the highest possible level of health. Health, as defined in the WHO constitution, is a state of complete physical, mental, and social well-being and not merely the absence of disease or infirmity.

Zero Population Growth, Inc. (ZPG)
1400 16th Street, NW, Suite 320
Washington, DC 20036
(202) 332-2200
(800) 767-1956
Fax: (202) 332-2302
E-mail: info@zpg.org
http://www.zpg.org

ZPG's mission is to slow population growth and achieve a sustainable balance between the Earth's people and its resources. ZPG seeks to protect the environment and ensure a high quality of life for present and future generations. Its education and advocacy programs aim to influence public policies, attitudes, and behavior on national and global population issues and related concerns.

Index

Index

F

Health Reference Series

COMPLETE CATALOG

AIDS Sourcebook, 1st Edition

Basic Information about AIDS and HIV Infection, Featuring Historical and Statistical Data, Current Research, Prevention, and Other Special Topics of Interest for Persons Living with AIDS

Along with Source Listings for Further Assistance

Edited by Karen Bellenir and Peter D. Dresser. 831 pages. 1995. 0-7808-0031-1. $78.

"One strength of this book is its practical emphasis. The intended audience is the lay reader . . . useful as an educational tool for health care providers who work with AIDS patients. Recommended for public libraries as well as hospital or academic libraries that collect consumer materials."
— Bulletin of the Medical Library Association, Jan '96

"This is the most comprehensive volume of its kind on an important medical topic. Highly recommended for all libraries." *— Reference Book Review, '96*

"Very useful reference for all libraries."
— Choice, Association of College and Research Libraries, Oct '95

"There is a wealth of information here that can provide much educational assistance. It is a must book for all libraries and should be on the desk of each and every congressional leader. Highly recommended."
— AIDS Book Review Journal, Aug '95

"Recommended for most collections."
— Library Journal, Jul '95

■

AIDS Sourcebook, 2nd Edition

Basic Consumer Health Information about Acquired Immune Deficiency Syndrome (AIDS) and Human Immunodeficiency Virus (HIV) Infection, Featuring Updated Statistical Data, Reports on Recent Research and Prevention Initiatives, and Other Special Topics of Interest for Persons Living with AIDS, Including New Antiretroviral Treatment Options, Strategies for Combating Opportunistic Infections, Information about Clinical Trials, and More

Along with a Glossary of Important Terms and Resource Listings for Further Help and Information

Edited by Karen Bellenir. 751 pages. 1999. 0-7808-0225-X. $78.

"Highly recommended."
—American Reference Books Annual, 2000

"Excellent sourcebook. This continues to be a highly recommended book. There is no other book that provides as much information as this book provides."
— AIDS Book Review Journal, Dec-Jan 2000

"Recommended reference source."
—Booklist, American Library Association, Dec '99

"A solid text for college-level health libraries."
—The Bookwatch, Aug '99

Cited in *Reference Sources for Small and Medium-Sized Libraries, American Library Association, 1999*

■

Alcoholism Sourcebook

Basic Consumer Health Information about the Physical and Mental Consequences of Alcohol Abuse, Including Liver Disease, Pancreatitis, Wernicke-Korsakoff Syndrome (Alcoholic Dementia), Fetal Alcohol Syndrome, Heart Disease, Kidney Disorders, Gastrointestinal Problems, and Immune System Compromise and Featuring Facts about Addiction, Detoxification, Alcohol Withdrawal, Recovery, and the Maintenance of Sobriety

Along with a Glossary and Directories of Resources for Further Help and Information

Edited by Karen Bellenir. 613 pages. 2000. 0-7808-0325-6. $78.

"Recommended reference source."
—Booklist, American Library Association, Dec '00

"Presents a wealth of information on alcohol use and abuse and its effects on the body and mind, treatment, and prevention." *— SciTech Book News, Dec '00*

"Important new health guide which packs in the latest consumer information about the problems of alcoholism." *— Reviewer's Bookwatch, Nov '00*

SEE ALSO *Drug Abuse Sourcebook, Substance Abuse Sourcebook*

■

Allergies Sourcebook

Basic Information about Major Forms and Mechanisms of Common Allergic Reactions, Sensitivities, and Intolerances, Including Anaphylaxis, Asthma, Hives and Other Dermatologic Symptoms, Rhinitis, and Sinusitis

Along with Their Usual Triggers Like Animal Fur, Chemicals, Drugs, Dust, Foods, Insects, Latex, Pollen, and Poison Ivy, Oak, and Sumac; Plus Information on Prevention, Identification, and Treatment

Edited by Allan R. Cook. 611 pages. 1997. 0-7808-0036-2. $78.

■

Alternative Medicine Sourcebook

Basic Consumer Health Information about Alternatives to Conventional Medicine, Including Acupressure, Acupuncture, Aromatherapy, Ayurveda, Bioelectromagnetics, Environmental Medicine, Essence

Therapy, Food and Nutrition Therapy, Herbal Therapy, Homeopathy Imaging, Massage, Naturopathy, Reflexology, Relaxation and Meditation, Sound Therapy, Vitamin and Mineral Therapy, and Yoga, and More

Edited by Allan R. Cook. 737 pages. 1999. 0-7808-0200-4. $78.

"Recommended reference source."
—*Booklist, American Library Association, Feb '00*

"A great addition to the reference collection of every type of library." —*American Reference Books Annual, 2000*

■

Alzheimer's, Stroke & 29 Other Neurological Disorders Sourcebook, 1st Edition

Basic Information for the Layperson on 31 Diseases or Disorders Affecting the Brain and Nervous System, First Describing the Illness, Then Listing Symptoms, Diagnostic Methods, and Treatment Options, and Including Statistics on Incidences and Causes

Edited by Frank E. Bair. 579 pages. 1993. 1-55888-748-2. $78.

"Nontechnical reference book that provides reader-friendly information."
—*Family Caregiver Alliance Update, Winter '96*

"Should be included in any library's patient education section." —*American Reference Books Annual, 1994*

"Written in an approachable and accessible style. Recommended for patient education and consumer health collections in health science center and public libraries." —*Academic Library Book Review, Dec '93*

"It is very handy to have information on more than thirty neurological disorders under one cover, and there is no recent source like it." —*Reference Quarterly, American Library Association, Fall '93*

SEE ALSO *Brain Disorders Sourcebook*

■

Alzheimer's Disease Sourcebook, 2nd Edition

Basic Consumer Health Information about Alzheimer's Disease, Related Disorders, and Other Dementias, Including Multi-Infarct Dementia, AIDS-Related Dementia, Alcoholic Dementia, Huntington's Disease, Delirium, and Confusional States

Along with Reports Detailing Current Research Efforts in Prevention and Treatment, Long-Term Care Issues, and Listings of Sources for Additional Help and Information

Edited by Karen Bellenir. 524 pages. 1999. 0-7808-0223-3. $78.

"Provides a wealth of useful information not otherwise available in one place. This resource is recommended for all types of libraries."
—*American Reference Books Annual, 2000*

"Recommended reference source."
—*Booklist, American Library Association, Oct '99*

Arthritis Sourcebook

Basic Consumer Health Information about Specific Forms of Arthritis and Related Disorders, Including Rheumatoid Arthritis, Osteoarthritis, Gout, Polymyalgia Rheumatica, Psoriatic Arthritis, Spondyloarthropathies, Juvenile Rheumatoid Arthritis, and Juvenile Ankylosing Spondylitis

Along with Information about Medical, Surgical, and Alternative Treatment Options, and Including Strategies for Coping with Pain, Fatigue, and Stress

Edited by Allan R. Cook. 550 pages. 1998. 0-7808-0201-2. $78.

". . . accessible to the layperson."
—*Reference and Research Book News, Feb '99*

■

Asthma Sourcebook

Basic Consumer Health Information about Asthma, Including Symptoms, Traditional and Nontraditional Remedies, Treatment Advances, Quality-of-Life Aids, Medical Research Updates, and the Role of Allergies, Exercise, Age, the Environment, and Genetics in the Development of Asthma

Along with Statistical Data, a Glossary, and Directories of Support Groups, and Other Resources for Further Information

Edited by Annemarie S. Muth. 628 pages. 2000. 0-7808-0381-7. $78.

"Highly recommended." —*The Bookwatch, Jan '01*

■

Back & Neck Disorders Sourcebook

Basic Information about Disorders and Injuries of the Spinal Cord and Vertebrae, Including Facts on Chiropractic Treatment, Surgical Interventions, Paralysis, and Rehabilitation

Along with Advice for Preventing Back Trouble

Edited by Karen Bellenir. 548 pages. 1997. 0-7808-0202-0. $78.

"The strength of this work is its basic, easy-to-read format. Recommended."
—*Reference and User Services Quarterly, American Library Association, Winter '97*

■

Blood & Circulatory Disorders Sourcebook

Basic Information about Blood and Its Components, Anemias, Leukemias, Bleeding Disorders, and Circulatory Disorders, Including Aplastic Anemia, Thalassemia, Sickle-Cell Disease, Hemochromatosis, Hemophilia, Von Willebrand Disease, and Vascular Diseases

Along with a Special Section on Blood Transfusions and Blood Supply Safety, a Glossary, and Source Listings for Further Help and Information

Edited by Karen Bellenir and Linda M. Shin. 554 pages. 1998. 0-7808-0203-9. $78.

"Recommended reference source."
—Booklist, American Library Association, Feb '99

"An important reference sourcebook written in simple language for everyday, non-technical users. "
— Reviewer's Bookwatch, Jan '99

■

Brain Disorders Sourcebook

Basic Consumer Health Information about Strokes, Epilepsy, Amyotrophic Lateral Sclerosis (ALS/Lou Gehrig's Disease), Parkinson's Disease, Brain Tumors, Cerebral Palsy, Headache, Tourette Syndrome, and More

Along with Statistical Data, Treatment and Rehabilitation Options, Coping Strategies, Reports on Current Research Initiatives, a Glossary, and Resource Listings for Additional Help and Information

Edited by Karen Bellenir. 481 pages. 1999. 0-7808-0229-2. $78.

"Belongs on the shelves of any library with a consumer health collection." *— E-Streams, Mar '00*

"Recommended reference source."
— Booklist, American Library Association, Oct '99

SEE ALSO *Alzheimer's, Stroke & 29 Other Neurological Disorders Sourcebook, 1st Edition*

■

Breast Cancer Sourcebook

Basic Consumer Health Information about Breast Cancer, Including Diagnostic Methods, Treatment Options, Alternative Therapies, Self-Help Information, Related Health Concerns, Statistical and Demographic Data, and Facts for Men with Breast Cancer

Along with Reports on Current Research Initiatives, a Glossary of Related Medical Terms, and a Directory of Sources for Further Help and Information

Edited by Edward J. Prucha and Karen Bellenir. 600 pages. 2001. 0-7808-0244-6. $78.

SEE ALSO *Cancer Sourcebook for Women, 1st and 2nd Editions, Women's Health Concerns Sourcebook*

■

Burns Sourcebook

Basic Consumer Health Information about Various Types of Burns and Scalds, Including Flame, Heat, Cold, Electrical, Chemical, and Sun Burns

Along with Information on Short-Term and Long-Term Treatments, Tissue Reconstruction, Plastic Surgery, Prevention Suggestions, and First Aid

Edited by Allan R. Cook. 604 pages. 1999. 0-7808-0204-7. $78.

"This key reference guide is an invaluable addition to all health care and public libraries in confronting this ongoing health issue."
—American Reference Books Annual, 2000

"This is an exceptional addition to the series and is highly recommended for all consumer health collections, hospital libraries, and academic medical centers." *—E-Streams, Mar '00*

"Recommended reference source."
—Booklist, American Library Association, Dec '99

SEE ALSO *Skin Disorders Sourcebook*

■

Cancer Sourcebook, 1st Edition

Basic Information on Cancer Types, Symptoms, Diagnostic Methods, and Treatments, Including Statistics on Cancer Occurrences Worldwide and the Risks Associated with Known Carcinogens and Activities

Edited by Frank E. Bair. 932 pages. 1990. 1-55888-888-8. $78.

Cited in *Reference Sources for Small and Medium-Sized Libraries, American Library Association, 1999*

"Written in nontechnical language. Useful for patients, their families, medical professionals, and librarians."
—Guide to Reference Books, 1996

"Designed with the non-medical professional in mind. Libraries and medical facilities interested in patient education should certainly consider adding the *Cancer Sourcebook* **to their holdings. This compact collection of reliable information . . . is an invaluable tool for helping patients and patients' families and friends to take the first steps in coping with the many difficulties of cancer."**
—Medical Reference Services Quarterly, Winter '91

"Specifically created for the nontechnical reader . . . an important resource for the general reader trying to understand the complexities of cancer."
—American Reference Books Annual, 1991

"This publication's nontechnical nature and very comprehensive format make it useful for both the general public and undergraduate students."
—Choice, Association of College and Research Libraries, Oct '90

■

New Cancer Sourcebook, 2nd Edition

Basic Information about Major Forms and Stages of Cancer, Featuring Facts about Primary and Secondary Tumors of the Respiratory, Nervous, Lymphatic, Circulatory, Skeletal, and Gastrointestinal Systems, and Specific Organs; Statistical and Demographic Data; Treatment Options; and Strategies for Coping

Edited by Allan R. Cook. 1,313 pages. 1996. 0-7808-0041-9. $78.

"An excellent resource for patients with newly diagnosed cancer and their families. The dialogue is simple, direct, and comprehensive. Highly recommended for patients and families to aid in their understanding of cancer and its treatment."
—Booklist Health Sciences Supplement, American Library Association, Oct '97

"The amount of factual and useful information is extensive. The writing is very clear, geared to general readers. Recommended for all levels."
— *Choice, Association of College and Research Libraries, Jan '97*

Cancer Sourcebook, 3rd Edition

Basic Consumer Health Information about Major Forms and Stages of Cancer, Featuring Facts about Primary and Secondary Tumors of the Respiratory, Nervous, Lymphatic, Circulatory, Skeletal, and Gastrointestinal Systems, and Specific Organs

Along with Statistical and Demographic Data, Treatment Options, Strategies for Coping, a Glossary, and a Directory of Sources for Additional Help and Information

Edited by Edward J. Prucha. 1,069 pages. 2000. 0-7808-0227-6. $78.

"Recommended reference source."
— *Booklist, American Library Association, Dec '00*

Cancer Sourcebook for Women, 1st Edition

Basic Information about Specific Forms of Cancer That Affect Women, Featuring Facts about Breast Cancer, Cervical Cancer, Ovarian Cancer, Cancer of the Uterus and Uterine Sarcoma, Cancer of the Vagina, and Cancer of the Vulva; Statistical and Demographic Data; Treatments, Self-Help Management Suggestions, and Current Research Initiatives

Edited by Allan R. Cook and Peter D. Dresser. 524 pages. 1996. 0-7808-0076-1. $78.

". . . written in easily understandable, non-technical language. Recommended for public libraries or hospital and academic libraries that collect patient education or consumer health materials."
— *Medical Reference Services Quarterly, Spring '97*

"Would be of value in a consumer health library. . . . written with the health care consumer in mind. Medical jargon is at a minimum, and medical terms are explained in clear, understandable sentences."
— *Bulletin of the Medical Library Association, Oct '96*

"The availability under one cover of all these pertinent publications, grouped under cohesive headings, makes this certainly a most useful sourcebook."
— *Choice, Association of College and Research Libraries, Jun '96*

"Presents a comprehensive knowledge base for general readers. Men and women both benefit from the gold mine of information nestled between the two covers of this book. Recommended."
— *Academic Library Book Review, Summer '96*

"This timely book is highly recommended for consumer health and patient education collections in all libraries." — *Library Journal, Apr '96*

SEE ALSO *Breast Cancer Sourcebook, Women's Health Concerns Sourcebook*

Cancer Sourcebook for Women, 2nd Edition

Basic Consumer Health Information about Specific Forms of Cancer That Affect Women, Including Cervical Cancer, Ovarian Cancer, Endometrial Cancer, Uterine Sarcoma, Vaginal Cancer, Vulvar Cancer, and Gestational Trophoblastic Tumor; and Featuring Statistical Information, Facts about Tests and Treatments, a Glossary of Cancer Terms, and an Extensive List of Additional Resources

Edited by Karen Bellenir. 600 pages. 2001. 0-7808-0226-8. $78.

SEE ALSO *Breast Cancer Sourcebook, Women's Health Concerns Sourcebook*

Cardiovascular Diseases & Disorders Sourcebook, 1st Edition

Basic Information about Cardiovascular Diseases and Disorders, Featuring Facts about the Cardiovascular System, Demographic and Statistical Data, Descriptions of Pharmacological and Surgical Interventions, Lifestyle Modifications, and a Special Section Focusing on Heart Disorders in Children

Edited by Karen Bellenir and Peter D. Dresser. 683 pages. 1995. 0-7808-0032-X. $78.

". . . comprehensive format provides an extensive overview on this subject."
— *Choice, Association of College and Research Libraries, Jun '96*

". . . an easily understood, complete, up-to-date resource. This well executed public health tool will make valuable information available to those that need it most, patients and their families. The typeface, sturdy non-reflective paper, and library binding add a feel of quality found wanting in other publications. Highly recommended for academic and general libraries. "
— *Academic Library Book Review, Summer '96*

SEE ALSO *Healthy Heart Sourcebook for Women, Heart Diseases & Disorders Sourcebook, 2nd Edition*

Caregiving Sourcebook

Basic Consumer Health Information for Caregivers, Including a Profile of Caregivers, Caregiving Responsibilities, Tips for Specific Conditions, Care Environments, and the Effects of Caregiving

Along with Legal Issues, Financial Concerns, Future Planning, a Glossary, and a Listing of Additional Resources

Edited by Joyce Brennfleck Shannon. 550 pages. 2001. 0-7808-0331-0. $78.

Colds, Flu & Other Common Ailments Sourcebook

Basic Consumer Health Information about Common Ailments and Injuries, Including Colds, Coughs, the Flu, Sinus Problems, Headaches, Fever, Nausea and Vomiting, Menstrual Cramps, Diarrhea, Constipation, Hemorrhoids, Back Pain, Dandruff, Dry and Itchy Skin, Cuts, Scrapes, Sprains, Bruises, and More

Along with Information about Prevention, Self-Care, Choosing a Doctor, Over-the-Counter Medications, Folk Remedies, and Alternative Therapies, and Including a Glossary of Important Terms and a Directory of Resources for Further Help and Information

Edited by Chad T. Kimball. 600 pages. 2001. 0-7808-0435-X. $78.

■

Communication Disorders Sourcebook

Basic Information about Deafness and Hearing Loss, Speech and Language Disorders, Voice Disorders, Balance and Vestibular Disorders, and Disorders of Smell, Taste, and Touch

Edited by Linda M. Ross. 533 pages. 1996. 0-7808-0077-X. $78.

"This is skillfully edited and is a welcome resource for the layperson. It should be found in every public and medical library." *— Booklist Health Sciences Supplement, American Library Association, Oct '97*

■

Congenital Disorders Sourcebook

Basic Information about Disorders Acquired during Gestation, Including Spina Bifida, Hydrocephalus, Cerebral Palsy, Heart Defects, Craniofacial Abnormalities, Fetal Alcohol Syndrome, and More

Along with Current Treatment Options and Statistical Data

Edited by Karen Bellenir. 607 pages. 1997. 0-7808-0205-5. $78.

"Recommended reference source." *— Booklist, American Library Association, Oct '97*

SEE ALSO *Pregnancy & Birth Sourcebook*

■

Consumer Issues in Health Care Sourcebook

Basic Information about Health Care Fundamentals and Related Consumer Issues, Including Exams and Screening Tests, Physician Specialties, Choosing a Doctor, Using Prescription and Over-the-Counter Medications Safely, Avoiding Health Scams, Managing Common Health Risks in the Home, Care Options for Chronically or Terminally Ill Patients, and a List of Resources for Obtaining Help and Further Information

Edited by Karen Bellenir. 618 pages. 1998. 0-7808-0221-7. $78.

"Both public and academic libraries will want to have a copy in their collection for readers who are interested in self-education on health issues." *—American Reference Books Annual, 2000*

"The editor has researched the literature from government agencies and others, saving readers the time and effort of having to do the research themselves. Recommended for public libraries." *— Reference and User Services Quarterly, American Library Association, Spring '99*

"Recommended reference source." *— Booklist, American Library Association, Dec '98*

■

Contagious & Non-Contagious Infectious Diseases Sourcebook

Basic Information about Contagious Diseases like Measles, Polio, Hepatitis B, and Infectious Mononucleosis, and Non-Contagious Infectious Diseases like Tetanus and Toxic Shock Syndrome, and Diseases Occurring as Secondary Infections Such as Shingles and Reye Syndrome

Along with Vaccination, Prevention, and Treatment Information, and a Section Describing Emerging Infectious Disease Threats

Edited by Karen Bellenir and Peter D. Dresser. 566 pages. 1996. 0-7808-0075-3. $78.

■

Death & Dying Sourcebook

Basic Consumer Health Information for the Layperson about End-of-Life Care and Related Ethical and Legal Issues, Including Chief Causes of Death, Autopsies, Pain Management for the Terminally Ill, Life Support Systems, Insurance, Euthanasia, Assisted Suicide, Hospice Programs, Living Wills, Funeral Planning, Counseling, Mourning, Organ Donation, and Physician Training

Along with Statistical Data, a Glossary, and Listings of Sources for Further Help and Information

Edited by Annemarie S. Muth. 641 pages. 1999. 0-7808-0230-6. $78.

"Recommended reference source." *—Booklist, American Library Association, Aug '00*

"This book is a definite must for all those involved in end-of-life care." *— Doody's Review Service, 2000*

■

Diabetes Sourcebook, 1st Edition

Basic Information about Insulin-Dependent and Non-insulin-Dependent Diabetes Mellitus, Gestational Diabetes, and Diabetic Complications, Symptoms, Treatment, and Research Results, Including Statistics on Prevalence, Morbidity, and Mortality

Along with Source Listings for Further Help and Information

Edited by Karen Bellenir and Peter D. Dresser. 827 pages. 1994. 1-55888-751-2. $78.

". . . very informative and understandable for the layperson without being simplistic. It provides a comprehensive overview for laypersons who want a general understanding of the disease or who want to focus on various aspects of the disease."
— *Bulletin of the Medical Library Association, Jan '96*

■

Diabetes Sourcebook, 2nd Edition

Basic Consumer Health Information about Type 1 Diabetes (Insulin-Dependent or Juvenile-Onset Diabetes), Type 2 (Noninsulin-Dependent or Adult-Onset Diabetes), Gestational Diabetes, and Related Disorders, Including Diabetes Prevalence Data, Management Issues, the Role of Diet and Exercise in Controlling Diabetes, Insulin and Other Diabetes Medicines, and Complications of Diabetes Such as Eye Diseases, Periodontal Disease, Amputation, and End-Stage Renal Disease

Along with Reports on Current Research Initiatives, a Glossary, and Resource Listings for Further Help and Information

Edited by Karen Bellenir. 688 pages. 1998. 0-7808-0224-1. $78.

"This comprehensive book is an excellent addition for high school, academic, medical, and public libraries. This volume is highly recommended."
— *American Reference Books Annual, 2000*

"An invaluable reference." — *Library Journal, May '00*

Selected as one of the 250 "Best Health Sciences Books of 1999." — *Doody's Rating Service, Mar-Apr 2000*

"Recommended reference source."
— *Booklist, American Library Association, Feb '99*

". . . provides reliable mainstream medical information . . . belongs on the shelves of any library with a consumer health collection." — *E-Streams, Sep '99*

"Provides useful information for the general public."
— *Healthlines, University of Michigan Health Management Research Center, Sep/Oct '99*

■

Diet & Nutrition Sourcebook, 1st Edition

Basic Information about Nutrition, Including the Dietary Guidelines for Americans, the Food Guide Pyramid, and Their Applications in Daily Diet, Nutritional Advice for Specific Age Groups, Current Nutritional Issues and Controversies, the New Food Label and How to Use It to Promote Healthy Eating, and Recent Developments in Nutritional Research

Edited by Dan R. Harris. 662 pages. 1996. 0-7808-0084-2. $78.

"Useful reference as a food and nutrition sourcebook for the general consumer." — *Booklist Health Sciences Supplement, American Library Association, Oct '97*

"Recommended for public libraries and medical libraries that receive general information requests on nutrition. It is readable and will appeal to those interested in learning more about healthy dietary practices."
— *Medical Reference Services Quarterly, Fall '97*

"An abundance of medical and social statistics is translated into readable information geared toward the general reader." — *Bookwatch, Mar '97*

"With dozens of questionable diet books on the market, it is so refreshing to find a reliable and factual reference book. Recommended to aspiring professionals, librarians, and others seeking and giving reliable dietary advice. An excellent compilation." — *Choice, Association of College and Research Libraries, Feb '97*

SEE ALSO *Digestive Diseases & Disorders Sourcebook, Gastrointestinal Diseases & Disorders Sourcebook*

■

Diet & Nutrition Sourcebook, 2nd Edition

Basic Consumer Health Information about Dietary Guidelines, Recommended Daily Intake Values, Vitamins, Minerals, Fiber, Fat, Weight Control, Dietary Supplements, and Food Additives

Along with Special Sections on Nutrition Needs throughout Life and Nutrition for People with Such Specific Medical Concerns as Allergies, High Blood Cholesterol, Hypertension, Diabetes, Celiac Disease, Seizure Disorders, Phenylketonuria (PKU), Cancer, and Eating Disorders, and Including Reports on Current Nutrition Research and Source Listings for Additional Help and Information

Edited by Karen Bellenir. 650 pages. 1999. 0-7808-0228-4. $78.

"This book is an excellent source of basic diet and nutrition information." — *Booklist Health Sciences Supplement, American Library Association, Dec '00*

"This reference document should be in any public library, but it would be a very good guide for beginning students in the health sciences. If the other books in this publisher's series are as good as this, they should all be in the health sciences collections."
— *American Reference Books Annual, 2000*

"This book is an excellent general nutrition reference for consumers who desire to take an active role in their health care for prevention. Consumers of all ages who select this book can feel confident they are receiving current and accurate information."
— *Journal of Nutrition for the Elderly, Vol. 19, No. 4, '00*

"Recommended reference source."
— *Booklist, American Library Association, Dec '99*

SEE ALSO *Digestive Diseases & Disorders Sourcebook, Gastrointestinal Diseases & Disorders Sourcebook*

■

Digestive Diseases & Disorders Sourcebook

Basic Consumer Health Information about Diseases and Disorders that Impact the Upper and Lower Digestive System, Including Celiac Disease, Constipation, Crohn's Disease, Cyclic Vomiting Syndrome, Diarrhea, Diverticulosis and Diverticulitis, Gallstones, Heart-

510

burn, Hemorrhoids, Hernias, Indigestion (Dyspepsia), Irritable Bowel Syndrome, Lactose Intolerance, Ulcers, and More

Along with Information about Medications and Other Treatments, Tips for Maintaining a Healthy Digestive Tract, a Glossary, and Directory of Digestive Diseases Organizations

Edited by Karen Bellenir. 335 pages. 1999. 0-7808-0327-2. $48.

"This title is recommended for public, hospital, and health sciences libraries with consumer health collections." — E-Streams, Jul-Aug '00

"Recommended reference source." —Booklist, American Library Association, May '00

SEE ALSO Diet & Nutrition Sourcebook, 1st and 2nd Editions, Gastrointestinal Diseases & Disorders Sourcebook

---

Disabilities Sourcebook

Basic Consumer Health Information about Physical and Psychiatric Disabilities, Including Descriptions of Major Causes of Disability, Assistive and Adaptive Aids, Workplace Issues, and Accessibility Concerns

Along with Information about the Americans with Disabilities Act, a Glossary, and Resources for Additional Help and Information

Edited by Dawn D. Matthews. 616 pages. 2000. 0-7808-0389-2. $78.

"An excellent source book in easy-to-read format covering many current topics; highly recommended for all libraries." — Choice, Association of College and Research Libraries, Jan '01

"Recommended reference source." —Booklist, American Library Association, Jul '00

"An involving, invaluable handbook." —The Bookwatch, May '00

Domestic Violence & Child Abuse Sourcebook

Basic Consumer Health Information about Spousal/ Partner, Child, Sibling, Parent, and Elder Abuse, Covering Physical, Emotional, and Sexual Abuse, Teen Dating Violence, and Stalking; Includes Information about Hotlines, Safe Houses, Safety Plans, and Other Resources for Support and Assistance, Community Initiatives, and Reports on Current Directions in Research and Treatment

Along with a Glossary, Sources for Further Reading, and Governmental and Non-Governmental Organizations Contact Information

Edited by Helene Henderson. 1,064 pages. 2000. 0-7808-0235-7. $78.

Drug Abuse Sourcebook

Basic Consumer Health Information about Illicit Substances of Abuse and the Diversion of Prescription Medications, Including Depressants, Hallucinogens, Inhalants, Marijuana, Narcotics, Stimulants, and Anabolic Steroids

Along with Facts about Related Health Risks, Treatment Issues, and Substance Abuse Prevention Programs, a Glossary of Terms, Statistical Data, and Directories of Hotline Services, Self-Help Groups, and Organizations Able to Provide Further Information

Edited by Karen Bellenir. 629 pages. 2000. 0-7808-0242-X. $78.

"Highly recommended." — The Bookwatch, Jan '01

SEE ALSO Alcoholism Sourcebook, Substance Abuse Sourcebook

Ear, Nose & Throat Disorders Sourcebook

Basic Information about Disorders of the Ears, Nose, Sinus Cavities, Pharynx, and Larynx, Including Ear Infections, Tinnitus, Vestibular Disorders, Allergic and Non-Allergic Rhinitis, Sore Throats, Tonsillitis, and Cancers That Affect the Ears, Nose, Sinuses, and Throat

Along with Reports on Current Research Initiatives, a Glossary of Related Medical Terms, and a Directory of Sources for Further Help and Information

Edited by Karen Bellenir and Linda M. Shin. 576 pages. 1998. 0-7808-0206-3. $78.

"Overall, this sourcebook is helpful for the consumer seeking information on ENT issues. It is recommended for public libraries." —American Reference Books Annual, 1999

"Recommended reference source." —Booklist, American Library Association, Dec '98

Endocrine & Metabolic Disorders Sourcebook

Basic Information for the Layperson about Pancreatic and Insulin-Related Disorders Such as Pancreatitis, Diabetes, and Hypoglycemia; Adrenal Gland Disorders Such as Cushing's Syndrome, Addison's Disease, and Congenital Adrenal Hyperplasia; Pituitary Gland Disorders Such as Growth Hormone Deficiency, Acromegaly, and Pituitary Tumors; Thyroid Disorders Such as Hypothyroidism, Graves' Disease, Hashimoto's Disease, and Goiter; Hyperparathyroidism; and Other Diseases and Syndromes of Hormone Imbalance or Metabolic Dysfunction

Along with Reports on Current Research Initiatives

Edited by Linda M. Shin. 574 pages. 1998. 0-7808-0207-1. $78.

"Omnigraphics has produced another needed resource for health information consumers." —American Reference Books Annual, 2000

"Recommended reference source." — Booklist, American Library Association, Dec '98

Environmentally Induced Disorders Sourcebook

Basic Information about Diseases and Syndromes Linked to Exposure to Pollutants and Other Substances in Outdoor and Indoor Environments Such as Lead, Asbestos, Formaldehyde, Mercury, Emissions, Noise, and More

Edited by Allan R. Cook. 620 pages. 1997. 0-7808-0083-4. $78.

"Recommended reference source."
— *Booklist, American Library Association, Sep '98*

"This book will be a useful addition to anyone's library." — *Choice Health Sciences Supplement, Association of College and Research Libraries, May '98*

". . . a good survey of numerous environmentally induced physical disorders . . . a useful addition to anyone's library."
— *Doody's Health Sciences Book Reviews, Jan '98*

". . . provide[s] introductory information from the best authorities around. Since this volume covers topics that potentially affect everyone, it will surely be one of the most frequently consulted volumes in the *Health Reference Series*." — *Rettig on Reference, Nov '97*

∎

Ethnic Diseases Sourcebook

Basic Consumer Health Information for Ethnic and Racial Minority Groups in the United States, Including General Health Indicators and Behaviors, Ethnic Diseases, Genetic Testing, the Impact of Chronic Diseases, Women's Health, Mental Health Issues, and Preventive Health Care Services

Along with a Glossary and a Listing of Additional Resources

Edited by Joyce Brennfleck Shannon. 600 pages. 2001. 0-7808-0336-1. $78.

∎

Family Planning Sourcebook

Basic Consumer Health Information about Planning for Pregnancy and Contraception, Including Traditional Methods, Barrier Methods, Hormonal Methods, Permanent Methods, Future Methods, Emergency Contraception, and Birth Control Choices for Women at Each Stage of Life

Along with Statistics, a Glossary, and Sources of Additional Information

Edited by Amy Marcaccio Keyzer. 520 pages. 2001. 0-7808-0379-5. $78.

SEE ALSO *Pregnancy & Birth Sourcebook*

Fitness & Exercise Sourcebook, 1st Edition

Basic Information on Fitness and Exercise, Including Fitness Activities for Specific Age Groups, Exercise for People with Specific Medical Conditions, How to Begin a Fitness Program in Running, Walking, Swimming, Cycling, and Other Athletic Activities, and Recent Research in Fitness and Exercise

Edited by Dan R. Harris. 663 pages. 1996. 0-7808-0186-5. $78.

"A good resource for general readers."
— *Choice, Association of College and Research Libraries, Nov '97*

"The perennial popularity of the topic . . . make this an appealing selection for public libraries."
— *Rettig on Reference, Jun/Jul '97*

∎

Fitness & Exercise Sourcebook, 2nd Edition

Basic Consumer Health Information about the Fundamentals of Fitness and Exercise, Including How to Begin and Maintain a Fitness Program, Fitness as a Lifestyle, the Link between Fitness and Diet, Advice for Specific Groups of People, Exercise as It Relates to Specific Medical Conditions, and Recent Research in Fitness and Exercise

Along with a Glossary of Important Terms and Resources for Additional Help and Information

Edited by Kristen M. Gledhill. 600 pages. 2001. 0-7808-0334-5. $78.

∎

Food & Animal Borne Diseases Sourcebook

Basic Information about Diseases That Can Be Spread to Humans through the Ingestion of Contaminated Food or Water or by Contact with Infected Animals and Insects, Such as Botulism, E. Coli, Hepatitis A, Trichinosis, Lyme Disease, and Rabies

Along with Information Regarding Prevention and Treatment Methods, and Including a Special Section for International Travelers Describing Diseases Such as Cholera, Malaria, Travelers' Diarrhea, and Yellow Fever, and Offering Recommendations for Avoiding Illness

Edited by Karen Bellenir and Peter D. Dresser. 535 pages. 1995. 0-7808-0033-8. $78.

"Targeting general readers and providing them with a single, comprehensive source of information on selected topics, this book continues, with the excellent caliber of its predecessors, to catalog topical information on health matters of general interest. Readable and thorough, this valuable resource is highly recommended for all libraries."
— *Academic Library Book Review, Summer '96*

"A comprehensive collection of authoritative information." — *Emergency Medical Services, Oct '95*

Food Safety Sourcebook

Basic Consumer Health Information about the Safe Handling of Meat, Poultry, Seafood, Eggs, Fruit Juices, and Other Food Items, and Facts about Pesticides, Drinking Water, Food Safety Overseas, and the Onset, Duration, and Symptoms of Foodborne Illnesses, Including Types of Pathogenic Bacteria, Parasitic Protozoa, Worms, Viruses, and Natural Toxins

Along with the Role of the Consumer, the Food Handler, and the Government in Food Safety; a Glossary, and Resources for Additional Help and Information

Edited by Dawn D. Matthews. 339 pages. 1999. 0-7808-0326-4. $48.

"This book is recommended for public libraries and universities with home economic and food science programs." —*E-Streams, Nov '00*

"This book takes the complex issues of food safety and foodborne pathogens and presents them in an easily understood manner. [It does] an excellent job of covering a large and often confusing topic."
—*American Reference Books Annual, 2000*

"Recommended reference source."
—*Booklist, American Library Association, May '00*

■

Forensic Medicine Sourcebook

Basic Consumer Information for the Layperson about Forensic Medicine, Including Crime Scene Investigation, Evidence Collection and Analysis, Expert Testimony, Computer-Aided Criminal Identification, Digital Imaging in the Courtroom, DNA Profiling, Accident Reconstruction, Autopsies, Ballistics, Drugs and Explosives Detection, Latent Fingerprints, Product Tampering, and Questioned Document Examination

Along with Statistical Data, a Glossary of Forensics Terminology, and Listings of Sources for Further Help and Information

Edited by Annemarie S. Muth. 574 pages. 1999. 0-7808-0232-2. $78.

"There are several items that make this book attractive to consumers who are seeking certain forensic data. . . . This is a useful current source for those seeking general forensic medical answers."
—*American Reference Books Annual, 2000*

"Recommended for public libraries."
—*Reference & User Services Quarterly, American Library Association, Spring 2000*

"Recommended reference source."
—*Booklist, American Library Association, Feb '00*

"A wealth of information, useful statistics, references are up-to-date and extremely complete. This wonderful collection of data will help students who are interested in a career in any type of forensic field. It is a great resource for attorneys who need information about types of expert witnesses needed in a particular case. It also offers useful information for fiction and nonfiction writers whose work involves a crime. A fascinating compilation. All levels." —*Choice, Association of College and Research Libraries, Jan 2000*

Gastrointestinal Diseases & Disorders Sourcebook

Basic Information about Gastroesophageal Reflux Disease (Heartburn), Ulcers, Diverticulosis, Irritable Bowel Syndrome, Crohn's Disease, Ulcerative Colitis, Diarrhea, Constipation, Lactose Intolerance, Hemorrhoids, Hepatitis, Cirrhosis, and Other Digestive Problems, Featuring Statistics, Descriptions of Symptoms, and Current Treatment Methods of Interest for Persons Living with Upper and Lower Gastrointestinal Maladies

Edited by Linda M. Ross. 413 pages. 1996. 0-7808-0078-8. $78.

". . . very readable form. The successful editorial work that brought this material together into a useful and understandable reference makes accessible to all readers information that can help them more effectively understand and obtain help for digestive tract problems."
—*Choice, Association of College and Research Libraries, Feb '97*

SEE ALSO *Diet & Nutrition Sourcebook, 1st and 2nd Editions, Digestive Diseases & Disorders Sourcebook*

■

Genetic Disorders Sourcebook, 1st Edition

Basic Information about Heritable Diseases and Disorders Such as Down Syndrome, PKU, Hemophilia, Von Willebrand Disease, Gaucher Disease, Tay-Sachs Disease, and Sickle-Cell Disease, Along with Information about Genetic Screening, Gene Therapy, Home Care, and Including Source Listings for Further Help and Information on More Than 300 Disorders

Edited by Karen Bellenir. 642 pages. 1996. 0-7808-0034-6. $78.

"Recommended for undergraduate libraries or libraries that serve the public."
—*Science & Technology Libraries, Vol. 18, No. 1, '99*

"Provides essential medical information to both the general public and those diagnosed with a serious or fatal genetic disease or disorder."
—*Choice, Association of College and Research Libraries, Jan '97*

"Geared toward the lay public. It would be well placed in all public libraries and in those hospital and medical libraries in which access to genetic references is limited." —*Doody's Health Sciences Book Review, Oct '96*

■

Genetic Disorders Sourcebook, 2nd Edition

Basic Consumer Health Information about Hereditary Diseases and Disorders, Including Cystic Fibrosis, Down Syndrome, Hemophilia, Huntington's Disease, Sickle Cell Anemia, and More; Facts about Genes, Gene Research and Therapy, Genetic Screening, Ethics of Gene Testing, Genetic Counseling, and Advice on Coping and Caring

Along with a Glossary of Genetic Terminology and a Resource List for Help, Support, and Further Information

Edited by Kathy Massimini. 768 pages. 2001. 0-7808-0241-1. $78.

■

Head Trauma Sourcebook

Basic Information for the Layperson about Open-Head and Closed-Head Injuries, Treatment Advances, Recovery, and Rehabilitation

Along with Reports on Current Research Initiatives

Edited by Karen Bellenir. 414 pages. 1997. 0-7808-0208-X. $78.

■

Health Insurance Sourcebook

Basic Information about Managed Care Organizations, Traditional Fee-for-Service Insurance, Insurance Portability and Pre-Existing Conditions Clauses, Medicare, Medicaid, Social Security, and Military Health Care

Along with Information about Insurance Fraud

Edited by Wendy Wilcox. 530 pages. 1997. 0-7808-0222-5. $78.

"Particularly useful because it brings much of this information together in one volume. This book will be a handy reference source in the health sciences library, hospital library, college and university library, and medium to large public library."
— Medical Reference Services Quarterly, Fall '98

Awarded "Books of the Year Award"
— American Journal of Nursing, 1997

"The layout of the book is particularly helpful as it provides easy access to reference material. A most useful addition to the vast amount of information about health insurance. The use of data from U.S. government agencies is most commendable. Useful in a library or learning center for healthcare professional students."
— Doody's Health Sciences Book Reviews, Nov '97

■

Healthy Aging Sourcebook

Basic Consumer Health Information about Maintaining Health through the Aging Process, Including Advice on Nutrition, Exercise, and Sleep, Help in Making Decisions about Midlife Issues and Retirement, and Guidance Concerning Practical and Informed Choices in Health Consumerism

Along with Data Concerning the Theories of Aging, Different Experiences in Aging by Minority Groups, and Facts about Aging Now and Aging in the Future; and Featuring a Glossary, a Guide to Consumer Help, Additional Suggested Reading, and Practical Resource Directory

Edited by Jenifer Swanson. 536 pages. 1999. 0-7808-0390-6. $78.

"Recommended reference source."
—Booklist, American Library Association, Feb '00

SEE ALSO *Physical & Mental Issues in Aging Sourcebook*

Healthy Heart Sourcebook for Women

Basic Consumer Health Information about Cardiac Issues Specific to Women, Including Facts about Major Risk Factors and Prevention, Treatment and Control Strategies, and Important Dietary Issues

Along with a Special Section Regarding the Pros and Cons of Hormone Replacement Therapy and Its Impact on Heart Health, and Additional Help, Including Recipes, a Glossary, and a Directory of Resources

Edited by Dawn D. Matthews. 336 pages. 2000. 0-7808-0329-9. $48.

"Contains very important information about coronary artery disease that all women should know. The information is current and presented in an easy-to-read format. The book will make a good addition to any library."
— American Medical Writers Association Journal, Summer '00

"Important, basic reference."
—Reviewer's Bookwatch, Jul '00

SEE ALSO *Cardiovascular Diseases & Disorders Sourcebook, 1st Edition, Heart Diseases & Disorders Sourcebook, 2nd Edition, Women's Health Concerns Sourcebook*

■

Heart Diseases & Disorders Sourcebook, 2nd Edition

Basic Consumer Health Information about Heart Attacks, Angina, Rhythm Disorders, Heart Failure, Valve Disease, Congenital Heart Disorders, and More, Including Descriptions of Surgical Procedures and Other Interventions, Medications, Cardiac Rehabilitation, Risk Identification, and Prevention Tips

Along with Statistical Data, Reports on Current Research Initiatives, a Glossary of Cardiovascular Terms, and Resource Directory

Edited by Karen Bellenir. 612 pages. 2000. 0-7808-0238-1. $78.

"Recommended reference source."
—Booklist, American Library Association, Dec '00

"Provides comprehensive coverage of matters related to the heart. This title is recommended for health sciences and public libraries with consumer health collections."
— E-Streams, Oct '00

SEE ALSO *Cardiovascular Diseases & Disorders Sourcebook, 1st Edition, Healthy Heart Sourcebook for Women*

■

Immune System Disorders Sourcebook

Basic Information about Lupus, Multiple Sclerosis, Guillain-Barré Syndrome, Chronic Granulomatous Disease, and More

Along with Statistical and Demographic Data and Reports on Current Research Initiatives

Edited by Allan R. Cook. 608 pages. 1997. 0-7808-0209-8. $78.

Infant & Toddler Health Sourcebook

Basic Consumer Health Information about the Physical and Mental Development of Newborns, Infants, and Toddlers, Including Neonatal Concerns, Nutrition Recommendations, Immunization Schedules, Common Pediatric Disorders, Assessments and Milestones, Safety Tips, and Advice for Parents and Other Caregivers

Along with a Glossary of Terms and Resource Listings for Additional Help

Edited by Jenifer Swanson. 585 pages. 2000. 0-7808-0246-2. $78.

■

Kidney & Urinary Tract Diseases & Disorders Sourcebook

Basic Information about Kidney Stones, Urinary Incontinence, Bladder Disease, End Stage Renal Disease, Dialysis, and More

Along with Statistical and Demographic Data and Reports on Current Research Initiatives

Edited by Linda M. Ross. 602 pages. 1997. 0-7808-0079-6. $78.

■

Learning Disabilities Sourcebook

Basic Information about Disorders Such as Dyslexia, Visual and Auditory Processing Deficits, Attention Deficit/Hyperactivity Disorder, and Autism

Along with Statistical and Demographic Data, Reports on Current Research Initiatives, an Explanation of the Assessment Process, and a Special Section for Adults with Learning Disabilities

Edited by Linda M. Shin. 579 pages. 1998. 0-7808-0210-1. $78.

Named "Outstanding Reference Book of 1999."
— *New York Public Library, Feb 2000*

"An excellent candidate for inclusion in a public library reference section. It's a great source of information. Teachers will also find the book useful. Definitely worth reading."
— *Journal of Adolescent & Adult Literacy, Feb 2000*

"Readable . . . provides a solid base of information regarding successful techniques used with individuals who have learning disabilities, as well as practical suggestions for educators and family members. Clear language, concise descriptions, and pertinent information for contacting multiple resources add to the strength of this book as a useful tool."
— *Choice, Association of College and Research Libraries, Feb '99*

"Recommended reference source."
— *Booklist, American Library Association, Sep '98*

"This is a useful resource for libraries and for those who don't have the time to identify and locate the individual publications."
— *Disability Resources Monthly, Sep '98*

Liver Disorders Sourcebook

Basic Consumer Health Information about the Liver and How It Works; Liver Diseases, Including Cancer, Cirrhosis, Hepatitis, and Toxic and Drug Related Diseases; Tips for Maintaining a Healthy Liver; Laboratory Tests, Radiology Tests, and Facts about Liver Transplantation

Along with a Section on Support Groups, a Glossary, and Resource Listings

Edited by Joyce Brennfleck Shannon. 591 pages. 2000. 0-7808-0383-3. $78.

"This title is recommended for health sciences and public libraries with consumer health collections."
— *E-Streams, Oct '00*

"Recommended reference source."
— *Booklist, American Library Association, Jun '00*

■

Medical Tests Sourcebook

Basic Consumer Health Information about Medical Tests, Including Periodic Health Exams, General Screening Tests, Tests You Can Do at Home, Findings of the U.S. Preventive Services Task Force, X-ray and Radiology Tests, Electrical Tests, Tests of Blood and Other Body Fluids and Tissues, Scope Tests, Lung Tests, Genetic Tests, Pregnancy Tests, Newborn Screening Tests, Sexually Transmitted Disease Tests, and Computer Aided Diagnoses

Along with a Section on Paying for Medical Tests, a Glossary, and Resource Listings

Edited by Joyce Brennfleck Shannon. 691 pages. 1999. 0-7808-0243-8. $78.

"A valuable reference guide."
— *American Reference Books Annual, 2000*

"Recommended for hospital and health sciences libraries with consumer health collections."
— *E-Streams, Mar '00*

"This is an overall excellent reference with a wealth of general knowledge that may aid those who are reluctant to get vital tests performed."
— *Today's Librarian, Jan 2000*

■

Men's Health Concerns Sourcebook

Basic Information about Health Issues That Affect Men, Featuring Facts about the Top Causes of Death in Men, Including Heart Disease, Stroke, Cancers, Prostate Disorders, Chronic Obstructive Pulmonary Disease, Pneumonia and Influenza, Human Immunodeficiency Virus and Acquired Immune Deficiency Syndrome, Diabetes Mellitus, Stress, Suicide, Accidents and Homicides; and Facts about Common Concerns for Men, Including Impotence, Contraception, Circumcision, Sleep Disorders, Snoring, Hair Loss, Diet, Nutrition, Exercise, Kidney and Urological Disorders, and Backaches

Edited by Allan R. Cook. 738 pages. 1998. 0-7808-0212-8. $78.

■

Mental Health Disorders Sourcebook, 1st Edition

Basic Information about Schizophrenia, Depression, Bipolar Disorder, Panic Disorder, Obsessive-Compulsive Disorder, Phobias and Other Anxiety Disorders, Paranoia and Other Personality Disorders, Eating Disorders, and Sleep Disorders

Along with Information about Treatment and Therapies

Edited by Karen Bellenir. 548 pages. 1995. 0-7808-0040-0. $78.

■

Mental Health Disorders Sourcebook, 2nd Edition

Basic Consumer Health Information about Anxiety Disorders, Depression and Other Mood Disorders, Eating Disorders, Personality Disorders, Schizophrenia, and More, Including Disease Descriptions, Treatment Options, and Reports on Current Research Initiatives

Along with Statistical Data, Tips for Maintaining Mental Health, a Glossary, and Directory of Sources for Additional Help and Information

Edited by Karen Bellenir. 605 pages. 2000. 0-7808-0240-3. $78.

Mental Retardation Sourcebook

Basic Consumer Health Information about Mental Retardation and Its Causes, Including Down Syndrome, Fetal Alcohol Syndrome, Fragile X Syndrome, Genetic Conditions, Injury, and Environmental Sources

Along with Preventive Strategies, Parenting Issues, Educational Implications, Health Care Needs, Employment and Economic Matters, Legal Issues, a Glossary, and a Resource Listing for Additional Help and Information

Edited by Joyce Brennfleck Shannon. 642 pages. 2000. 0-7808-0377-9. $78.

■

Obesity Sourcebook

Basic Consumer Health Information about Diseases and Other Problems Associated with Obesity, and Including Facts about Risk Factors, Prevention Issues, and Management Approaches

Along with Statistical and Demographic Data, Information about Special Populations, Research Updates, a Glossary, and Source Listings for Further Help and Information

Edited by Wilma Caldwell and Chad T. Kimball. 376 pages. 2001. 0-7808-0333-7. $48.

■

Ophthalmic Disorders Sourcebook

Basic Information about Glaucoma, Cataracts, Macular Degeneration, Strabismus, Refractive Disorders, and More

Along with Statistical and Demographic Data and Reports on Current Research Initiatives

Edited by Linda M. Ross. 631 pages. 1996. 0-7808-0081-8. $78.

■

Oral Health Sourcebook

Basic Information about Diseases and Conditions Affecting Oral Health, Including Cavities, Gum Disease, Dry Mouth, Oral Cancers, Fever Blisters, Canker Sores, Oral Thrush, Bad Breath, Temporomandibular Disorders, and other Craniofacial Syndromes

Along with Statistical Data on the Oral Health of Americans, Oral Hygiene, Emergency First Aid, Information on Treatment Procedures and Methods of Replacing Lost Teeth

Edited by Allan R. Cook. 558 pages. 1997. 0-7808-0082-6. $78.

"Unique source which will fill a gap in dental sources for patients and the lay public. A valuable reference tool even in a library with thousands of books on dentistry. Comprehensive, clear, inexpensive, and easy to read and use. It fills an enormous gap in the health care literature." — *Reference and User Services Quarterly, American Library Association, Summer '98*

"Recommended reference source."
— *Booklist, American Library Association, Dec '97*

■

Osteoporosis Sourcebook

Basic Consumer Health Information about Primary and Secondary Osteoporosis and Juvenile Osteoporosis and Related Conditions, Including Fibrous Dysplasia, Gaucher Disease, Hyperthyroidism, Hypophosphatasia, Myeloma, Osteopetrosis, Osteogenesis Imperfecta, and Paget's Disease

Along with Information about Risk Factors, Treatments, Traditional and Non-Traditional Pain Management, a Glossary of Related Terms, and a Directory of Resources

Edited by Allan R. Cook. 584 pages. 2001. 0-7808-0239-X. $78.

SEE ALSO *Women's Health Concerns Sourcebook*

■

Pain Sourcebook

Basic Information about Specific Forms of Acute and Chronic Pain, Including Headaches, Back Pain, Muscular Pain, Neuralgia, Surgical Pain, and Cancer Pain

Along with Pain Relief Options Such as Analgesics, Narcotics, Nerve Blocks, Transcutaneous Nerve Stimulation, and Alternative Forms of Pain Control, Including Biofeedback, Imaging, Behavior Modification, and Relaxation Techniques

Edited by Allan R. Cook. 667 pages. 1997. 0-7808-0213-6. $78.

"The text is readable, easily understood, and well indexed. This excellent volume belongs in all patient education libraries, consumer health sections of public libraries, and many personal collections."
— *American Reference Books Annual, 1999*

"A beneficial reference." — *Booklist Health Sciences Supplement, American Library Association, Oct '98*

"The information is basic in terms of scholarship and is appropriate for general readers. Written in journalistic style ... intended for non-professionals. Quite thorough in its coverage of different pain conditions and summarizes the latest clinical information regarding pain treatment." — *Choice, Association of College and Research Libraries, Jun '98*

"Recommended reference source."
— *Booklist, American Library Association, Mar '98*

Pediatric Cancer Sourcebook

Basic Consumer Health Information about Leukemias, Brain Tumors, Sarcomas, Lymphomas, and Other Cancers in Infants, Children, and Adolescents, Including Descriptions of Cancers, Treatments, and Coping Strategies

Along with Suggestions for Parents, Caregivers, and Concerned Relatives, a Glossary of Cancer Terms, and Resource Listings

Edited by Edward J. Prucha. 587 pages. 1999. 0-7808-0245-4. $78.

"A valuable addition to all libraries specializing in health services and many public libraries."
— *American Reference Books Annual, 2000*

"Recommended reference source."
— *Booklist, American Library Association, Feb '00*

"An excellent source of information. Recommended for public, hospital, and health science libraries with consumer health collections." — *E-Streams, Jun '00*

■

Physical & Mental Issues in Aging Sourcebook

Basic Consumer Health Information on Physical and Mental Disorders Associated with the Aging Process, Including Concerns about Cardiovascular Disease, Pulmonary Disease, Oral Health, Digestive Disorders, Musculoskeletal and Skin Disorders, Metabolic Changes, Sexual and Reproductive Issues, and Changes in Vision, Hearing, and Other Senses

Along with Data about Longevity and Causes of Death, Information on Acute and Chronic Pain, Descriptions of Mental Concerns, a Glossary of Terms, and Resource Listings for Additional Help

Edited by Jenifer Swanson. 660 pages. 1999. 0-7808-0233-0. $78.

"Recommended for public libraries."
— *American Reference Books Annual, 2000*

"This is a treasure of health information for the layperson." — *Choice Health Sciences Supplement, Association of College & Research Libraries, May 2000*

"Recommended reference source."
— *Booklist, American Library Association, Oct '99*

SEE ALSO *Healthy Aging Sourcebook*

■

Podiatry Sourcebook

Basic Consumer Health Information about Foot Conditions, Diseases, and Injuries, Including Bunions, Corns, Calluses, Athlete's Foot, Plantar Warts, Hammertoes and Clawtoes, Club Foot, Heel Pain, Gout, and More

Along with Facts about Foot Care, Disease Prevention, Foot Safety, Choosing a Foot Care Specialist, a Glossary of Terms, and Resource Listings for Additional Information

Edited by M. Lisa Weatherford. 600 pages. 2001. 0-7808-0215-2. $78.

517

Pregnancy & Birth Sourcebook

Basic Information about Planning for Pregnancy, Maternal Health, Fetal Growth and Development, Labor and Delivery, Postpartum and Perinatal Care, Pregnancy in Mothers with Special Concerns, and Disorders of Pregnancy, Including Genetic Counseling, Nutrition and Exercise, Obstetrical Tests, Pregnancy Discomfort, Multiple Births, Cesarean Sections, Medical Testing of Newborns, Breastfeeding, Gestational Diabetes, and Ectopic Pregnancy

Edited by Heather E. Aldred. 737 pages. 1997. 0-7808-0216-0. $78.

"A well-organized handbook. Recommended."
— *Choice, Association of College and Research Libraries, Apr '98*

"Recommended reference source."
— *Booklist, American Library Association, Mar '98*

"Recommended for public libraries."
— *American Reference Books Annual, 1998*

SEE ALSO *Congenital Disorders Sourcebook, Family Planning Sourcebook*

■

Public Health Sourcebook

Basic Information about Government Health Agencies, Including National Health Statistics and Trends, Healthy People 2000 Program Goals and Objectives, the Centers for Disease Control and Prevention, the Food and Drug Administration, and the National Institutes of Health

Along with Full Contact Information for Each Agency

Edited by Wendy Wilcox. 698 pages. 1998. 0-7808-0220-9. $78.

"Recommended reference source."
— *Booklist, American Library Association, Sep '98*

"This consumer guide provides welcome assistance in navigating the maze of federal health agencies and their data on public health concerns."
— *SciTech Book News, Sep '98*

■

Reconstructive & Cosmetic Surgery Sourcebook

Basic Consumer Health Information on Cosmetic and Reconstructive Plastic Surgery, Including Statistical Information about Different Surgical Procedures, Things to Consider Prior to Surgery, Plastic Surgery Techniques and Tools, Emotional and Psychological Considerations, and Procedure-Specific Information

Along with a Glossary of Terms and a Listing of Resources for Additional Help and Information

Edited by M. Lisa Weatherford. 374 pages. 2001. 0-7808-0214-4. $48.

Rehabilitation Sourcebook

Basic Consumer Health Information about Rehabilitation for People Recovering from Heart Surgery, Spinal Cord Injury, Stroke, Orthopedic Impairments, Amputation, Pulmonary Impairments, Traumatic Injury, and More, Including Physical Therapy, Occupational Therapy, Speech/ Language Therapy, Massage Therapy, Dance Therapy, Art Therapy, and Recreational Therapy

Along with Information on Assistive and Adaptive Devices, a Glossary, and Resources for Additional Help and Information

Edited by Dawn D. Matthews. 531 pages. 1999. 0-7808-0236-5. $78.

"Recommended reference source."
— *Booklist, American Library Association, May '00*

■

Respiratory Diseases & Disorders Sourcebook

Basic Information about Respiratory Diseases and Disorders, Including Asthma, Cystic Fibrosis, Pneumonia, the Common Cold, Influenza, and Others, Featuring Facts about the Respiratory System, Statistical and Demographic Data, Treatments, Self-Help Management Suggestions, and Current Research Initiatives

Edited by Allan R. Cook and Peter D. Dresser. 771 pages. 1995. 0-7808-0037-0. $78.

"Designed for the layperson and for patients and their families coping with respiratory illness. . . . an extensive array of information on diagnosis, treatment, management, and prevention of respiratory illnesses for the general reader."
— *Choice, Association of College and Research Libraries, Jun '96*

"A highly recommended text for all collections. It is a comforting reminder of the power of knowledge that good books carry between their covers."
— *Academic Library Book Review, Spring '96*

"A comprehensive collection of authoritative information presented in a nontechnical, humanitarian style for patients, families, and caregivers."
— *Association of Operating Room Nurses, Sep/Oct '95*

■

Sexually Transmitted Diseases Sourcebook, 1st Edition

Basic Information about Herpes, Chlamydia, Gonorrhea, Hepatitis, Nongonoccocal Urethritis, Pelvic Inflammatory Disease, Syphilis, AIDS, and More

Along with Current Data on Treatments and Preventions

Edited by Linda M. Ross. 550 pages. 1997. 0-7808-0217-9. $78.

Sexually Transmitted Diseases Sourcebook, 2nd Edition

Basic Consumer Health Information about Sexually Transmitted Diseases, Including Information on the Diagnosis and Treatment of Chlamydia, Gonorrhea, Hepatitis, Herpes, HIV, Mononucleosis, Syphilis, and Others

Along with Information on Prevention, Such as Condom Use, Vaccines, and STD Education; And Featuring a Section on Issues Related to Youth and Adolescents, a Glossary, and Resources for Additional Help and Information

Edited by Dawn D. Matthews. 538 pages. 2001. 0-7808-0249-7. $78.

Skin Disorders Sourcebook

Basic Information about Common Skin and Scalp Conditions Caused by Aging, Allergies, Immune Reactions, Sun Exposure, Infectious Organisms, Parasites, Cosmetics, and Skin Traumas, Including Abrasions, Cuts, and Pressure Sores

Along with Information on Prevention and Treatment

Edited by Allan R. Cook. 647 pages. 1997. 0-7808-0080-X. $78.

"... comprehensive, easily read reference book."
— *Doody's Health Sciences Book Reviews, Oct '97*

SEE ALSO Burns Sourcebook

Sleep Disorders Sourcebook

Basic Consumer Health Information about Sleep and Its Disorders, Including Insomnia, Sleepwalking, Sleep Apnea, Restless Leg Syndrome, and Narcolepsy

Along with Data about Shiftwork and Its Effects, Information on the Societal Costs of Sleep Deprivation, Descriptions of Treatment Options, a Glossary of Terms, and Resource Listings for Additional Help

Edited by Jenifer Swanson. 439 pages. 1998. 0-7808-0234-9. $78.

"This text will complement any home or medical library. It is user-friendly and ideal for the adult reader."
— *American Reference Books Annual, 2000*

"Recommended reference source."
— *Booklist, American Library Association, Feb '99*

"A useful resource that provides accurate, relevant, and accessible information on sleep to the general public. Health care providers who deal with sleep disorders patients may also find it helpful in being prepared to answer some of the questions patients ask."
— *Respiratory Care, Jul '99*

Sports Injuries Sourcebook

Basic Consumer Health Information about Common Sports Injuries, Prevention of Injury in Specific Sports, Tips for Training, and Rehabilitation from Injury

Along with Information about Special Concerns for Children, Young Girls in Athletic Training Programs, Senior Athletes, and Women Athletes, and a Directory of Resources for Further Help and Information

Edited by Heather E. Aldred. 624 pages. 1999. 0-7808-0218-7. $78.

"Public libraries and undergraduate academic libraries will find this book useful for its nontechnical language." — *American Reference Books Annual, 2000*

"While this easy-to-read book is recommended for all libraries, it should prove to be especially useful for public, high school, and academic libraries; certainly it should be on the bookshelf of every school gymnasium." — *E-Streams, Mar '00*

Substance Abuse Sourcebook

Basic Health-Related Information about the Abuse of Legal and Illegal Substances Such as Alcohol, Tobacco, Prescription Drugs, Marijuana, Cocaine, and Heroin; and Including Facts about Substance Abuse Prevention Strategies, Intervention Methods, Treatment and Recovery Programs, and a Section Addressing the Special Problems Related to Substance Abuse during Pregnancy

Edited by Karen Bellenir. 573 pages. 1996. 0-7808-0038-9. $78.

"A valuable addition to any health reference section. Highly recommended."
— *The Book Report, Mar/Apr '97*

"... a comprehensive collection of substance abuse information that's both highly readable and compact. Families and caregivers of substance abusers will find the information enlightening and helpful, while teachers, social workers and journalists should benefit from the concise format. Recommended."
— *Drug Abuse Update, Winter '96/'97*

SEE ALSO Alcoholism Sourcebook, Drug Abuse Sourcebook

Traveler's Health Sourcebook

Basic Consumer Health Information for Travelers, Including Physical and Medical Preparations, Transportation Health and Safety, Essential Information about Food and Water, Sun Exposure, Insect and Snake Bites, Camping and Wilderness Medicine, and Travel with Physical or Medical Disabilities

Along with International Travel Tips, Vaccination Recommendations, Geographical Health Issues, Disease Risks, a Glossary, and a Listing of Additional Resources

Edited by Joyce Brennfleck Shannon. 613 pages. 2000. 0-7808-0384-1. $78.

Women's Health Concerns Sourcebook

Basic Information about Health Issues That Affect Women, Featuring Facts about Menstruation and Other Gynecological Concerns, Including Endometriosis, Fibroids, Menopause, and Vaginitis; Reproductive Concerns, Including Birth Control, Infertility, and Abortion; and Facts about Additional Physical, Emotional, and Mental Health Concerns Prevalent among Women Such as Osteoporosis, Urinary Tract Disorders, Eating Disorders, and Depression

Along with Tips for Maintaining a Healthy Lifestyle

Edited by Heather E. Aldred. 567 pages. 1997. 0-7808-0219-5. $78.

"Handy compilation. There is an impressive range of diseases, devices, disorders, procedures, and other physical and emotional issues covered . . . well organized, illustrated, and indexed." — *Choice, Association of College and Research Libraries, Jan '98*

SEE ALSO Breast Cancer Sourcebook, Cancer Sourcebook for Women, 1st and 2nd Editions, Healthy Heart Sourcebook for Women, Osteoporosis Sourcebook

■

Workplace Health & Safety Sourcebook

Basic Consumer Health Information about Workplace Health and Safety, Including the Effect of Workplace Hazards on the Lungs, Skin, Heart, Ears, Eyes, Brain, Reproductive Organs, Musculoskeletal System, and Other Organs and Body Parts

Along with Information about Occupational Cancer, Personal Protective Equipment, Toxic and Hazardous Chemicals, Child Labor, Stress, and Workplace Violence

Edited by Chad T. Kimball. 626 pages. 2000. 0-7808-0231-4. $78.

"Highly recommended." — *The Bookwatch, Jan '01*

■

Worldwide Health Sourcebook

Basic Information about Global Health Issues, Including Malnutrition, Reproductive Health, Disease Dispersion and Prevention, Emerging Diseases, Risky Health Behaviors, and the Leading Causes of Death

Along with Global Health Concerns for Children, Women, and the Elderly, Mental Health Issues, Research and Technology Advancements, and Economic, Environmental, and Political Health Implications, a Glossary, and a Resource Listing for Additional Help and Information

Edited by Joyce Brennfleck Shannon. 500 pages. 2001. 0-7808-0330-2. $78.

Health Reference Series Cumulative Index 1999

A Comprehensive Index to the Individual Volumes of the Health Reference Series, Including a Subject Index, Name Index, Organization Index, and Publication Index

Along with a Master List of Acronyms and Abbreviations

Edited by Edward J. Prucha, Anne Holmes, and Robert Rudnick. 990 pages. 2000. 0-7808-0382-5. $78.

"Essential for collections that hold any of the numerous *Health Reference Series* titles."
— *Choice, Association of College and Research Libraries, Nov '00*